PROMOTING SCHOOL READINESS AND EARLY LEARNING

Also from Karen L. Bierman

Aggression, Antisocial Behavior, and Violence among Girls: A Developmental Perspective
Martha Putallaz and Karen L. Bierman, Editors

Peer Rejection: Developmental Processes and Intervention Strategies
Karen L. Bierman

Promoting School Readiness and Early Learning

IMPLICATIONS OF DEVELOPMENTAL RESEARCH FOR PRACTICE

EDITED BY

Michel Boivin
Karen L. Bierman

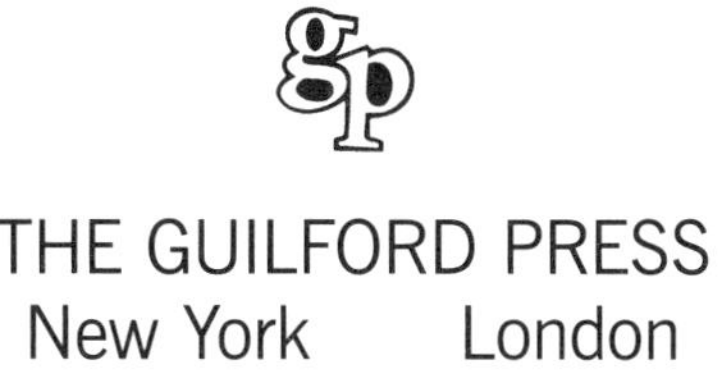

THE GUILFORD PRESS
New York London

A Division of Guilford Publications, Inc.
72 Spring Street, New York, NY 10012
www.guilford.com

Printed in the United States of America

This book is printed on acid-free paper.

Last digit is print number: 9 8 7 6 5 4 3 2 1

Library of Congress Cataloging-in-Publication Data

Promoting school readiness and early learning : implications of developmental research for practice / edited by Michel Boivin, Karen L. Bierman.
pages cm
Includes bibliographical references and index.
ISBN 978-1-4625-1145-7 (hardback)
1. Readiness for school. I. Boivin, Michel, 1953– editor of compilation. II. Bierman, Karen L., editor of compilation.
LB1132.P76 2014
372.21–dc23
2013021214

About the Editors

Michel Boivin, PhD, is Professor of Psychology and Canada Research Chair in Child Social Development at Laval University in Quebec. He is director of Laval University's Research Unit on Children's Psychosocial Maladjustment and of the Strategic Knowledge Cluster on Early Child Development, a pan-Canadian consortium. Dr. Boivin is a Fellow of the Royal Society of Canada. His research focuses on the biological, psychological, and social components of child development. He has played a central role in the creation and follow-up of large population-based longitudinal studies of children, including the Quebec Newborn Twin Study and the Quebec Longitudinal Study of Child Development.

Karen L. Bierman, PhD, is Distinguished Professor of Psychology and Director of the Child Study Center at The Pennsylvania State University (Penn State). She was the founding director of the Children, Youth, and Families Consortium at Penn State, and has also served as director of Penn State's Social Science Research Institute. Dr. Bierman's research focuses on child social-emotional development and the design and evaluation of school- and community-based prevention programs that promote social-emotional learning and school readiness. She has served as an educational advisor to a number of organizations devoted to improving early education for disadvantaged children, including Head Start and Sesame Workshop.

Contributors

Karen L. Bierman, PhD, Child Study Center, The Pennsylvania State University, University Park, Pennsylvania

Michel Boivin, PhD, Research Unit on Children's Psychosocial Maladjustment, School of Psychology, Laval University, Quebec City, Quebec, Canada

Mara Brendgen, PhD, Research Unit on Children's Psychosocial Maladjustment, Department of Psychology, University of Quebec in Montreal, Montreal, Quebec, Canada

Monique Brodeur, PhD, Department of Special Education and Training, University of Quebec in Montreal, Montreal, Quebec, Canada

Dillon Browne, PhD, Ontario Institute for Studies in Education, Toronto, Ontario, Canada

France Capuano, PhD, Department of Special Education and Training, University of Quebec in Montreal, Montreal, Quebec, Canada

Sylvana M. Côté, PhD, Department of Social and Preventive Medicine, University of Montreal, Montreal, Quebec, Canada

Lydia DeFlorio, PhD, College of Education, University of Nevada, Reno, Reno, Nevada

Hélène Desrosiers, MA, Social and Longitudinal Surveys, Quebec Institute of Statistics, Montreal, Quebec, Canada

Ginette Dionne, PhD, Research Unit on Children's Psychosocial Maladjustment, School of Psychology, Laval University, Quebec City, Quebec, Canada

Celene E. Domitrovich, PhD, Prevention Research Center, The Pennsylvania State University, University Park, Pennsylvania

Valerie Flores, MA, doctoral student, Department of Psychology, Loyola University Chicago, Chicago, Illinois

Nadine Forget-Dubois, PhD, Research Unit on Children's Psychosocial Maladjustment, School of Psychology, Laval University, Quebec City, Quebec, Canada

Marie-Claude Geoffroy, PhD, MRC Center of Epidemiology for Child Health/Centre for Paediatric Epidemiology and Biostatistics, University College London, London, United Kingdom

Scott D. Gest, PhD, Department of Human Development and Family Studies, The Pennsylvania State University, University Park, Pennsylvania

Jacinthe Giroux, PhD, Department of Special Education and Training, University of Quebec in Montreal, Montreal, Quebec, Canada

Kelly Haas, PhD, Department of Psychology, Loyola University Chicago, Chicago, Illinois

Annemarie H. Hindman, PhD, College of Education, Temple University, Philadelphia, Pennsylvania

Angela Howell-Moneta, PhD, Department of Psychology, Queen's University, Kingston, Ontario, Canada

Jennifer M. Jenkins, PhD, Department of Human Development and Applied Psychology, University of Toronto, Toronto, Ontario, Canada

Alice Klein, PhD, STEM Program, WestEd, Oakland, California

Jean-Pascal Lemelin, PhD, Department of Psychoeducation, Faculty of Education, University of Sherbrooke, Sherbrooke, Quebec, Canada

Jaclyn Lennon, BS, doctoral student, Department of Psychology, Loyola University Chicago, Chicago, Illinois

Christine Pajunar Li-Grining, PhD, Department of Psychology, Loyola University Chicago, Chicago, Illinois

Maria Marcus, BS, doctoral student, Department of Psychology, Loyola University Chicago, Chicago, Illinois

Emylie Mathieu, BA, doctoral student, Research Unit on Children's Psychosocial Maladjustment, School of Psychology, Laval University, Quebec City, Quebec, Canada

Erin T. Mathis, MS, doctoral student, Child Study Center, The Pennsylvania State University, University Park, Pennsylvania

Catherine Mimeau, BA, doctoral student, Research Unit on Children's Psychosocial Maladjustment, School of Psychology, Laval University, Quebec City, Quebec, Canada

Robert L. Nix, PhD, Prevention Research Center, The Pennsylvania State University, University Park, Pennsylvania

Ray DeV. Peters, PhD, Department of Psychology, Queen's University, Kingston, Ontario, Canada

Jean-Baptiste Pingault, PhD, Research Unit on Children's Psychosocial Maladjustment, University of Montreal, Sainte-Justine Hospital Research Center, Montreal, Quebec, Canada

Heather Prime, PhD, Ontario Institute for Studies in Education, Toronto, Ontario, Canada

François Poulin, PhD, Department of Psychology, University of Quebec in Montreal, Montreal, Quebec, Canada

Rob Santos, PhD, Healthy Child Manitoba Office, Healthy Child Committee of Cabinet, Government of Manitoba; and Department of Community Health Sciences, Faculty of Medicine, University of Manitoba, Winnipeg, Manitoba, Canada

Prentice Starkey, PhD, STEM Program, WestEd, Oakland, California

Richard E. Tremblay, PhD, Research Unit on Children's Psychosocial Maladjustment, University of Montreal, Montreal, Quebec, Canada; School of Public Health and Population Sciences, University College Dublin, Dublin, Ireland

Pierrette Verlaan, PhD, School of Psychoeducation, University of Sherbrooke, Sherbrooke, Quebec, Canada

Frank Vitaro, PhD, Research Unit on Children's Psychosocial Maladjustment, School of Psychoeducation, University of Montreal, Montreal, Quebec, Canada

Mark Wade, PhD, Ontario Institute for Studies in Education, Toronto, Ontario, Canada

Barbara A. Wasik, PhD, College of Education, Temple University, Philadelphia, Pennsylvania

Janet A. Welsh, PhD, Prevention Research Center, The Pennsylvania State University, University Park, Pennsylvania

Preface

In the context of fast-growing technical, economic, and social changes, contemporary societies are confronted with the enduring challenge of caring for, educating, and training new generations of children. This ambitious and complex endeavor is all the more pressing in countries such as Canada and the United States, where low birth rates and aging populations compress the pyramid of age, and where a growing, progressively retiring senior population will rely on a shrinking (relatively speaking) working-age population for maintaining a knowledge-based economy and providing the means for public services.

This challenge is further amplified by the increasing demands put on the child care and education systems. It is generally expected that these systems will provide children with the intellectual tools, skills, attitudes, and values required to understand and expand their views of the world, as well as to adjust and innovate in a rapidly changing social and economic landscape. But these systems were also conceived to serve the ethics and ideals of a society; they are expected to diminish social inequalities and to foster in children and youth a humanist value system that will lead them to respect and express concern for others, appreciate diversity in society, act responsibly, and potentially work toward the pursuit of social justice and the collective good. The UNESCO Task Force on Education for the Twenty-First Century has elegantly summarized these overarching education goals in its four pillars of learning: learning to know, learning to do, learning to be, and learning to live together (Delors et al., 1996).

It is now clear that this ambitious task has to start very early in life, at a time when the brain is characterized by unparalleled growth and plasticity. At this stage, the brain allows for the rapid acquisition of foundational cognitive and emotional skills as the basis for the ability to learn, achieve self-control, set and meet goals, and relate to others and actively participate in society. Early child development and population well-being are clearly interlocked. Understanding and promoting the early pathways toward optimal development, and preventing the establishment of unhealthy developmental trajectories, is a *passage obligé* for the further improvement of human and social capital.

This developmental landscape is the leitmotif underlying the present work. Borrowing from cutting-edge developmental research, the goal of this volume is to present in an integrated way what school readiness entails and how it can be improved. The focus on school readiness is intended to unite the burgeoning scientific evidence about the factors and conditions under which early learning takes place and how optimal early development can be fostered by appropriate services and programs. Thus, the notion of school readiness is really meant as a multifaceted developmental construct. Accordingly, this volume aims large. The relevant knowledge is organized in a logical order, from basic research centering on prediction and developmental process to applied research aimed at preventing difficulties in school. The book identifies the cognitive, language, behavioral, motor, and social-emotional skills that enable young children to function successfully in school contexts. It presents compelling longitudinal findings on the benefits of early programs and interventions for preschoolers at risk due to poverty and other factors. It explores specific ways in which school- and family-based interventions–including programs that target reading and language, math, self-regulation, and social-emotional development–can contribute to school readiness. The book also addresses challenges in the large-scale dissemination of evidence-based practices.

There is a story to every book and this one is no exception. Its birth can be traced back to an international conference on "School Readiness and School Success: From Research to Policy and Practice," held in Quebec City in November 2009. Organized under the joint auspices of the Strategic Knowledge Cluster on Early Child Development and the Centre of Excellence for Early Childhood Development, the conference brought leading figures in the field of early learning to present their work. The success of the conference made it clear that there was an appetite for further knowledge dissemination about the importance of school readiness and the ways it could be improved. This book is intended to fulfill this need.

This conference was made possible by the generous support of partners who truly believed in the importance of the early years. We would like to thank the Lucie et André Chagnon Foundation, the Margaret and

Wallace McCain Family Foundation, Laval University, and the Social Sciences and Humanities Research Council of Canada for their financial support in organizing this initial conference. A special thanks to Claire Gascon-Giard and Kristell Le Martret, who masterminded the organization of the conference, and to Jocelyne Désy, for keeping my (i.e., M. B.) feet on the ground and for not having rebutted the idea of this book one sleepless night in Barcelona.

We would like to dedicate this book to the people—practitioners, stakeholders, policymakers, and scientists—who tirelessly commit their time and effort to the improvement of young children's lives and development. Canada has recently lost two pioneer thinkers and advocates, Fraser Mustard and Clyde Hertzman, who both combined their science, conviction, and determination to promote the idea that a healthy society is defined by how well it treats and prepares young children. Their talent and dedication were an inspiration for many of us. We hope this edited book will contribute further to this mission by informing evidence-based practice, service planning, and public policy to optimize support for children and families, especially those in need.

MICHEL BOIVIN and KAREN L. BIERMAN

REFERENCE

Delors, J., Al Mufti, I., Amagi, I., Carneiro, R., Chung, F., Geremek, B., et al. (1996). *Learning: The treasure within.* Paris: UNESCO.

Contents

PART II. Determinants of School Readiness

PART III. Supporting School Readiness with Evidence-Based Programs and Practices

PART IV. Going to Scale with Evidence-Based Programs: Sustaining High-Quality Practice

PROMOTING SCHOOL READINESS AND EARLY LEARNING

PART I

SETTING THE STAGE

The Importance of School Readiness for School Success

CHAPTER 1

School Readiness

Introduction to a Multifaceted and Developmental Construct

MICHEL BOIVIN and KAREN L. BIERMAN

As stated in the preface of this book, modern democracies must increasingly rely on an integrated care-and-education system that provides their future citizens with the intellectual skills required to understand the world, adapt to constantly evolving socioeconomic conditions, and succeed in the workplace. At the same time, this system is also expected to nurture the social-emotional attitudes and values that help them reconcile the pursuit of individual happiness with that of the collective good. This is quite a challenge.

Clearly, the stakes and hopes are high but, unfortunately, the results do not always meet the expectations; many children and youth experience school difficulties. For instance, in 2007–2008, 28% of Québec youth less than 20 years of age had not yet graduated from secondary school and were not attending a secondary school (Ministère de l'Éducation, du Loisir et du Sport, 2010). In the United States, 22% of youth fail to complete high school, with rates much higher among minority groups, averaging 47% for Hispanic students and 50% for African American students (Children's Defense Fund, 2004).

School dropout is a significant national problem in Canada and in the United States (HRSDC-Statistics Canada, 2011; U.S. Department of

Education, 2012), as it may set individuals on a life trajectory marked by employment upheavals, as well as physical and mental health adversities (see Vitaro, Brendgen, & Tremblay, Chapter 2, this volume). This phenomenon also extends beyond high school. For instance, in 2007–2008 in Québec, dropout rates in college (2 years of postsecondary schooling) reached almost 30% in preuniversity programs, and were above 40% in technical programs (Ministère de l'Éducation, du Loisir et du Sport, 2010). Low levels of schooling in turn create significant challenges for youth in the workplace. For example, among teens and young adults (ages 16–24) in the United States, unemployment rates exceed 50% for those without a high school education, relative to 75% among high school graduates, 86% among youth with 1–3 years of postsecondary schooling, and 95% among those with a 4-year college degree (Sum, Khatiwada, & McLaughlin, 2009).

Despite the clear long-term financial advantages of higher education, many youth do not pursue postsecondary education or they drop out before completion. To some extent, students are deterred by challenges associated with access or financing, but in addition, many fail to move forward because of professional indecisiveness and poor readiness, resulting from a lack of academic preparation, motivation, and achievement (Howell, Kurlaender, & Grodsky, 2010). The general hypothesis underlying this volume is that these various forms of school disengagement reflect personal "risk" factors that are partly rooted in early childhood experiences.

Clearly, school dropout (or nongraduation) is a major problem for any society that increasingly relies on a knowledge-based economy. However, because school dropout rates are crude estimates, they barely reflect the "tip of the iceberg" in terms of society's shortcomings in building human capital. Indeed, a broader concern is that the level and quality of learning and training of society's children and youth are compromised by weak educational experiences. For instance, in 2007, it was estimated that more than 40% of the labor force in Canada (i.e., the population ages 16–65) lacked the literacy skills (i.e., the ability to find, synthetize, and use written information), and that 50% lacked the basic math abilities (i.e., managing numbers) needed to succeed in today's economy (Canadian Council on Learning, 2007). Similarly, in a 2003 national study of the U.S. population, 14% emerged as functionally illiterate, and an additional 29% had only the basic level of literacy skills needed for everyday activities (National Center for Educational Statistics, 2003). These figures raise concerns about the number of children and youth who are not learning the skills needed to function adequately in a knowledge-based economy. These educational deficits also jeopardize the capacity of many citizens to critically appraise policies and politics, one of the keystones of a healthy democracy.

School Readiness and School Achievement

In recent years, efforts have focused increasingly on improving long-term educational outcomes by improving early learning, based on research suggesting that school readiness and initial school learning set the pace for later school attainment (Zaslow, Tout, Halle, Vick, & Lavelle, 2010). There is little doubt that over the course of schooling, achievement results from complex transactions among personal, familial, social, and school factors operating over time, and that the early learning years lay a critical foundation for these later developmental transactions and trajectories. For example, recipients of high-quality early childhood education tend to show long-term benefits in areas of achievement, grade progression, and high school graduation (Stegelin, 2004; Vandel et al., 2010), but these general trends must be qualified (see Côté, Geoffroy, & Pingault, Chapter 6, this volume). Accordingly, a thorough understanding of the origin and development of school trajectories commands an integrated longitudinal approach that starts in early childhood and considers a variety of behavioral, familial, relational, and societal antecedents (Barclay & Doll, 2001; Doll & Hess, 2001).

The search for the developmental roots of school achievement has generated a surge of interest in the construct of school readiness (Pianta, Cox, & Snow, 2007; Rimm-Kaufman & Pianta, 2000). According to the most common view, *school readiness* refers to the basic skills that children need to possess at school entry in order to adapt successfully to the school environment and to learn and achieve at a satisfying level (Forget-Dubois et al., 2007). It may be defined as a threshold, that is, the minimum developmental level allowing the child to respond adequately to school demands (Carlton & Winsler, 1999), but it is more often used as a relative term; a child may be more or less likely to make the transition into grade school successfully and thrive as a function of a variety of cognitive and social-emotional skills and characteristics.

There is no consensus on a precise content definition of school readiness. For example, teachers and parents may have different views regarding the child characteristics that make him or her "ready for school." Whereas parents define readiness in terms of academic abilities (i.e., literacy and numeracy), teachers more often emphasize health conditions (i.e., being rested and well fed), communication skills, and attitudes (i.e., curiosity and motivation) toward scholastic activities (Rimm-Kaufman, 2004; Rimm-Kaufman, Pianta, & Cox, 2000). In general, however, researchers and stakeholders agree that school readiness should be defined multidimensionally, with a consideration of the multiple health, cognitive, emotional, and social characteristics that reflect the child's ability to function successfully in school contexts. According to this child-centered, multifactor view, measures of school readiness generally assess a variety of cognitive, language, behavioral, motor, and social-emotional skills. For instance, readiness to achieve in school depends on self-regulation skills, such as the capacity to focus attention, follow the teacher's instruction, persist in learning tasks (Blair, 2002; Bierman, Nix, Greenberg, Blair, & Domitrovich, 2008), and the social-emotional skills needed to integrate harmoniously with the peer and school milieu, cooperate, and get along well with peers and teachers (Ladd, Herald, & Kochel, 2006; Parker & Asher, 1987), as well as the cognitive skills and knowledge components necessary to achieve adequately in school (LaParo & Pianta, 2000; Scarpati & Silver, 1999). These various components are correlated, but each contributes in some significant and unique ways to school readiness.

The Relevance of School Readiness for School Achievement and Developmental Health

Fueled by a growing awareness of the importance of school readiness, and the sizable number of children who start school without it, interest in early childhood education has surged during the past two decades (Pianta et al., 2007). Research documenting the developmental experiences that promote school readiness, as well as the consequences of poor school readiness, has proliferated. As indicated previously, one of the major reasons underlying the growing interest in school readiness lies in its potential to provide information about the future school trajectories, or, stated otherwise, in its predictive validity regarding future school achievement and overall adjustment. To the extent that school success may depend on entering school "ready to learn," achieving school readiness prior to school entry should be considered one of the most important developmental tasks facing preschool-age children (LaParo & Pianta, 2000).

This burgeoning field of research has shed light on the multifaceted nature of school readiness. Several longitudinal datasets are now available, following children in the United States and Canada from school entry through high school completion. Results from these developmental studies underscore the importance of initial school adjustment, and its predictive significance. For example, there is cumulating evidence that cognitive skills assessed in late preschool and at school entry predict later school achievement. Fluid cognitive skills, such as executive functions and memory, are seen as prerequisites of future school achievement (Blair, 2006), but more crystallized preacademic knowledge components, such as knowledge about letters and numbers, have also been shown to predict early school achievement over and above general cognitive ability (Hess, Holloway, Dickson, & Price, 1984; Lemelin et al., 2007). A meta-analysis by LaParo and Pianta (2000), based on 70 independent studies, revealed that preschool and kindergarten cognitive readiness measures, especially those targeting literacy and numeracy, predicted early school achievement in a moderate-to-strong way. A recent study conducted in six different samples in the United States, the United Kingdom, and Canada showed that the strongest predictors of later school achievement (i.e., in math and reading) were school-entry math and reading, as well as attention skills (Duncan et al., 2007). This study was especially noteworthy for raising awareness that early math skills and knowledge play a particularly important role for later school achievement. While the strong predictive validity supports the use of such measures for screening purposes (i.e., the identification of children at risk), at the same time, it also indicates that other, noncognitive factors are involved.

Early disparities in school readiness associated with socioeconomic disadvantage are particularly striking and widespread, with approximately 1 in 5 children entering school with low academic readiness and elevated emotional or behavior problems that reduce their capacity to engage and learn at school (Rimm-Kaufman et al., 2000). Over 40% of children growing up in poverty demonstrate delayed language skills and social skills at school entry, and over 20% exhibit high rates of disruptive behavior problems that undermine school adjustment (Macmillan, McMorris, & Kruttschnitt, 2004). Longitudinal studies show that at least half of the long-term educational achievement gaps between poor and nonpoor children exist at school entry, and this "achievement gap" associated with poverty widens over time (Ryan, Fauth, & Brooks-Gunn, 2006). Yet socioeconomic factors only partially account for school readiness and the lack thereof, and research has started to uncover other personal and familial risk factors that need to be considered to explain more fully why so many children lack the academic and social-emotional skills to connect and learn in school.

Research documents the powerful impact social environments may have on developmental processes early in life. Recent advances in developmental neuroscience have illuminated the importance of the early childhood years for the development of the neural architecture for learning–the cognitive structures that support the regulation of attention, behavior, and emotion (Hughes, 2011). We now understand how early experiences influence these important aspects of brain development, fostering the neural connections that provide the foundation for learning, reasoning, problem solving, social skills, and school success. However, there are no fixed paths. The early phases of brain organization are characterized by high levels of plasticity. Early experiences provoke changes that may become embedded in the neurobiological systems, but these changes often combine with a cascade of environmental events and contexts to influence future cognitive, emotional, and behavioral development (Hughes & Ensor, 2009). Unpacking the personal, familial, and socioeconomic factors that contribute to school readiness and account for disparities within populations is of critical importance to inform early intervention and prevention programs. From a prevention perspective, the capacity to identify before school entry and, inasmuch as is possible, earlier in the preschool period, specific risk markers of future, school-related problems offers considerable potential for providing at-risk individuals or groups of children with early interventions that reduce their later risks (Bierman, Domitrovich, Nix, Welsh, & Gest, Chapter 10, this volume; Blair & Diamond, 2008; Duncan et al., 2007).

Interventions to Promote School Readiness and Early Learning

Parallel to this growing base of developmental research, recent years have witnessed a great increase in early intervention research focused on understanding optimal early childhood educational practices and beneficial methods of early intervention for at-risk children. The good news is that positive change is possible when the efforts are intense and lasting. Long-term assessments of early preventive interventions, such as home visitation programs and early childhood education programs, document the potential for long-lasting positive effects for children, families, and society (Barnett, 1995). We now know that interventions fostering positive, nurturing experiences in the early years of childhood can have lifelong benefits, including increased learning abilities, school success, involvement in community activities, active participation in the labor market, and quality of life.

Despite these research advances, which broaden our understanding of school readiness and strategies to enhance it, a significant gap exists between the guidelines and programming implemented by school districts, and the research base. Developmental and intervention research provides rich working models to support early learning and improve school readiness. However, this information only trickles down slowly to potential users, perhaps because it is not easily accessible to practitioners or policymakers, or because this knowledge basis has tended to develop in silos, that is, with little connection across domains. For instance, findings from the field of developmental science have not been effectively integrated with findings from the field of education. Little has been done to bring these research areas together to form a comprehensive picture aimed at developing an understanding of school readiness, early school achievement, and later school success.

This volume is intended to bring together these complementary interdisciplinary efforts spanning the domains of theory, research, practice, and policy. It is organized into four sections: Part I—Setting the Stage: The Importance of School Readiness for School Success; Part II—Determinants of School Readiness; Part III—Supporting School Readiness with Evidence-Based Programs and Practices; and Part IV—Going to Scale with Evidence-Based Programs: Sustaining High-Quality Practice. The volume starts with this overview chapter along with three chapters that review longitudinal research and underscore the importance of focusing on school readiness as a predictor of later school success. Taking advantage of various population-based longitudinal studies spanning the different periods of development, these studies "set the stage" for the following chapters, by identifying the child characteristics, as well as school, family, and community risk and protective factors that predict the course of schooling and adolescent outcomes from the preschool years and school entry. In these three chapters, important issues concerning the conceptualization and measurement of school readiness are discussed, and the determinants and impact of school readiness on later schooling outcomes are informed by a broad range of developmental literatures and longitudinal study analyses. In Chapter 2, Vitaro, Brendgen, and Tremblay document the longitudinal associations between disruptive behaviors at school entry, such as inattention–hyperactivity and aggression–opposition, and the later course of academic achievement, school motivation and high school graduation. In Chapter 3, Boivin, Desrosiers, Lemelin, and Forget-Dubois describe how multifaceted school readiness measures suitable to a population-based approach substantially predict early school achievement, and significantly mediate the contribution of a variety of early childhood risk indicators to early school achievement difficulties. Using a twin design approach, they also show that familywide environments underlie these strong predictions.

The chapters in Part II build upon the developmental framework, and fill in the earlier phase of development for two specific classes of personal and environmental determinants of school readiness: language and nonparental care. These chapters feature the early developmental predictors and trajectories leading to school readiness using shorter-term, process-oriented approaches. Chapter 4, by Wade, Prime, Browne, and Jenkins, presents a multilevel perspective to examine the relative contributions of different types of risk in explaining early cognitive school readiness. The focus here is really on the early years (0–3), and on the interplay of individual characteristics (early language) and family and neighborhood experiences in the predicting early reading and expressive language. In Chapter 5, Dionne, Mimeau, and Mathieu focus on the role of early language development and language stimulation in the family setting for children's readiness to read at the formal entry into school. Drawing from results in two population-based longitudinal studies, the chapter describes the mechanisms linking predictors of reading readiness over time, including genetic liabilities and early literacy practices in the home. Finally, in Chapter 6, Coté, Geoffroy, and Pingault review the empirical evidence regarding the putative role of early child care experiences in promoting cognitive school readiness. The review covers and distinguishes population-based studies, which typically compare children and families who use different type of child care settings at various intensities, to smaller studies, which provide for more fine-grained analyses of the quality of the child care settings.

Part III includes five chapters focused on evidence-based programs that have demonstrated improved school readiness in rigorous randomized or quasi-experimental designs. Chapter 7, by Wasik and Hindman, describes and discusses factors that influence the development of reading skills, with a special focus on children who experience academic difficulties. This chapter also reviews the intervention research on language, especially early vocabulary-focused interventions and professional development models for teachers, and discusses the implication of this knowledge basis for early education. The chapter also describes one successful intervention: *Ex*ceptional *C*oaching for *E*arly *L*anguage and *L*iteracy (ExCELL).

Chapter 8, by Starkey, Klein, and DeFlorio, begins with an overview of early mathematical development, describing developmental processes that span the age period from birth through kindergarten. It also describes recent intervention research, namely, an early math home and classroom intervention program, Pre-K Mathematics, illustrating how mathematical knowledge can be enhanced in economically disadvantaged children by math enrichments in their classroom and home learning environments.

Chapter 9, by Li-Grining, Lennon, Marcus, Flores, and Haas, describes the development of the executive control skills, a major component of self-regulation skills associated with the maturation of the prefrontal cortex, and the socialization experiences that foster or impede its development. Sometimes described as the "neural architecture for learning," these skills figure centrally in school readiness; they support sustained attention, as well as behavioral and emotional regulation, fostering the self-control needed for school success. A central focus of the chapter is the Chicago School Readiness Project (CSRP), an intervention program designed to improve low-income children's readiness for school by fostering their self-regulation.

In Chapter 10, Bierman, Domitrovich, Nix, Welsh, and Gest present empirical evidence supporting a focus on social-emotional development during the preschool years as a method for enhancing school readiness.

Interventions with documented effects on improving social-emotional school readiness are reviewed. The chapter also describes the theoretical foundations, the curriculum materials, and the teaching strategies of the REDI program, and reviews results from a randomized evaluation trial. The chapter terminates with a discussion of implications for professional development and practice. Finally, in Chapter 11, Welsh, Bierman, and Mathis review the developmental research that documents the role parents play in supporting child cognitive and social-emotional school readiness, as well as intervention studies that use parent education and home visiting to support parenting skills and reduce school readiness delays.

Efficacy studies of programs that have promoted school readiness provide guidance on how to close the socioeconomic gap in school achievement. However, to have substantial impact at the population level, larger-scale efforts are needed to promote the national dissemination of evidence-based school readiness programming. The chapters in Part IV examine the challenges associated with "going to scale" with evidence-based early childhood programs, and disseminating and sustaining high-quality practices on a broad, national basis. In Chapter 12, Peters and Howell-Moneta review the current research literature on school readiness and early child development programs, then describe the Better Beginnings, Better Futures program, a large-scale, community-based prevention designed to facilitate school readiness and successful transition into school. Developed for families with young children, and implemented in eight disadvantaged neighborhoods in Ontario, this primary prevention program provides a model for engaging communities in the development and implementation of evidence-based early childhood programs. In Chapter 13, Poulin, Capuano, Vitaro, Verlaan, Brodeur, and Giroux provide an overview of the Fluppy prevention program's history and content, and a summary of the results of an initial evaluation trial. Widely implemented in the province of Québec, the Fluppy program is offered to children in kindergarten and consists of several types of intervention that engage parents, teachers, and classmates. The authors describe its dissemination across Québec, document a number of implementation issues, and discuss the results from a recent impact study. The chapter illustrates a range of implementation issues that emerged during the period of provincewide dissemination.

The volume concludes with a commentary on policy implications provided by Santos, and a final summation by Bierman and Boivin. These chapters integrate findings and articulate important general implications of the groundbreaking research described in this book. The advances in conceptualization and methodology, the discovery of malleable antecedents and mediators of school readiness, and the new data on the efficacy of evidence-based practice all create a solid foundation for improving current early childhood programs and practices. If we can surmount the challenges of going to scale, we have the potential to close the achievement gap associated with poverty and promote the school readiness of all children, giving them a strong starting base for future achievement. In the final chapter, we summarize the implications the volume holds for future research, for future directions and priorities in early childhood practice, preventive intervention, and policy.

REFERENCES

Barclay, J. R., & Doll, B. (2001). Early prospective studies of the high school dropout. *School Psychology Quarterly, 16,* 357–369.

Barnett, S. (1995). Long-term effects of early childhood programs on cognitive and school outcomes. *The Future of Children, 5,* 25–50.

Bierman, K. L., Nix, R. L., Greenberg, M. T., Blair, C., & Domitrovich, C. E. (2008). Executive functions and school readiness intervention: Impact, moderation, and mediation in the Head Start REDI Program. *Development and Psychopathology, 20,* 821–843.

Blair, C. (2002). School readiness: Integrating cognition and emotion in a neurobiological conceptualization of children's functioning at school entry. *American Psychologist, 57*(2), 111–127.

Blair, C. (2006). How similar are fluid cognition and general intelligence?: A developmental neuroscience perspective on fluid cognition as an aspect of human cognitive ability. *Behavioral and Brain Sciences, 29,* 109–125.

Blair, C., & Diamond, A. (2008). Biological processes in prevention and intervention: Promotion of self-regulation and the prevention of early school failure. *Development and Psychopathology, 20,* 899–911.

Canadian Council on Learning. (2007). State of learning in Canada: No time for complacency. In *Report on Learning in Canada 2007.* Ottawa: Author.

Carlton, M. P., & Winsler, A. (1999). School readiness: The need for a paradigm shift. *School Psychology Review, 28*(3), 338–352.

Children's Defense Fund. (2004, June). The road to dropping out: Minority students and academic factors correlated with failure to complete high school. Retrieved October 21, 2012, from *www.childrensdefense.org/child-research-data-publications/data/education-dropping-out-facts-2004.pdf.*

Doll, B., & Hess, R. (2001). Through a new lens: Contemporary psychological perspectives on school completion and dropping out of high school. *School Psychology Quarterly, 16,* 350–356.

Duncan, G. J., Dowsett, C. J., Claessens, A., Magnuson, K., Huston, A. C., Klebanov, P., et al. (2007). School readiness and later achievement. *Developmental Psychology, 43,* 1428–1446.

Forget-Dubois, N., Lemelin, J.-P., Boivin, M., Dionne, G., Séguin, J. R., Vitaro, F., et al. (2007). Predicting early school achievement with the EDI: A longitudinal population-based study. *Early Education and Development, 18,* 405–426.

Hess, R. D., Holloway, S. D., Dickson, W. P., & Price, G. G. (1984). Maternal preschool variables as predictors of children's school readiness and later achievement in vocabulary and mathematics in sixth grade. *Child Development, 55*, 1902–1912.

Howell, J., Kurlaender, M., & Grodsky, E. (2010). Postsecondary preparation and remediation: Examing the effect of the early assessment program at California State University. *Journal of Policy Analysis and Management, 29*, 726–748.

HRSDC-Statistics Canada. (2011). *Labour force survey estimates, by educational attainment, sex and age group*. Ottawa, ON: Statistics Canada.

Hughes, C. (2011). Changes and challenges in 20 years of research into the development of executive functions. *Infant and Child Development, 20*, 251–271.

Hughes, C. H., & Ensor, R. A. (2009). How do families help or hinder the emergence of early executive function? In C. Lewis & J. M. Carpendale (Eds.), Social interaction and the development of executive function. *New Directions in Child and Adolescent Development, 123*, 35–50.

Institut de la Statistique du Québec. (2009). *Perspectives démographiques du Québec et des regions* [Demographic perspectives of Québec and regions], *2006–2056*. Québec: Author.

Kausler, D. H., & Kausler, B. C. (2001). *The graying of America: An encyclopedia of aging, health, mind, and behavior* (2nd ed.). Champaign: University of Illinois Press.

Ladd, G. W., Herald, S. L., & Kochel, K. P. (2006). School readiness: Are there social prerequisites? *Early Education and Development, 17*(1), 115–150.

LaParo, K. M., & Pianta, R. C. (2000). Predicting children's competence in the early school years: A meta-analytic review. *Review of Educational Research, 70*, 443–484.

Lemelin, J.-P., Boivin, M., Forget-Dubois, N., Dionne, G., Séguin, J. R., Brendgen, M., et al. (2007). The genetic–environmental etiology of cognitive school readiness in early childhood. *Child Development, 78*(6), 1855–1869.

Macmillan, R., McMorris, B. J., & Kruttschnitt, C. (2004). Linked lives: Stability and change in maternal circumstances trajectories of antisocial behavior in children. *Child Development, 75*, 205–220.

Ministère de l'Éducation, du Loisir et du Sport. (2010). *Indicateur de l'Éducation–Édition 2010* [Education Indicators–Édition 2010]. Québec: Gouvernement du Québec.

National Center for Educational Statistics. (2003). *The 2003 National Assessment of Adult Literacy*. Retrieved October 23, 2012, from *http://nces.ed.gov/pubs2003/2003495rev.pdf*.

Parker, J. G., & Asher, S. R. (1987). Peer relations and later personal adjustment: Are low-accepted children at risk? *Psychological Bulletin, 102*(3), 357–389.

Pianta, R., Cox, M., & Snow, K. (2007). *School readiness and the transition to kindergarten in the era of accountability*. Baltimore: Brookes.

Rimm-Kaufman, S. (2004). School transition and school readiness: An outcome of early childhood development. In R. E. Tremblay, R. DeV. Peters, & M. Boivin (Eds.), *Encyclopedia on early childhood development* (pp. 1–7). Montréal, Québec: Centre of Excellence for Early Childhood Development. Retrieved from *www.child-encyclopedia.com/documents/rimm-kaufmanangxp.pdf*.

Rimm-Kaufman, S. E., & Pianta, R. C. (2000). An ecological perspective on the transition to kindergarten: A theoretical framework to guide empirical research. *Journal of Applied Developmental Psychology, 21*(5), 491–511.

Rimm-Kaufman, S., Pianta, R. C., & Cox, M. (2000). Teachers' judgments of problems in the transition to school. *Early Childhood Research Quarterly, 15*, 147–166.

Ryan, R. M., Fauth, R. C., & Brooks-Gunn, J. (2006). Childhood poverty: Implications for school readiness and early childhood education. In B. Spodek & O.N. Saracho (Eds.), *Handbook of research on the education of children* (2nd ed., pp. 323–346). Mahwah, NJ: Erlbaum.

Scarpati, S., & Silver, P. G. (1999). Readiness for academic achievement in preschool children. In E. V. Nuttall & I. Romero (Eds.), *Assessing and screening preschoolers: Psychological and educational dimensions* (pp. 262–280). Boston: Allyn & Bacon.

Stegelin, D. (2004). Early childhood education. In F. P. Schargel & J. Smink (Eds.), *Helping students graduate: A strategic approach to dropout prevention* (pp. 115–123). Larchmont, NY: Eye on Education.

Sum, A., Khatiwada, I., & McLaughlin, J. (2009). The consequences of dropping out of high school: Joblessness and jailing for high school dropouts and the high cost for taxpayers. *Center for Labor Market Studies Publication*, Paper 23. Available online at *http://hdl.handle.net/2047/d20000596.*

Vandell, D. L., Belsky, J., Burchinal, M., Steinberg, L., & Vandergrift, N. (2010). Do effects of early child care extend to age 15 years?: Results from the NICHD Study of Early Child Care and Youth Development. *Child Development, 81*(3), 737–756.

U.S. Department of Education, National Center for Education Statistics. (2012). *The Condition of Education 2012* (NCES 2012-045). Retrieved from *http://nces.ed.gov/programs/coe/tables/table-sde-1.asp.*

Zaslow, M., Tout, K., Halle, T., Vick, J., & Lavelle, B. (2010). *Towards the identification of features of effective professional development for early childhood educators: A review of the literature.* Washington, DC: U.S. Department of Education.

CHAPTER 2

Early Predictors of High School Completion

The Developmental Interplay between Behavior, Motivation, and Academic Performance

FRANK VITARO, MARA BRENDGEN, and RICHARD E. TREMBLAY

In industrialized countries, not achieving at least a high school diploma may entail dire consequences for both individuals and the society (Cohen, 1998). Adults without a high school diploma are more likely to be recipients of welfare and unemployment insurance (Rumberger, 1987). They also experience more physical and mental health problems, are more likely to engage in illegal activities, and are more prone to psychoactive substance abuse. Finally, they are less involved in their communities, and when they become parents, their own children are at increased risk of having similar limited academic trajectories (McCaul, Donaldson, Coladarci, & Davis, 1992; Serbin & Stack, 1998).

As in many other industrialized countries, failure to achieve a high school diploma in Canada or the United States is a nationally recognized problem (HRSDC-Statistics Canada, 2011; U.S. Department of Education, 2008). In the previous decade, one Canadian or American youth out of five had not graduated from high school by age 20 years. The proportion of young adults without a high school diploma is even higher in the province of Québec, with a little more than one out of four youth without a high school diploma by age 20 years (Québec Ministry of Education, 2010). If not corrected soon, this situation will be exacerbated by the demographic curve showing a decline of the youth strata and an increase of the senior strata over the next decade in Western countries. A larger aging portion of the population will depend on a smaller number of young individuals in the work force. Consequently, an industrialized society cannot afford to have many of its young citizens minimally educated and less competitive on the labor market.

Graduation (or the failure thereof) from school should be distinguished from school persistence and its opposite, school interruption (i.e., school dropout) (Christenson, Sinclair, Lehr, & Godber, 2001). *Graduation* refers to the completion of the school program as attested to by a diploma, whereas *school dropout* refers to an interruption of school attendance, which may be definitive (i.e., permanent dropout) or followed by a return to school (i.e., temporary dropout). This distinction is crucial given results showing that "temporary dropouts" who eventually graduate usually become well-adjusted adults, whereas "permanent dropouts" (i.e., those who never graduate) often suffer from psychosocial problems (Entwisle, Alexander, & Olson, 2004). In other words, it is not the interruption of school attendance per se, but rather the failure to complete the full academic program that forecasts adjustment problems.

In order to avert school failure and promote high school completion, many suggestions have been made to improve children's readiness for school as a first step for school success (Blair & Diamond, 2008; Duncan et al., 2007). It remains unclear, however, which specific skills and knowledge should be emphasized during the crucial period covering the years right before and right after school entry in order to promote later high school completion. Our goal in this chapter is to shed light on this issue by presenting results from a large, population-based sample of Québec children followed from kindergarten entry through early adulthood. This study provides a unique opportunity to examine the predictive value of a variety of academic and behavioral skills at school entry with respect to high school completion.

Children's Abilities

Emerging literacy and numeracy in kindergarten or grade 1 have been shown to be good predictors of school achievement in primary and secondary school (Ensminger & Slusarcick, 1992). In contrast, it is still unclear whether behavioral skills or difficulties make an additional, unique contribution to high school achievement. Two behavioral dimensions have been linked to school achievement: inattention–hyperactivity and aggression–opposition. In the school readiness literature, inattention–hyperactivity refers to difficulties focusing and sustaining attention and inhibiting impulsive actions, reflecting low levels of behavioral self-regulation (McClelland & Cameron, 2011) and associated with deficits in developing executive function skills (flexible attention, inhibitory control, and working memory) (Garon, Bryson, & Smith, 2008; Hughes, Ensor, Wilson, & Graham, 2010). In contrast, aggressive–oppositional behaviors, including fighting, arguing, and failing to follow rules, reflect individual differences in social-emotional arousal and reactivity, linked with temperament and social learning experiences (Blair & Diamond, 2008).

Central to this chapter is the question of whether the two behavioral dimensions, inattention–hyperactivity and aggression–opposition, make independent and additive contributions to predicting high school completion. Some research has revealed that early aggression–opposition predicted early academic functioning and, in some cases, later school achievement (Ensminger & Slusarcick, 1992; Masten et al., 2005; Moilanen, Shaw, & Maxwell, 2010; Obradovic, Burt, & Masten, 2010). These studies generally controlled for children's academic and family background characteristics. However, most studies did not take into account children's inattention–hyperactivity, despite its well-documented overlap with aggression–opposition and its known association with children's classroom participation and achievement, as well as with school noncompletion (Bierman, Torres, Domitrovich, Welsh, & Gest, 2009; Pingault et al., 2011; Vitaro, Brendgen, Larose, & Tremblay, 2005). The few studies that examined both early aggression–opposition and early inattention–hyperactivity found that only the latter predicted later academic achievement and school noncompletion, thus suggesting that early aggression–opposition is related to scholastic outcomes through its association with inattention–hyperactivity (Breslau et al., 2009; Burt & Roisman, 2010; Duncan et al., 2007; Rapport, Scanlan, & Denney, 1999; Vitaro et al., 2005). In one study, however, conduct disorders (i.e., aggression and rule violations) in late childhood predicted later academic difficulties and high school nongraduation, above and beyond inattention–hyperactivity (Galéra, Melchior, Chastang, Bouvard, & Fombonne, 2009). This study assessed conduct problems in late childhood, whereas studies that found no specific contribution of aggression–opposition rather focused on young children, typically between 6 and 8 years of age. It could be that aggression–opposition starts playing a role in academic achievement only in late childhood, whereas inattention–hyperactivity matters early on and throughout primary school (see Hinshaw, 1992).

INDIRECT PATHWAYS

Why would inattention–hyperactivity at school entry predict high school nongraduation above and beyond academic abilities, and why should aggression–opposition add to this prediction only at a later stage? Inattention–hyperactivity could predict high school nongraduation because it impedes classroom participation and interferes with academic performance. Children who are inattentive and hyperactive tend to disobey or ignore teachers' instructions, thus limiting directly their opportunities for learning, especially in crucial areas such as reading (Chen, Rubin, & Li, 1995). This negative disposition toward the classroom activities may operate already at school entry, and persist throughout primary school. It is unlikely that aggression–opposition operates in a similar way. Instead, childhood conduct problems could contribute to later academic achievement through indirect pathways that involve a series of negative social experiences that become important by middle or late childhood. For example, aggressive–oppositional children tend to be rejected by their normative peers (Dodge, Coie, Pettit, & Price, 1990). However, this is not necessarily the case at school entry, especially if the group norms are supportive or neutral in regard to aggressive–oppositional behaviors (Boivin, Dodge, & Coie, 1995). Hence, aggressive–oppositional behaviors may be met with peer rejection more systematically or more intensively during the second part of primary school than at school entry (Younger, Schwartzman, & Ledingham, 1986). On the other hand, aggressive–oppositional children progressively tend to affiliate with other aggressive–oppositional children, partly by choice and partly by default (Boivin, Vitaro, & Poulin, 2005). The cliques thus formed may cultivate anti-school norms, increasing the likelihood that youth who affiliate with them will get involved in deviant activities that are incompatible with school-related work (Dishion, Veronneau, & Myers, 2010). This process may not be clearly in place before middle childhood, at which point the networks of aggressive–oppositional children become increasingly exclusive. Starting in middle childhood, cliques likely become increasingly homogeneous with respect to behavior and academic performance, increasing the pressure on members to act according to clique norms. These social experiences at the group level can reduce aggressive–oppositional children's motivation toward school.

Aggressive–oppositional children are also at risk of experiencing conflicts with their teachers, resulting in some cases in highly negative sanctions from teachers (e.g., school suspension or public humiliation), and further increasing the likelihood of rejection by normative peers and affiliation with non-normative classmates (Brendgen, Wanner, Vitaro, Bukowski, & Tremblay, 2007; Hughes, Luo, Kwok, & Loyd, 2008; Pianta & Stuhlman, 2004). These additional negative experiences with the teacher can further reduce aggressive–oppositional children's classroom engagement and achievement motivation (Erath, Flanagan, & Bierman, 2008; Ladd, Kochenderfer, & Coleman, 1997; Stipek & Miles, 2008; Wentzel, 2009). Thus, unlike inattention–hyperactivity, aggression–opposition may not impact school completion through reduced school performance, but rather through a decrease in school motivation (Ladd & Dinella, 2009; see Figure 2.1 for an illustration). Given that motivation during primary school is as important a predictor of future high school completion as school performance (Spinath, Spinath, Harlaar, & Plomin, 2006; Véronneau, Vitaro, Pedersen, & Tremblay, 2008), aggression–opposition can have a long-term effect on high school achievement that is as strong as the effect of early inattention–hyperactivity. However, given that the negative social experiences encountered by aggressive–oppositional children with their peers and teachers do not crystallize before the middle of primary school, it is likely that their possible consequences for school motivation and, indirectly, school completion will not be apparent before this period. Hence, the first objective of the current study was to examine, through a transactional model whether primary school students' inattention–hyperactivity and aggression–opposition uniquely predict high school graduation either directly or indirectly through changes in academic performance or school motivation. The second objective was to evaluate whether the associations between behavior problems (i.e., inattention–hyperactivity and aggression–opposition), academic achievement, and school motivation vary developmentally across primary school.

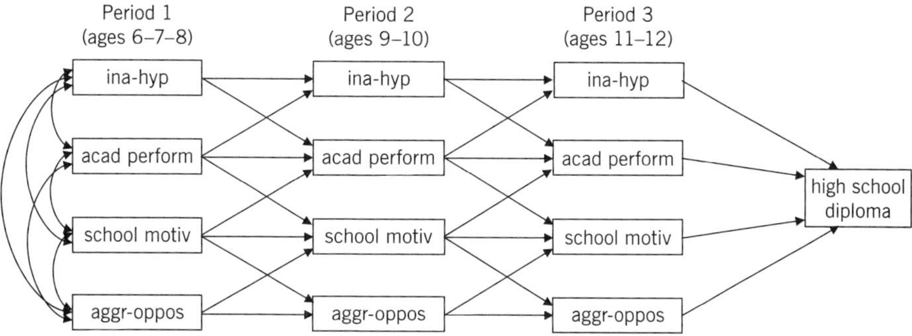

FIGURE 2.1. Transactional model tested. Cross-sectional links among study variables are illustrated for period 1 only but are included also for periods 2 and 3 in the tested model. Control variables (sex, mother's occupational prestige, child's anxiety–depressive symptoms at each time period), as well as cross-lagged links between aggression–opposition and inattention–hyperactivity, are also included in the tested model but omitted in the figure for the sake of parsimony.

Directional and Bidirectional Effects

The proposed model speculates that both inattention–hyperactivity and aggression–opposition contribute, through various pathways, to academic difficulties and nongraduation. These pathways may also be recursive. For example, academic difficulties and low school motivation might aggravate behavior problems and precipitate negative outcomes (Dishion, Patterson, Stoolmiller, & Skinner, 1991; Moffitt, 1990; Morgan, Farkas, Tufis, & Sperling, 2008; Williams & McGee, 1994). Conversely, early school difficulties could foster an increase in behavior problems, which in turn could foster an increase in academic difficulties over time (Miles & Stipek, 2006). Bidirectional (i.e., reciprocal, transactional) links may exist not only between the behavioral dimensions and school performance but also between the behavioral dimensions and school motivation, possibly mediated by reduced school performance (Ladd & Dinella, 2009). Finally, directional (i.e., sequential) as well as bidirectional links between school performance and school motivation also ought to exist (Véronneau et al., 2008) such that, for example, behavior problems influence school motivation, which in turn influences academic performance (and vice versa). As illustrated in Figure 2.1, the third objective of this study was to test for bidirectional links: (1) between externalizing behavior problems (i.e., inattention–hyperactivity, aggression–opposition) and academic difficulties (i.e., low academic performance and school motivation), and (2) between academic difficulties and school motivation.

It was expected that inattention–hyperactivity would predict decreased academic performance starting in kindergarten and throughout primary school and, conversely, decreased academic performance would predict an increase in inattention–hyperactivity over time. For aggression–opposition, transactional interplay was expected during the second part of primary school but not during the first part. Similarly, it was expected that low academic performance would predict decreased school motivation in kindergarten and throughout primary school, and conversely, decreased school motivation would predict decreased academic performance.

Sex as Possible Moderator and Control Variable

In examining these issues, we also tested whether the model illustrated in Figure 2.1 applies equally to boys and girls. Because boys tend to be more aggressive–oppositional and more inattentive–hyperactive than girls, the links between the behavioral dimensions and non-high school graduation may be stronger for boys. In contrast, girls may be more negatively affected than boys by interpersonal stressors (peer rejection, teachers' sanctions) (Crick & Zahn-Waxler, 2003; Little & Garber, 2004). Girls' school motivation and school performance may also suffer more than boys as a consequence of such negative experiences. Social-familial adversity served as a control variable in this study given its relevance with regard to both the predictors, the intermediate variables (i.e., school motivation, school performance), and the distal outcome (i.e., high school graduation) (Brooks-Gunn & Duncan, 1997; Campbell, Spieker, Burchinal, Poe, & the NICHD Early Child Care Research Network, 2006; Ensminger & Slusarcick, 1992). Cross-sectional and cross-lagged links between the two externalizing behavioral dimensions (i.e., inattention–hyperactivity and aggression–opposition) were also controlled. Finally, because of the overlap and the reciprocal influence between externalizing (i.e., inattention–hyperactivity, aggression–opposition) and internalizing (i.e., anxiety–depression) behaviors (van Lier et al., 2012) and the possible links between internalizing behaviors and academic achievement (Duchesne, Vitaro, Larose, & Tremblay, 2008), we also controlled for children's anxious–depressed symptoms throughout primary school.

Method

Participants

Participants in the present study were part of a representative population-based sample (i.e., randomly selected from the list provided by the Ministry of Education) that initially included 6,397 kindergarten children throughout the Province of Québec in 1986–1987. The final sample included 4,090 children (2,090 boys) for whom ratings were available from teachers and parents at least two times during data collection and for whom official information on their high school diploma was not missing. By design, approximately one quarter of the final sample comprised children who scored at the 80th percentile or higher (with sex-specific cutoffs) on a disruptive behavior scale according to either the parent or teacher in kindergarten. More details about the sampling procedure can be found in Rouquette et al. (2012). The vast majority of participants were French-speaking white Canadian kindergartners (i.e., 95%), and most (i.e., 81%) were living with their two biological parents. Mothers had an average of 11.7 years of schooling (*SD* = 2.8), and fathers had an average of 11.9 years of schooling (*SD* = 3.5). A total of 2,307 children were lost through attrition or by design (not all participants were followed longitudinally). On the basis of high school completion data provided by the Ministry of Education, participants and nonparticipants did not differ with respect to the proportion of individuals who had not graduated from high school by ages 22–23.

Measures

Means, standard deviations, skewness and kurtosis for all study variables, except high school graduation (the dichotomous outcome variable) are presented in Table 2.1.

High School Graduation (Distal Outcome Variable)

Information about high school graduation was obtained through the Québec Ministry of Education in 2003 when the participants were ages 22–23 years. The measure differentiated between participants who had a high school diploma (coded 1; a high school diploma is normally reached by age 17 after 11 years of schooling) and participants who did not (coded 0, which included dropouts and people who were still attending school). This variable was available for 95% of all participants, of whom 68% had obtained their diploma by age 22–23 years. About half of the 32% who had not obtained a high school diploma by that age were enrolled in night courses or adult professional training. The percentage of participants with no high school diploma is higher than expected because of our over-sampling for at-risk children.

Child Behavioral Dimensions (Predictors)

Mothers and teachers rated children's behavior every year between the ages of 6 and 12 years using items from the Social Behavior Questionnaire (SBQ; Tremblay et al., 1991). Items were scored 0 (*never*) to 2 (*often*). To maximize measurement variance and reliability, the scores were averaged across three periods: first, across ages 6, 7, and 8 years (i.e., when children were typically in kindergarten, grade 1, and grade 2); second, across ages 9 and 10 (i.e., typically in grades 3 and 4), and finally, across ages 11 and 12 (i.e., typically in grades 5 and 6). The Inattention–Hyperactivity Scale included six items: (1) weak capacity for concentration, cannot maintain his or her attention for a long time on the same task; (2) easily distracted; (3) absentminded; (4) gives up easily; (5) restless, runs about, or jumps up and down, does not keep still; and (6) squirmy, fidgety child (alpha = 0.83–0.87 for teachers; alpha = 0.73–0.79 for mothers). Teacher and mother ratings were correlated, *r*s between .41 and .47 every year, and

TABLE 2.1. Means ($\overline{X}$) and Standard Deviations (*SD*) for Children's Inattention–Hyperactivity, Aggression–Opposition, Academic Performance, and School Motivation Scores

Variable		Development period		
		(6)-7-8	9-10	11-12
Inattention–hyperactivity	$\overline{X}$ (*SD*)	0.61 (0.38)	0.62 (0.44)	0.55 (0.43)
	Skewness	0.66	0.57	0.77
	Kurtosis	-0.12	-0.41	-0.05
Aggression–opposition	$\overline{X}$ (*SD*)	0.38 (0.28)	0.34 (0.24)	0.31 (0.28)
	Skewness	1.33	1.37	1.53
	Kurtosis	2.10	2.16	3.07
Academic performance	$\overline{X}$ (*SD*)	2.33 (1.06)	2.25 (1.02)	2.18 (1.01)
	Skewness	-0.19	-0.34	-0.02
	Kurtosis	-0.66	-0.60	-0.60
School motivation	$\overline{X}$ (*SD*)	0.89 (0.18)	0.92 (0.17)	0.87 (0.19)
	Skewness	-1.82	0.19	-1.43
	Kurtosis	3.23	12.87	1.39
Parent occupational prestige	$\overline{X}$ (*SD*)	42.48 (10.61)		
	Skewness	0.52		
	Kurtosis	0.04		
Anxiety–depressive symptoms	$\overline{X}$ (*SD*)	0.53 (0.28)	0.53 (0.32)	0.49 (0.30)
	Skewness	0.70	0.71	0.72
	Kurtosis	0.84	0.49	0.41

Note. The first developmental period includes age 6 years for hyperactivity–inattention and aggression–opposition (i.e., behavioral dimensions), whereas it does not for academic performance and school motivation (i.e., scholastic dimensions). Moreover, the behavioral dimensions were averaged at the item level across mothers and teachers, whereas the scholastic dimensions were rated only by teachers.

were averaged annually into a composite score meant to be a reliable and representative measure of children's inattention–hyperactivity.

The Aggression–Opposition scale included eight items: (1) fights with other children; (2) bullies other children; (3) kicks, bites, or hits other children; (4) irritable, quick to "fly off the handle"; (5) is disobedient; (6) doesn't share toys; (7) blames others; and (8) inconsiderate of others (alpha = 0.87–0.91 for teachers; alpha = 0.74–0.77 for mothers). Teacher and mother ratings were correlated, *r*s between .31 and .35 every year, and were averaged into a composite score.

Child Academic Achievement (Predictor and Putative Mediator)

Teachers rated each child's academic achievement each year when the child was between the ages of 7 and 12 years (the kindergarten assessment was not available) using three items to assess the child's writing, reading, and mathematics performance, and one item to measure the child's overall academic achievement. Teacher ratings of children's academic achievement have been shown to be valid and highly correlated with other, more objective, measures of school achievement (Demaray & Elliott, 1998; Feinberg & Shapiro, 2003). Each question had five response categories (0 = *considerably below the mean* to 4 = *considerably above the mean*). For each child, a composite academic achievement score was computed by averaging the four items at each time point, then averaging them over the same three periods as those for the behavioral dimensions (i.e., ages 7–8, ages 9–10, and ages 11–12). Annual Cronbach alphas were very high and stable (i.e., alpha = 0.95).

Child School Motivation (Predictor and Putative Mediator)

Teachers rated each child's school motivation each year when the child was between the ages of 7 and 12 years. Three items (likes school, shows interest toward school, lacks motivation to learn new material–reverse coded) were rated using a 2-point scale (yes–no; alpha = 0.66–0.69). A composite school motivation score was computed by summing the three items at each time point, and averaging them over the same three periods as for school performance (i.e., ages 7–8, ages 9–10, and ages 11–12).

Family Characteristics (Control Variable)

When the children were 6 years old, parents completed the Blishen, Carroll, and Moore (1987) Occupational Prestige Scale. This socioeconomic index classifies occupations by income and education in Canada. A mean score for both parents was used (mother: mean = 44.01; *SD* = 13.03, father: mean = 44.00; *SD* = 14.88).

Child Anxiety–Depressed Symptoms (Control Variable)

Mothers and teachers rated each child's internalizing behaviors (i.e., anxious–depressed symptoms) every year between the ages of 6 and 12 years, using five items from the SBQ (Tremblay et al., 1991): (1) is worried; worries about many things; (2) tends to play on his or her own, is rather solitary; (3) appears miserable, unhappy, tearful, or distressed; (4) tends to be fearful or afraid of new things or new situations; and (5) cries easily. Each item was scored 0 to 2 depending on how frequently the child manifested the behavior (alpha = 0.72–0.76 for teachers; alpha = 0.62–0.66 for mothers). Annual teacher and mother ratings were averaged into a composite score. Finally, the scores were averaged across the same three periods as for the other behavioral dimensions: across ages 6–8, 9–10, and 11–12 years.

Results

Descriptive Statistics and Bivariate Correlations

The descriptive statistics and distributional properties for all study variables are presented in Table 2.1. Kurtosis and skewness were within the acceptable range. Following recommendations by Schielzeth (2010), we standardized all independent variables prior to subsequent analysis. This strategy provided a uniform point of comparison for judging the relative importance of predictors within models (Gelman & Hill, 2007).

Table 2.2 presents the bivariate correlations between the study variables, including the control variables and the outcome variable (i.e., high school diploma). The correlation pattern illustrated in Table 2.2 revealed no collinearity problem. With few exceptions, all correlations were in the expected direction and significant. To illustrate, significant relations involving gender were found with respect to high school graduation, $\chi^2(1) = 106.29$, $p < .001$. Compared to boys, girls were more likely to graduate (74.6% for girls vs. 59.5% for boys). Girls were also less hyperactive–inattentive and less aggressive–oppositional throughout all the study periods. Finally, girls had higher academic achievement and school motivation than boys throughout the three study periods. However, they did not differ from boys on anxiety–depression symptoms. As expected, parent occupational prestige was positively related to high school graduation, as well as to children's academic achievement and school motivation, but negatively related to children's externalizing behavior problems (i.e., inattention–hyperactivity and aggression–opposition). In turn, children's externalizing behavior problems at each period were significantly and negatively related to high school diploma, whereas academic performance and school motivation at each period were positively related to high school diploma. Interestingly, the correlations between school motivation and high school diploma were the same magnitude as the correlations between academic performance and high school diploma (*r*s in the lower .40s). However, the correlations between inattention–hyperactivity and high school diploma tended to be higher than those between aggression–opposition (or anxiety–depression) and high school diploma (*r*s in the lower .40s for inattention–hyperactivity vs. *r*s in the higher .20s for aggression–opposition and *r*s of around .15 for anxiety–depression).

TABLE 2.2. Bivariate Correlations between Study Variables (i.e., Hyperactivity–Inattention, Aggression–Opposition, Academic Performance, and School Motivation), Control Variables (Anxiety–Depression, Parent Occupational Prestige, and Child Sex), and Outcome Variable (High School Diploma)

Variables	I-H(1)	I-H(2)	I-H(3)	A-O(1)	A-O(2)	A-O(3)	AP(1)	AP(2)	AP(3)	SM(1)	SM(2)	SM(3)	AD(1)	AD(2)	AD(3)	POP	Sex	HSD
Inattention–Hyperact: I-H(1)	1																	
Inattention–Hyperact: I-H (2)	.69	1																
Inattention–Hyperact: I-H (3)	.66	.73	1															
Aggression–Oppos: A-O(1)	.63	.47	.46	1														
Aggression–Oppos: A-O(2)	.48	.58	.45	.66	1													
Aggression–Oppos: A-O(3)	.44	.46	.59	.62	.66	1												
Academic Performance: AP(1)	–.53	–.47	–.44	–.25	–.21	–.20	1											
Academic Performance: AP(2)	–.49	–.57	–.50	–.26	–.24	–.23	.70	1										
Academic Performance: AP(3)	–.50	–.53	–.58	–.25	–.23	–.27	.70	.75	1									
School Motivation: SM(1)	–.54	–.46	–.47	–.35	–.30	–.30	.54	.45	.44	1								
School Motivation: SM(2)	–.37	–.54	–.47	–.24	–.33	–.29	.32	.41	.39	.55	1							
School Motivation: SM(3)	–.43	–.49	–.67	–.32	–.34	–.46	.40	.45	.54	.47	.57	1						
Anxiety–Depress: AD(1)	.32	.19	.18	.22	.13	.11	–.21	–.18	–.17	–.23	–.14	–.13	1					
Anxiety–Depress: AD(2)	.28	.41	.24	.18	.31	.17	–.20	–.24	–.21	–.20	–.28	–.15	.48	1				
Anxiety–Depress: AD(3)	.28	.29	.41	.20	.20	.31	–.19	–.19	–.24	–.22	–.23	–.28	.46	.50	1			
Parent Occupational Prestige (POP)	–.20	–.19	–.18	–.11	–.12	–.12	.23	.28	.28	.16	.12	.19	–.09	–.07	–.11	1		
Sex (girls = 1; boys = 0)	–.27	–.25	–.28	–.27	–.24	–.25	.12	.15	.16	.19	.10	.21	(–.04)	(.00)	(.01)	(.01)	1	
High School Diploma (HSD)	–.40	–.41	–.48	–.29	–.27	–.33	.43	.45	.49	.38	.35	.48	–.13	–.14	–.20	.25	.36	1

Note. All correlations are significant at $p < .05$ except for those in parentheses. (1) (2) (3) indicate the developmental periods: (1) ages 6–7–8; (2) ages 9–10; (3) ages 11–12.

Most notably, the correlations involving any of the predictors assessed during the first period (i.e., ages 6–8) were as strong as the correlations involving the same predictors during the subsequent two periods.

Results presented in Table 2.2 also reveal that all study variables were relatively stable from one period to the next. Stability, however, was far from perfect, with more than half of the variance unexplained by the same variable during the previous interval. The results in Table 2.2 also provide preliminary support for the hypothesis that both types of externalizing problems (i.e., inattention–hyperactivity and aggression–opposition) are related to changes in academic achievement and school motivation. In fact, each type of externalizing problem was correlated with participants' subsequent academic achievement and school motivation across all intervals. However, the reverse pattern (i.e., academic achievement and school motivation predicting externalizing problems) was not as systematic.

Model Testing

Structural equation modeling (SEM) analyses (Bollen, 1989) using the Mplus 6.01 software (Muthén & Muthén, 2010) were conducted to assess the fit of the transactional model depicted in Figure 2.1. Cross-sectional links among study variables for periods 2 and 3 as well as cross-lagged links between the two types of externalizing problems (i.e., inattention–hyperactivity and aggressiveness–opposition) were included in the tested model but are not illustrated in Figure 2.1 for the sake of parsimony. Because of the categorical nature of the outcome (i.e., high school graduation), the usual chi-square-based fit statistics proposed by Kline (2005) could not be used to assess adequate model fit. However, models could be compared to other, more or less complex models using the –2LL difference test, which is equivalent to a nested chi-square difference test (Purcell, 2002). The full information maximum likelihood (FIML) estimation procedure was used for the SEM analysis (Allison, 2003). With this method, the covariance matrix used to estimate model parameters is constructed from all available information for all participants, even those with some missing data. FIML estimation is deemed adequate when analyzing data with moderate levels of missingness even when data are not missing completely at random, provided the predictors of missingness are included in the model, as was the case here (Widaman, 2006).

Description of Significant Paths for the Whole Sample

A first set of analyses was performed to assess the transactional model using data from boys and girls together. The results from this model are depicted in Figure 2.2.

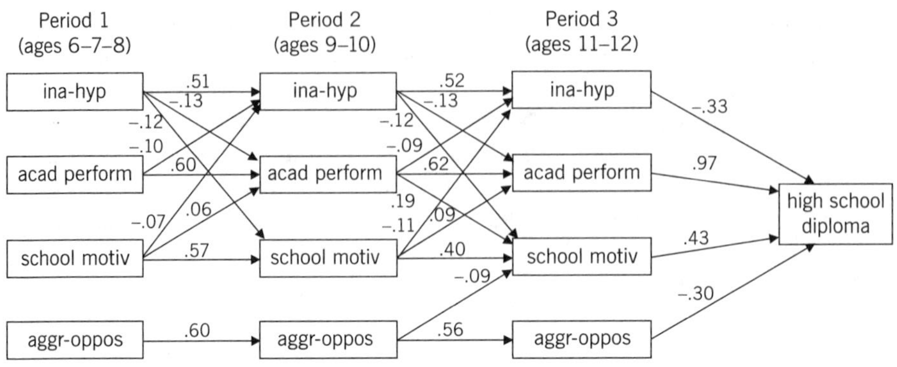

FIGURE 2.2. Significant stability and cross-lagged associations for boys and girls together, with cross-sectional links and control variables included but not illustrated.

Baseline Model, with Stability (Autoregressive) and Cross-Sectional Links Only

As shown in Figure 2.2, participants' academic achievement, school motivation, inattention–hyperactivity, and aggression–opposition were highly stable, with significant associations from one developmental period to the next. As expected, the direct positive links between academic performance and school motivation at the end of primary school and high school diploma were significant and moderately high (odds ratios = 2.65 and 1.54, respectively; $p < .05$). Interestingly, the direct negative links between inattention–hyperactivity and aggression–opposition at the end of primary school and high school diploma were also moderate and significant (odds ratios = 0.72 and 0.74, respectively; $p < .05$). Thus, it is a combination of behavioral, motivational, and achievement factors at the end of primary school that predicts high school diploma, and most of these predictions can be traced back to school entry.

Full Model, with the Addition of Cross-Lagged Links

As also depicted in Figure 2.2, participants' inattention–hyperactivity predicted changes in their academic performance and school motivation from the beginning to the middle of the primary school period and from the middle to the end of the primary school period. Conversely, both scholastic dimensions (i.e., academic performance and school motivation) systematically predicted changes in inattention–hyperactivity over both periods. In contrast, the predictive links involving aggression–opposition were few and nonsystematic. Nevertheless, aggression–opposition in the middle of the primary school period predicted a reduction in school motivation by the end of primary school, which, in turn, predicted high school diploma. No predictive links between aggression–opposition and academic performance or between academic performance and aggression–opposition were found. An examination of the indirect links of the predictor variables to high school diploma across all three developmental periods revealed several significant associations. Importantly, all the indirect (i.e., mediated) links involving inattention–hyperactivity and high school diploma through either academic performance or school motivation at intervening developmental periods were significant ($p < .05$), albeit modest. These included links to high school diploma from inattention–hyperactivity (Times 1 and 2) to academic performance (Times 2 and 3), betas ranging from –0.07 to –0.13, and links to high school diploma from inattention–hyperactivity (Times 1 and 2) to school motivation (Times 2 and 3), betas = –0.02 to –0.03. An additional link emerged between aggression–opposition (Time 2) and high school diploma through school motivation (Time 3), beta = –0.04.

There were also a number of transactional links between the two scholastic dimensions, independent of the behavioral dimensions. Specifically, school motivation predicted an improvement in academic performance across all three developmental periods, whereas academic performance predicted a moderate change in school motivation from period 2 to period 3 only. All the indirect links involving the scholastic dimensions predicting to high school diploma were significant at $p < .05$, albeit modest. Links to high school diploma included academic performance (Times 1 and 2) to school motivation (Time 3), beta = 0.05; school motivation (Time 1 and 2) to academic performance (Times 2 and 3), beta = 0.04 and beta = 0.03) and to school motivation (Time 3), beta = 0.01. In summary, the moderately high, direct pathways are complemented by indirect modest pathways that originate in the first developmental period, except for aggression–opposition. Some results varied according to gender as documented next.

Description of Significant Paths for the Boys and Girls Separately

In a second set of analyses, we performed a two-group analysis to examine whether the model parameters depicted in Figure 2.2 applied equally to male and female participants. To this end, we compared a model in which all regression and correlation coefficients were constrained to be equal across genders (i.e., the constrained model) to the same model in which those coefficients could freely vary across genders (i.e., the unconstrained model). The log likelihood difference test between the unconstrained model (log likelihood = –56,549.55) and the fully constrained model (log likelihood = –56,639.40) was significant, $\chi^2(52) = 179.71$; $p < .001$, suggesting that the constrained model did not fit the data well. Guided by the residual statistics and the Lagrange multipliers, we next freed as many parameters as necessary across the two sex-groups to obtain a parsimonious model that did not differ significantly in fit from the constrained model, $\chi^2(37) = 32.75$; $p = .67$. The results from this parsimonious best fitting model are illustrated in Figure 2.3a (for boys) and 2.3b (for girls).

The results illustrated in Figure 2.3a and 2.3b show that the majority of the cross-lagged links did not differ between boys and girls. The few differences were mostly differences in magnitude (i.e., links were significant for both sexes but stronger for one sex than the other). There were, however, three notable qualitative differences between boys and girls. First, inattention–hyperactivity at the end of primary school predicted non–high school graduation for girls but not for boys (for whom the link reached just a significant trend at $p = .06$). Second, academic performance in period 1 predicted an increase in school motivation from period 1 to period 2 for girls but not for boys. Third, aggression–opposition in period 1 predicted a decrease in school motivation from period 1 to period 2 for girls but an *increase* for boys. The indirect effects of aggression–opposition in period 1 to high school diploma through school motivation in period 2 and school motivation or academic performance in period 3 for boys were significant and positive (.02 and .03, respectively; $p < .05$). For girls, the indirect pathway through school motivation in periods 2 and 3 was also significant but negative (–.02, $p < .05$).

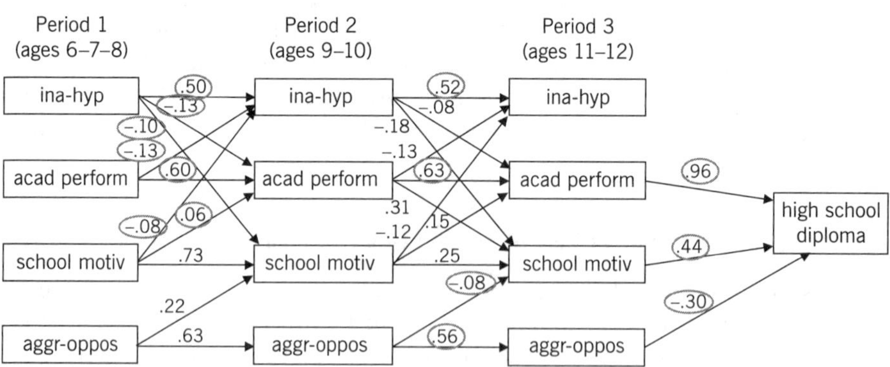

FIGURE 2.3a. Significant stability and cross-lagged associations for boys, with cross-sectional links and control variables included but not illustrated. Circled values are equal across genders.

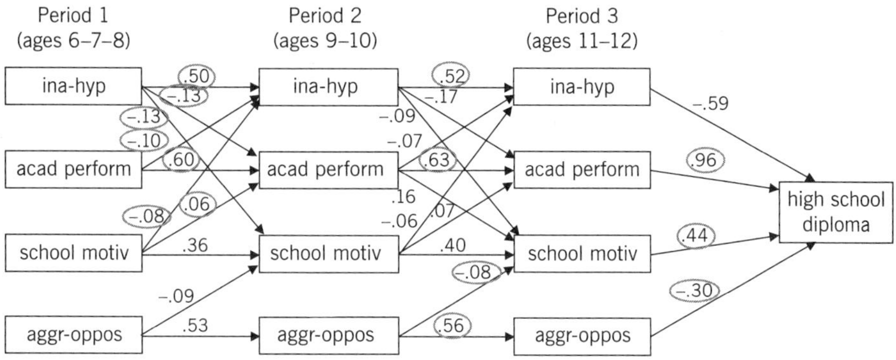

FIGURE 2.3b. Significant stability and cross-lagged associations for girls, with cross-sectional links and control variables included but not illustrated. Circled parameters are equal across genders.

Control Variables and Concurrent Links (Not Shown in Figure 2.2)

As predicted, boys were more at risk than girls for both types of externalizing behaviors across all three periods. They were also more at risk for lower academic achievement and school motivation during each developmental period (except at school entry in regard to school motivation) compared to girls. However, boys were not less likely to graduate from high school than girls once the behavioral and scholastic dimensions were accounted for (p = .08). In contrast, parent occupational prestige significantly predicted high school diploma independent of other study variables (beta = 0.41, SE = .05, p = .001). Anxious–depressed feelings also failed uniquely to predict high school diploma (beta = 0.01, p = .83), despite significant bivariate correlations. Finally, only one cross-lag link between aggression–opposition and inattention–hyperactivity was significant (beta = 0.06).

Discussion

The main objective of this study was to examine, through a transactional model, whether primary school students' inattention–hyperactivity and aggression–opposition uniquely predicted high school graduation either directly or indirectly through changes in academic performance or school motivation. The second objective was to test whether these associations varied across development, from the beginning to the end of primary school. The third objective was to examine possible reciprocal links between behavioral and scholastic dimensions. A final objective was to test whether the pattern of results differed for boys and girls.

To avoid spurious effects, parent occupational prestige, children's sex, and children's internalizing problems were included as control variables. Autoregressive (i.e., stability) links and concurrent links between study variables were also controlled in the transactional design. The need for such a stringent control in testing the main hypotheses proved necessary given the cross-sectional associations among most study variables and their moderate stability.

Indirect and Reciprocal Effects

Our first hypothesis, that a decrease in academic performance would account for (i.e., mediate) the predictive link between inattention–hyperactivity and high school graduation, was supported. Interestingly, reduced school motivation also played a mediating role between inattention–hyperactivity and high school graduation. Our second hypothesis, that aggression–opposition would predict graduating from high school through a decrease in school motivation was also partially supported. These findings are discussed in turn.

Inattention–Hyperactivity

As described earlier, inattentive–hyperactive behaviors can deter youth from achieving a high school diploma because they may interfere with academic tasks and self-regulated learning, and consequently with academic achievement (Erath et al., 2008; Ladd & Dinella, 2009). Inattention–hyperactivity also contributes to non-high school graduation because it reduces children's motivation toward school, possibly through social processes such as peer rejection and negative teacher–child interactions (McDougall, Hymel, Vaillancourt, & Mercer, 2001). Importantly, this dual process of academic failure and school disengagement associated with inattention–hyperactivity problems is already active in the early years of school (i.e., between ages 6 and 8 years). It is also cumulative, as indicated by unique contributions of inattention–hyperactivity to changes in both academic performance and school motivation across all three developmental periods considered in this study. Finally, this dual mediation process (through reduced academic performance and motivation) completely accounted for the link between inattention–hyperactivity and high school graduation for the boys. In other words, inattentive–hyperactive boys do not graduate because they get bad grades and lose interest in school. For girls, however, other processes seem to be involved during secondary school, given that the residual link between inattention–hyperactivity and high school graduation was still moderately high and significant even after accounting for reductions in academic performance and school motivation throughout primary school.

Aggression–Opposition

In contrast to inattention–hyperactivity, aggressive–oppositional behaviors contributed to high school graduation either directly or through school motivation. In the overall analysis that included both boys and girls, the indirect contribution of aggression–opposition through reduced school motivation was limited to the interval between the second and the third period. However, the lack of a significant contribution of aggression–opposition in period 1 in the whole sample masked an important difference between girls and boys: For girls, the contribution of aggression–opposition in period 1 was negative, whereas it was positive for boys. Hence, contrary to Hinshaw's speculations (Hinshaw, 1992), it is not only during the later childhood years that aggression–opposition interferes with later academic success. According to these findings, aggression–opposition also plays an important role during the first years of school, but in opposite directions for girls and boys. For girls, aggression–opposition negatively affects their attitude toward school, probably because it negatively affects their social relationships with their teacher and their peers (Izard et al., 2001) and consequently their opportunities for positive exchanges that promote cooperative learning and cognitive development (Buhs, Ladd, & Herald, 2006; Coolahan, Fantuzzo, Mendez, & McDermott, 2000). Perhaps because aggression–opposition is non-normative and not well tolerated for girls, it undermines school adjustment in kindergarten and throughout primary school. In contrast, for boys, aggression–opposition is better tolerated by teachers and peers during the initial school years, and does not undermine school adjustment until later (i.e., by middle childhood, periods 2 and 3 in the present study) when aggression–opposition becomes non-normative (Broidy et al., 2003). Existing research suggests that for boys, some aggressive–oppositional behaviors do not elicit social rebuff from peers at school entry, particularly if the norms are supportive or neutral in regard to aggressive behaviors (Boivin et al., 1995; Dodge et al., 1990; Vaughn, Vollenweider, Bost, Azria-Evans, & Snider, 2003). To illustrate, Dodge et al. (1990) looked at how different forms of aggressive behaviors (i.e., reactive–hostile aggression, instrumental–proactive aggression, bullying, rough-and-tumble play) related to peer status in first- and third-grade boys. They found that both reactive aggression and instrumental aggression, but not rough play, were associated with negative peer status at both ages. Bullying was also related to negative peer status, but only in the third-grade group. In the first-grade group, it was the more popular boys who displayed more bullying, as if to establish their dominance, whereas for older boys, social dominance was attained by more sophisticated strategies. The global measure of aggression–opposition used in this study included behaviors such as bullying, blurring the link between aggression–opposition and peer status during period 1 and, consequently, its role with respect to school motivation and high school completion: if indeed, our aggression–opposition measure was a proxy for bullying and a marker of social dominance, then it makes sense that its contribution to school motivation and high school graduation for boys was positive rather than negative. It is also possible that teachers devote special attention to aggressive–oppositional behaviors in boys during the first years of school in an attempt to change these behaviors (Goldstein, Arnold, Rosenberg, Stowe, & Ortiz, 2001). This increased attention might in some cases be successful in eliciting interest in and motivation for school-related activities in young aggressive–oppositional boys. Interestingly, Bierman et al. (2009) also reported that aggressive behavior enhanced the prediction of children's cognitive readiness during the preschool years, once deficits in prosocial behavior were controlled. As such, although the positive contribution of aggression–opposition in period 1 to boys' school motivation was unexpected and our explanations necessarily remain speculative, this association and possible underlying processes merit further investigation in future research.

Academic Achievement and School Motivation

Interestingly, in the early years of school, school motivation predicted an increase in academic achievement for both genders, whereas academic achievement predicted an increase in school motivation but only for boys. This result is in line with past research showing that attitude toward school at school entry is an important predictor of school functioning and academic performance, but not the other way around, at least for boys (Ladd, Buhs, & Seid, 2000). From the second to the third period, school motivation predicted an increase in academic performance and, reciprocally, academic achievement predicted a change in school motivation. These reciprocal links were significant for both genders but even more so in boys than in girls. These findings suggest that it is important to support children's (particularly boys') motivation and interest toward school, as much as their school performance throughout primary school. One way to achieve this goal is to foster positive relationships with teachers and peers (Baker, 2006; Brendgen, Wanner, & Vitaro, 2006; Buhs & Ladd, 2001; Buhs et al., 2006; Hamre & Pianta, 2001; Ladd et al., 1997). Children who have positive interactions with teachers and peers experience more positive emotions toward school than those who have negative interactions (Izard et al., 2001). In turn, positive emotions toward school foster learning. Indeed, these results clearly suggest that school motivation remains a significant predictor of sustained academic performance throughout primary school and ultimately of school completion, net of academic performance, behavioral difficulties and socioeconomic factors.

Scholastic and Behavioral Dimensions

These findings show that inattention–hyperactivity and, to a lesser degree, aggression–opposition contribute to academic difficulties or school motivation. In return, academic difficulties and low school motivation aggravate children's inattention–hyperactivity problems but not aggressive–oppositional behaviors. These findings are in line with other studies showing that early academic problems are related to an increase in externalizing behaviors (Dishion et al., 1991; Moffitt, 1990; Morgan et al., 2008; Williams & McGee, 1994). However, given that past studies did not distinguish between subtypes of externalizing problems or did not control for the overlap between them (Miles & Stipek, 2006), it is difficult to conclude whether the directional links between academic functioning and externalizing behaviors are limited to inattention–hyperactivity problems as suggested here. In any case, this study shows that low school motivation contributes to this process, independent of academic achievement.

Residual Direct Effects

The indirect and reciprocal effects reported in this study are important, especially in the context of a transactional model in which researchers control for autoregressive and concurrent links. However, they are modest compared to the residual direct effects of either the behavioral or the scholastic dimensions. The residual direct effect of aggression–opposition for both sexes deserves a particular mention given the ongoing debate about the contribution of social-emotional difficulties to high school completion. Contrary to inattention–hyperactivity, which triggers a series of scholastic consequences throughout primary school, aggression–opposition may affect high school graduation by processes that become increasingly important during the adolescent years. Affiliation of aggressive–oppositional boys and girls with peers outside the school system, some of whom are dropouts or deviant, may start a disengagement process throughout adolescence that culminates in nongraduation from high school (Kiesner, Poulin, & Nicotra, 2003; Véronneau et al., 2010). The residual link between aggression–oppositional behavior and nongraduation may thus not be direct after all, but mediated through these putative processes. Unfortunately, these possible mediation processes were not assessed in the present study.

To summarize, our findings are in line with studies showing that early inattention–hyperactivity (i.e., at ages 6, 7 and 8 years) uniquely predicts lack of school completion because it disrupts learning and motivation toward school (Breslau et al., 2009; Burt & Roisman, 2010; Duncan et al., 2007; Rapport et al., 1999; Vitaro et al., 2005). They are also in line with findings by Galéra and colleagues (2009) that conduct disorders by late childhood impede later academic performance and high school graduation, above and beyond inattention and hyperactivity. This is also the case at school entry, but for girls only. Contrary to the role of inattention–hyperactivity, which is explained by both reduced academic performance and school motivation, the contribution of aggression–opposition is partly explained by reduced school motivation (except from period 1 to period 2 for boys) and partly by other factors not measured in this study. Such factors might include rejection by normative peers and affiliation with deviant peers, both of which contribute to the involvement in behaviors that are incompatible with school achievement, such as drug use and delinquency (Vitaro, Pedersen, & Brendgen, 2007). These behaviors are not only well-established outcomes of aggressive–oppositional problems during adolescence but also well-known predictors of poor school success (Dishion et al., 2010).

Control Variables

Parent occupational prestige, an indicator of children's socioeconomic status, predicted high school completion independently of behavioral and scholastic variables. This result is in line with past studies (National Center for Education Statistics, 2008) and suggests that it may not be sufficient to improve children's self-regulatory and social-emotional skills to ensure school success. It may also be necessary to support parents and families by providing them with socioeconomic or educational solutions. Unexpectedly, gender did not predict high school graduation in the multivariate model, although it did in the bivariate analysis. This suggests that the link between gender and high school completion is explained by children's behavioral and scholastic performances throughout primary school. Finally, the third and final control variable (i.e., children's anxious–depressive symptoms) did not predict high school graduation in the multivariate analyses, although it was related to high school graduation at the bivariate level. Thus, it appears that the bivariate association between anxious–depressive symptoms at each period and graduating from high school is spurious and likely the consequence of its shared variance with the two behavioral predictors, that is, inattention-hyperactivity and aggression–opposition. Previous studies also reported that internalized problems do not predict later school achievement, when appropriate controls are included (Burt & Roisman, 2010; Duncan et al., 2007; Masten et al., 2005; Moilanen et al., 2010; Vitaro et al., 2005). It is still possible, however, that internalizing problems become linked to academic difficulties by early adolescence or for subgroups of anxious-depressed children (Duchesne et al., 2008; Moilanen et al., 2010), two aspects not examined in this study.

Strengths and Limitations

The current study presents several strengths. First, its longitudinal design, including repeated measures of all study variables over three developmental periods, made it possible to test for direct and indirect effects. As a consequence, the study afforded a better understanding of the dynamic processes that might explain changes in behavioral and academic adjustment over the primary school years and their long-term linkages with high school graduation. Although it is often acknowledged that interpersonal behavior problems and school-related behaviors mutually influence each other, very few empirical studies have modeled these complex relations. Second, all measures represented the point of view of several raters, as teachers changed from one year to the next. Hence, although we did not use latent scores to reduce measurement error, we increased reliability and validity by creating composite scores across several years. Finally, the use of a population-based sample with a low attrition rate on the outcome variable (i.e., high school graduation) is also worth mentioning.

Despite these strengths, the current study also has some limitations. First, although three developmental periods were covered (i.e., from ages 6–12 years), upward and downward extensions of the time frame would have yielded a more complete picture of the developmental processes involved. A second limitation is that, due to the complexity of the transactional model, further social or psychological experiences that could provide an even richer understanding of the processes linking the behavioral and scholastic functioning to high school completion could not be included. For example, more information about friends' characteristics, children's sociometric status within the classroom, the quality of the teacher–child relationship or children's academic self-perceptions would have contributed to a better understanding of the transactional or sequential links between children's behavioral, social, emotional, and academic achievement (Wentzel, 2009). A third limitation is the weakness of many of the indirect links, especially those including several intervening variables. However, weak indirect links can be expected in a complex transactional model where stability and cross-sectional links are controlled. Indeed, while stronger indirect links might be found in a less complex model, they might actually reflect partially spurious associations.

One last limitation relates to the generalizability of the current findings to other samples. As previously noted, the sample was relatively homogeneous in terms of ethnicity. Consequently, the results may not generalize to children from different social-demographic backgrounds. In future studies, special efforts should be devoted to recruiting a more ethnically diverse sample, in order to enhance the generalizability of the findings. Despite these limitations, this study makes an important contribution to our understanding of the interplay between externalizing behavior problems, academic achievement, and school motivation during the primary school years, and their long-term consequences for achieving a high school diploma.

Implications for Practice and Policy

Although only experimental studies can reveal causal relationships between variables, this longitudinal–transactional design provides valuable information on the possible direction of effects from kindergarten through grade 6. The present results suggest that extra academic support and interventions that decrease inattention–hyperactivity and aggression–opposition during primary school (e.g., via social and self-regulation skills training) may help at-risk students move away from a negative academic trajectory and eventually achieve a high school diploma. Present and past findings suggest that a priority for intervention at school entry should be inattention–hyperactivity because of its increasing entanglement with scholastic outcomes such as academic performance and school motivation. Given the negative direct and indirect effects of aggression–opposition on high school graduation for both boys and girls (except for boys from period 1 to period 2), it is also worth to reduce aggression–opposition by fostering social skills and social problem-solving skills. Blair and Diamond (2008) offered several useful suggestions to promote self-regulation (i.e., opposite of inattention–hyperactivity) and social-emotional competence (i.e., opposite of aggression–opposition). These preventive and promotional actions can be put in place at school entry. At this young age, when aggression–opposition is generally declining, it may be easier to affect the course of these behaviors than later on, when they tend to crystalize. There is evidence that an intervention targeting early aggression–opposition by teaching age 6- to 8-year-old children problem solving and social regulation skills will improve high school achievement (Boisjoli, Vitaro, Lacourse, Barker, & Tremblay, 2007).

Our findings also suggest that we need to distinguish between specific behavioral dimensions such as inattention–hyperactivity and aggression–opposition. It is even possible that we ought to split further between inattention and hyperactivity and between aggression and opposition, although the results at this moment are mixed in that regard. With respect to the inattention–hyperactivity/self-regulation skills construct, some authors found that hyperactivity but not inattention is associated with underachievement in young children (Friedman-Weieneth, Harvey, Youngwirth, & Goldstein, 2007). Others, however, found that inattention but not hyperactivity was uniquely associated with underachievement during adolescence (Pingault et al., 2011). As for the aggression–opposition/social-emotional skills construct, it may be that different forms (i.e., relational, physical, verbal) or different functions (i.e., reactive–hostile, proactive–instrumental, bullying) of aggressive behaviors may play different roles with respect to academic achievement as they do with respect to other domains of functioning (see Vitaro & Brendgen, 2012). Finally and most importantly, these findings suggest that social-emotional and self-regulation skills are equally important during the first school years and throughout primary school. In that sense, one should not be preferred over the other as indicators of school readiness or as targets for early interventions.

References

Allison, P. D. (2003). Missing data techniques for structural equation modeling. *Journal of Abnormal Psychology, 112*(4), 545–557.

Baker, J. A. (2006). Contributions of teacher–child relationships to positive school adjustment during elementary school. *Journal of School Psychology, 44*(3), 211–229.

Bierman, K. L., Torres, M. M., Domitrovich, C. E., Welsh, J. A., & Gest, S. D. (2009). Behavioral and cognitive readiness for school: Cross-domain associations for children attending Head Start. *Social Development, 18*(2), 305–323.

Blair, C., & Diamond, A. (2008). Biological processes in prevention and intervention: The promotion of self-regulation as a means of preventing school failure. *Development and Psychopathology, 20*(3), 899–911.

Blishen, B. R., Carroll, W. K., & Moore, C. (1987). The 1981 socioeconomic index for occupations in Canada. *Canadian Review of Sociology and Anthropology, 24*, 465–488.

Boisjoli, R., Vitaro, F., Lacourse, E., Barker, E. D., & Tremblay, R. E. (2007). Impact and clinical significance of a preventive intervention for disruptive boys: 15-year follow-up. *British Journal of Psychiatry, 191*(5), 415–419.

Boivin, M., Dodge, K. A., & Coie, J. D. (1995). Individual-group behavioral similarity and peer status in experimental play groups: The social misfit revisited. *Journal of Personality and Social Psychology, 69*(2), 269–279.

Boivin, M., Vitaro, F., & Poulin, F. (2005). Peer relationships and the development of aggressive behavior in early childhood. In R. E. Tremblay, W. W. Hartup, & J. Archer (Eds.), *Developmental origins of aggression* (pp. 376–397). New York: Guilford Press.

Bollen, K. A. (1989). *Structural equations with latent variables*. New York: Wiley.

Brendgen, M., Wanner, B., & Vitaro, F. (2006). Verbal abuse by the teacher and child adjustment from kindergarten through grade 6. *Pediatrics, 117*, 1585–1598.

Brendgen, M., Wanner, B., Vitaro, F., Bukowski, W. M., & Tremblay, R. E. (2007). Verbal abuse by the teacher during childhood and academic, behavioral, and emotional adjustment in young adulthood. *Journal of Educational Psychology, 99*, 26–38.

Breslau, J., Miller, E., Breslau, N., Bohnert, K., Lucia, V., & Schweitzer, J. (2009). The impact of early behavior disturbances on academic achievement in high school. *Pediatrics, 123*(6), 1472–1476.

Broidy, L. M., Nagin, D. S., Tremblay, R. E., Bates, J. E., Brame, B., Dodge, K. A., et al. (2003). Developmental trajectories of childhood disruptive behaviors and adolescent delinquency: A six-site, cross-national study. *Developmental Psychology, 39*, 222–245.

Brooks-Gunn, J., & Duncan, G. J. (1997). The effects of poverty on children. *The Future of Children, 7*(2), 55–71.

Buhs, E. S., & Ladd, G. W. (2001). Peer rejection as an antecedent of young children's school adjustment: An examination of mediating processes. *Developmental Psychology, 37*(4), 550–560.

Buhs, E. S., Ladd, G. W., & Herald, S. L. (2006). Peer exclusion and victimization: Processes that mediate the relation between peer group rejection and children's classroom engagement and achievement? *Journal of Educational Psychology, 98*, 1–13.

Burt, K. B., & Roisman, G. I. (2010). Competence and psychopathology: Cascade effects in the NICHD Study of Early Child Care and Youth Development. *Development and Psychopathology, 22*(3), 557–567.

Campbell, S. B., Spieker, S., Burchinal, M., Poe, M. D., & the NICHD Early Child Care Research Network. (2006). Trajectories of aggression from toddlerhood to age 9 predict academic and social functioning through age 12. *Journal of Child Psychology and Psychiatry, 47*(8), 791–800.

Chen, X., Rubin, K. H., & Li, Z.-Y. (1995). Social functioning and adjustment in Chinese children: A longitudinal study. *Developmental Psychology, 31*(4), 531–539.

Christenson, S. L., Sinclair, M. F., Lehr, C. A., & Godber, Y. (2001). Promoting successful school completion: Critical conceptual and methodological guidelines. *School Psychology Quarterly, 16*, 468–484.

Cohen, M. A. (1998). The monetary value of saving a high risk youth. *Journal of Quantitative Criminology, 4*, 5–33.

Coolahan, K., Fantuzzo, J., Mendez, J., & McDermott, P. (2000). Preschool peer interactions and readiness to learn: Relationships between classroom peer play and learning behaviors and conduct. *Journal of Educational Psychology, 92*(3), 458–465.

Crick, N. R., & Zahn-Waxler, C. (2003). The development of psychopathology in females and males: Current progress and future challenges. *Development and Psychopathology, 15*(3), 719–742.

Demaray, M. K., & Elliott, S. N. (1998). Teachers' judgments of students' academic functioning: A comparison of actual and predicted performances. *School Psychology Quarterly, 13*(1), 8–24.

Dishion, T. J., Patterson, G. R., Stoolmiller, M., & Skinner, M. L. (1991). Family, school, and behavioral antecedents to early adolescent involvement with antisocial peers. *Developmental Psychology, 27*(1), 172–180.

Dishion, T. J., Veronneau, M. H., & Myers, M. W. (2010). Cascading peer dynamics underlying the progression from problem behavior to violence in early to late adolescence. *Development and Psychopathology, 22*(3), 603–619.

Dodge, K. A., Coie, J. D., Pettit, G., & Price, J. (1990). Peer status and aggression in boys' groups: Developmental and contextual analyses. *Child Development, 61*, 1289–1309.

Duchesne, S., Vitaro, F., Larose, S., & Tremblay, R. E. (2008). Trajectories of anxiety during elementary-school years and the prediction of high school noncompletion. *Journal of Yourth and Adolescence, 37*(9), 1134–1146.

Duncan, G. J., Claessens, A., Huston, A. C., Pagani, L. S., Engel, M., Sexton, H. R., et al. (2007). School readiness and later achievement. *Developmental Psychology, 43*(6), 1428–1446.

Ensminger, M. E., & Slusarcick, A. L. (1992). Paths to high school graduation or dropout: A longitudinal study of a first-grade cohort. *Sociology of Education, 65*, 95–113.

Entwisle, D. R., Alexander, K. L., & Olson, L. S. (2004). Temporary as compared to permanent high school dropout. *Social Forces, 82*(3), 1181–1205.

Erath, S. A., Flanagan, K. S., & Bierman, K. L. (2008). Early adolescent school adjustment: Associations with friendship and peer victimization. *Social Development, 17*, 853–870.

Feinberg, A. B., & Shapiro, E. S. (2003). Accuracy of teacher judgments in predicting oral reading fluency. *School Psychology Quarterly, 18*(1), 52–65.

Friedman-Weieneth, J. L., Harvey, E. A., Youngwirth, S. D., & Goldstein, L. H. (2007). The relation between 3-year-old children's skills and their hyperactivity, inattention, and aggression. *Journal of Educational Psychology, 99*(3), 671–681.

Galéra, C., Melchior, M., Chastang, J.-F., Bouvard, M.-P., & Fombonne, E. (2009). Childhood and adolescent hyperactivity–inattention symptoms and academic achievement 8 years later: The GAZEL Youth Study. *Psychological Medicine, 39*(11), 1895–1906.

Garon, N., Bryson, S. E., & Smith, I. M. (2008). Executive function in preschoolers: A review using an integrative framework [Review]. *Psychological Bulletin, 134*(1), 31–60.

Gelman, A., & Hill, J. (2007). *Data analysis using regression and multilevel/hierarchical models.* Cambridge, UK: Cambridge University Press.

Goldstein, N. E., Arnold, D. H., Rosenberg, J. L., Stowe, R. M., & Ortiz, C. (2001). Contagion of aggression in day care classrooms as a function of peer and teacher responses. *Journal of Educational Psychology, 93*(4), 708–719.

Hamre, B. K., & Pianta, R. C. (2001). Early teacher–child relationships and the trajectory of children's school outcomes through the eighth grade. *Child Development, 72*, 625–638.

Hinshaw, S. P. (1992). Academic underachievement, attention deficits, and aggression: Comorbidity and implications for intervention. *Journal of Consulting and Clinical Psychology, 60*(6), 893–903.

HRSDC-Statistics Canada. (2011). *Labour force survey estimates, by educational attainment, sex and age group*. Ottawa, ON: Statistics Canada.

Hughes, C., Ensor, R., Wilson, A., & Graham, A. (2010). Tracking executive function across the transition to school: A latent variable approach. *Developmental Neuropsychology, 35*(1), 20–36.

Hughes, J. N., Luo, W., Kwok, O. M., & Loyd, L. K. (2008). Teacher–student support, effortful engagement, and achievement: A 3-year longitudinal study. *Journal of Educational Psychology, 100*(1), 1–14.

Izard, C., Fine, S., Schultz, D., Mostow, A., Ackerman, B., & Youngstrom, E. (2001). Emotion knowledge as a predictor of social behavior and academic competence in children at risk. *Psychological Science, 12*(1), 18–23.

Kiesner, J., Poulin, F., & Nicotra, E. (2003). Peer relations across contexts: Individual-network homophily and network inclusion in and after school. *Child Development, 74*, 1328–1343.

Kline, R. B. (2005). *Principles and practice of structural equation modeling*. New York: Guilford Press.

Ladd, G. W., Buhs, E. S., & Seid, M. (2000). Children's initial sentiments about kindergarten: Is school liking an antecedent of early classroom participation and achievement? *Merrill–Palmer Quarterly, 46*, 255–279.

Ladd, G. W., & Dinella, L. M. (2009). Continuity and change in early school engagement: Predictive of children's achievement trajectories from first to eighth grade? *Journal of Educational Psychology, 101*(1), 190–206.

Ladd, G. W., Kochenderfer, B. J., & Coleman, C. C. (1997). Classroom peer acceptance, friendship, and victimization: Distinct relational systems that contribute uniquely to children's school adjustment? *Child Development, 68*(6), 1181–1197.

Little, S. A., & Garber, J. (2004). Interpersonal and achievement orientations and specific stressors predict depressive and aggressive symptoms. *Journal of Adolescent Research, 19*(1), 63–84.

Masten, A. S., Roisman, G. I., Long, J. D., Burt, K. B., Obradovic, J., Riley, J. R., et al. (2005). Developmental cascades: Linking academic achievement and externalizing and internalizing symptoms over 20 years. *Developmental Psychology, 41*(5), 733–746.

McCaul, E. J., Donaldson, G. A., Coladarci, T., & Davis, W. E. (1992). Consequences of dropping out of school: Findings from high school and beyond. *Journal of Educational Research, 85*, 198–207.

McClelland, M. M., & Cameron, C. E. (2011). Self-regulation and academic achievement in elementary school children. In R. M. Lerner, J. V. Lerner, E. P. Bowers, S. Lewin-Bizan, S. Gestsdottir, & J. B. Urban (Eds.), Thriving in childhood and adolescence: The role of self-regulation processes. *New Directions for Child and Adolescent Development, 133*, 29–44.

McDougall, P., Hymel, S., Vaillancourt, T., & Mercer, L. (2001). The consequences of childhood peer rejection. In M. R. Leary (Ed.), *Interpersonal rejection* (pp. 213–247). New York: Oxford University Press.

Miles, S. B., & Stipek, D. (2006). Contemporaneous and longitudinal associations between social behavior and literacy achievement in a sample of low-income elementary school children. *Child Development, 77*(1), 103–117.

Moffitt, T. E. (1990). Juvenile delinquency and attention deficit disorder: Boys' developmental trajectories from age 3 to age 15. *Child Development, 61*(3), 893–910.

Moilanen, K. L., Shaw, D. S., & Maxwell, K. L. (2010). Developmental cascades: Externalizing, internalizing, and academic competence from middle childhood to early adolescence. *Development and Psychopathology, 22*(3), 635–653.

Morgan, P. L., Farkas, G., Tufis, P. A., & Sperling, R. A. (2008). Are reading and behavior problems risk factors for each other? *Journal of Learning Disabilities, 41*(5), 417–436.

Muthén, L. K., & Muthén, B. O. (2010). *MPlus users' guide* (6th ed.). Los Angeles: Authors.

National Center for Education Statistics. (2008). *Percentage of high school dropouts among persons 16 through 24 years old (status dropout rate), by income level, and percentage distribution of status dropouts, by labor force status and educational attainement: 1970 through 2007.* Retrieved from *http://nces.ed.gov/programs/digest/d08/tables/dt08_110.asp.*

Obradovic, J., Burt, K. B., & Masten, A. S. (2010). Testing a dual cascade model linking competence and symptoms over 20 years from childhood to adulthood. *Journal of Clinical Child and Adolescent Psychology, 39*(1), 90–102.

Pianta, R. C., & Stuhlman, M. W. (2004). Teacher–child relationships and children's success in the first years of school. *School Psychology Review, 33*(3), 444–458.

Pingault, J.-B., Tremblay, R. E., Vitaro, F., Carbonneau, R., Genolini, C., Falissard, B., et al. (2011). Childhood trajectories of inattention and hyperactivity and prediction of educational attainment in early adulthood: A 16-year longitudinal population-based study. *American Journal of Psychiatry, 168*(11), 1164–1170.

Purcell, S. (2002). Variance components models for gene–environment interaction in twin analysis. *Twin Research, 5*(6), 554–571.

Québec Ministry of Education. (2010). *Indicateurs de l'éducation. Gouvernement du Québec* [Education Indicators: Governement of Québec]. Québec City, Canada: Government of Québec Press.

Rapport, M. D., Scanlan, S. W., & Denney, C. B. (1999). Attention-deficit/hyperactivity disorder and scholastic achievement: A model of dual developmental pathways. *Journal of Child Psychology and Psychiatry and Allied Disciplines, 40*(8), 1169–1183.

Rouquette, A., Côté, S., Pryor, L., Carbonneau, R., Vitaro, F., & Tremblay, R. E. (2012) Cohort profile: The Quebec Longitudinal Study of Kindergarten Children (QLSKC). *International Journal of Epidemiology.* Advance online publication.

Rumberger, R. W. (1987). High school dropouts: A review of issues and evidence. *Review of Educational Research, 57*(2), 101–121.

Schielzeth, H. (2010). Simple means to improve the interpretability of regression coefficients. *Methods in Ecology and Evolution, 1*(2), 103–113.

Serbin, L. A., & Stack, D. M. (1998). Introduction to the special section: Studying intergeneration continuity and the transfer of risk. *Developmental Psychology, 34,* 1159–1161.

Spinath, B., Spinath, F. M., Harlaar, N., & Plomin, R. (2006). Predicting school achievement from general cognitive ability, self-perceived ability, and intrinsic value. *Intelligence, 34*(4), 363–374.

Stipek, D., & Miles, S. (2008). Effects of aggression on achievement: Does conflict with the teacher make it worse? *Child Development, 79*(6), 1721–1735.

Tremblay, R. E., Loeber, R., Gagnon, C., Charlebois, P., Larivée, S., & LeBlanc, M. (1991). Disruptive boys with stable and unstable high fighting behavior patterns during junior elementary school. *Journal of Abnormal Child Psychology, 19,* 285–300.

U.S. Department of Education. (2008). *National Center for Education Statistics, Digest of Education Statistics 2007* (NCESS-2008-022). Washington, DC: U.S. Government Printing Office.

van Lier, P. A. C., Vitaro, F., Barker, E. D., Brendgen, M., Tremblay, R. E., & Boivin, M. (2012). Peer victimization, poor academic achievement and the link between childhood externalizing and internalizing problems. *Child Development, 83*(5), 1775–1788.

Vaughn, B. E., Vollenweider, M., Bost, K. K., Azria-Evans, M. R., & Snider, J. B. (2003). Negative interactions and social competence for preschool children in two samples: Reconsidering the interpretation of aggressive behavior for young children. *Merrill–Palmer Quarterly, 49*(3), 245–278.

Véronneau, M.-H., Vitaro, F., Brendgen, M., Dishion, T. J., & Tremblay, R. E. (2010). Transactional analysis of the reciprocal links between peer experiences and academic achievement from middle childhood to early adolescence. *Developmental Psychology, 46*(4), 773–790.

Véronneau, M.-H., Vitaro, F., Pedersen, S., & Tremblay, R. E. (2008). Do peers contribute to the likelihood of secondary school graduation among disadvantaged boys? *Journal of Educational Psychology, 100*(2), 429–442.

Vitaro, F., & Brendgen, M. (2012). Subtypes of aggressive behaviors: Etiologies, development, and consequences. In T. Bliesener, A. Beelmann, & M. Stemmler (Eds.), *Antisocial behavior and crime: Contributions of developmental and evaluation research to prevention and intervention* (pp. 17–38). Cambridge, MA: Hogrefe.

Vitaro, F., Brendgen, M., Larose, S., & Tremblay, R. E. (2005). Kindergarten disruptive behaviors, protective factors, and educational achievement by early adulthood. *Journal of Educational Psychology, 97*(4), 617–629.

Vitaro, F., Pedersen, S., & Brendgen, M. (2007). Children's disruptiveness, peer rejection, friends' deviancy, and delinquent behaviors: A process-oriented approach. *Development and Psychopathology, 19,* 433–453.

Wentzel, K. R. (2009). Peers and academic functionning at school. In K. H.

Rubin, W. M. Bukowski, & B. Laursen (Eds.), *Handbook of peer interactions, relationships, and groups* (pp. 531–547). New York: Guilford Press.

Widaman, K. F. (2006). Missing data: What to do with or without them? *Monographs of the Society for Research in Child Development, 71*(3), 42–64.

Williams, S., & McGee, R. (1994). Reading attainment and juvenile delinquency. *Journal of Child Psychology and Psychiatry, 35*(3), 441–450.

Younger, A. J., Schwartzman, A. E., & Ledingham, J. E. (1986). Age-related differences in children's perceptions of social deviance: Changes in behavior or in perspective? *Developmental Psychology, 22*, 531–542.

CHAPTER 3

Assessing the Predictive Validity and Early Determinants of School Readiness Using a Population-Based Approach

MICHEL BOIVIN, HÉLÈNE DESROSIERS, JEAN-PASCAL LEMELIN, and NADINE FORGET-DUBOIS

Succeeding in school is an important milestone of human development and a key marker of society's human capital development. Thus, it is not surprising to witness a generalized concern among the civil society, the media, and politicians alike for the persistent rates of children dropping out of school before the end of high school (or failing to receive a diploma). Clearly, early school dropout is a dramatic culmination of school disengagement, which may have dire consequences for the individual and society (see Vitaro et al., Chapter 2, this volume). For these reasons, it is often described as a barometer of society's stumbling achievements in educating and training the next generation of children. However, as argued below, school dropout is only a crude indicator of learning for both the individual and the society, and we need a developmental approach to learning that takes into account achievements over time to more precisely assess their developmental trajectories, and then look at their determinants.

Although academic achievement and school dropout are related, they differ in many respects. Dropping out of school depends on a variety of personal, familial, school, and societal risk factors. Poor academic achievement is one of its most central predictors, and partly captures (i.e., mediates) the contributions of other important risk factors, such as poverty, disengagement, truancy, and grade retention (Battin-Pearson et al., 2000; Christenson, Sinclair, Lehr, & Godber, 2001; Garnier, Stein, & Jacobs, 1997; Worrell, 1997). Therefore, a focus on school achievement not only encompasses an important precursor of school dropout, but it also provides a more comprehensive and nuanced appraisal of the state of learning in a population than does a narrow focus on school dropout alone. More importantly, whereas school dropout is an outcome defined as an event that comes late in development, academic achievement is a developmental construct that shows change and trend over time. By examining the development of academic achievement, it is possible to describe more fully how trajectories of school achievement are established over time, to examine the extent to which, and conditions under which they forecast negative outcomes such as dropping out of school, and also to document the early predictors. Our aim in this chapter is to document the latter.

School Readiness and School Achievement Trajectories

School achievement trajectories likely result from complex interactions among personal, familial, social, and school factors operating over time. For instance, the achievement trajectories in the early school grades are likely affected by not only the degree of support from the family and the child care and school systems (e.g., the degree of literacy in preschool) but also the cognitive and social-emotional dispositions in the child, such as the capacity to focus one's attention, to self-control, and to integrate harmoniously with the peer and school milieu (Blair, 2002; Bierman, Nix, Greenberg, Blair, & Domitrovich, 2008; Ladd, Herald, & Kochel, 2006). It is assumed that these interactions start to shape children's dispositions toward school in a multifaceted way long before school entry.

From a prevention perspective, the capacity to identify, before school entry and, inasmuch as possible, earlier in the preschool period, specific risk markers of future school-related problems offers considerable potential for providing at-risk individuals or groups of children with early interventions that reduce their later risks (Blair & Diamond, 2008; Duncan et al., 2007). Accumulating evidence suggests that cognitive skills assessed in late preschool and at school entry predict later school achievement, at least during the early years of school. For example, Chew and colleagues (Chew & Lang, 1990; Chew & Morris, 1989) found significant predictive associations between prekindergarten and kindergarten cognitive school readiness and academic achievement between kindergarten and fourth grade. Similarly, Kurdek and Sinclair (2000) showed that cognitive school readiness in kindergarten predicted several academic outcomes, including teacher-rated verbal and mathematical skills from first to fifth grades.

These results were clearly confirmed by reviews and meta-analyses conducted more than a decade ago (LaParo & Pianta, 2000; Tramontana, Hooper, & Selzer, 1988). For instance, a meta-analysis by LaParo and Pianta (2000), based on 70 independent studies, revealed that preschool and kindergarten cognitive readiness measures predicted early school achievement in a moderate-to-strong way, accounting for about 25% of the variance. While this strong predictive validity is clearly sufficient to support the early identification of children at risk, at the same time, it also indicates that other, nonscholastic factors could be involved. For instance, a recent multinational study revealed that the best predictors of later school achievement were not only school-entry math and reading but also attention skills (Duncan et al., 2007).

Because school readiness is a multidimensional construct, its predictive validity regarding future school achievement tends to vary greatly as a function of the content of the assessment (LaParo & Pianta, 2000). Although literacy and numeracy in the first years of school are strong predictors of school performance during primary and secondary school (Duncan et al., 2007; Ensminger & Slusarcick, 1992; Vitaro et al., Chapter 2, this volume), assessments of behaviors and social skills do not show the same predictive validity with respect to later achievement scores, after accounting for early achievement, attention skills, and family factors. However, there is parallel evidence that externalizing behaviors, such inattentive–hyperactive behaviors and aggressive–oppositional behaviors, may indirectly alter school outcomes, such as graduating from high school, by interfering with self-regulated learning and motivation (Vitaro et al., Chapter 2, this volume).

It seems that predictions to later school achievement and attainment can be successfully extended downward from measures of preschool skills and adjustment. Over and above literacy and numeracy knowledge and skills, child characteristics such as self-control, emotion regulation, and social-emotional behaviors measured in preschool have indeed been found to predict participation and academic achievement (Bierman, Torres, Domitrovich, Welsh, & Gest, 2009; Galéra et al., 2011; Moffit et al., 2011; Normandeau & Guay, 1998; Pingault et al., 2012). However, given the mixed results (Duncan et al., 2007), it is unclear whether this prediction is robust enough to motivate the use of social-emotional and behavioral factors in preschool as significant risk factors for later school achievement. In order to do so more decisively, it is important to consider fully the multidimensional nature of school readiness in the predictions, which has not been always taken into account in previous studies. For example, it is not clear whether preschool behavioral/social skills contribute to later academic achievement over and above the contribution of preschool cognitive skills, whether preschool cognitive/language and behavioral/social skills differentially predict later school achievement, and whether some cognitive components are more important than others for later academic achievement. There is indeed much to be learned about the basic requirements and the specific developmental and social processes underlying school readiness and school achievement in the critical early years of schools.

With this in mind, we have initiated a program of research on the early determinants of school readiness and achievement. This program of research involves two population-based birth cohorts followed longitudinally since age 5 months, the Québec Longitudinal Study of Child Development, and the Québec Newborn Twin Study (described below), and is guided by a series of overarching principles and objectives. First, in both cohorts, we assessed school readiness in a multidimensional way, with the goal of documenting the predictive validity of the various components in terms of short-, medium-, and long-term academic and social outcomes. School readiness has been assessed in various ways over the years, but often using assessments of limited scope that did not reflect the multifactorial nature of school readiness. Some studies used direct but general assessments of cognitive and language skills, such as IQ tests and verbal proficiency measures, while others used specific ad hoc ratings, such as ratings of aggressive behaviors used as proxies for social adjustment (Blair, 2002; LaParo & Pianta, 2000). In our program of research, we wanted to provide distinct coverage of relevant cognitive, language, motor, social-emotional skills, and knowledge components, and prospectively document the extent to which these various components predicted relevant school outcomes, including school achievement.

Second, we also aimed to document the early determinants of school readiness by considering a host of early child, family, and social antecedents, including their genetic and environmental underpinnings through the use of a twin design in the Québec Newborn Twin Study (see below). This meant starting early in child's life (i.e., at age 5 months) to prospectively document the relevant factors forecasting school readiness at the end of the preschool period, just before school entry. These early determinants were considered within a developmental longitudinal framework in order to ponder their relative weights as predictors, but more importantly, with the goal of examining the biosocial developmental processes leading to school readiness and achievement.

Finally, we adopted a population approach (i.e., used population-based samples) in order to inform services and policies, and provide tools for monitoring early childhood development in a population. There are indeed operational constraints on the choice of a school readiness measure in the context of a population approach. Given the multidimensional nature of the school readiness construct, the use of time-consuming, extensive batteries is nonoptimal, if not precluded, in evaluating school readiness in a large population of children, when the time of contact with individual children may be limited. In such a context, direct assessments of school readiness should be short and easy to administer.

GOALS OF THIS CHAPTER

Our goals in this chapter were threefold. First, we wanted to document the combined predictive validity of two multidimensional measures of school readiness with respect to early school trajectories. We focused on two instruments, the Early Development Instrument (EDI; Janus & Offord, 2007 and the Lollipop Test (Chew & Morris, 1984), both designed to assess school readiness in a populationwide context at the end of the preschool years. The EDI is a teacher-rated questionnaire targeting five areas of school readiness: physical health and well-being, social competence, emotional maturity, language and cognitive development, and communication skills and general knowledge. The Lollipop Test is a multidimensional measure of cognitive school readiness that directly assesses, through a series of short tests and questions put to the child, aspects seen as central to early success in school (Chew, 1987), including the identification of letters, numbers, colors, shapes, and spatial notions. Together, the EDI and the Lollipop instruments are suitable for a populationwide assessment and provide extensive coverage of the relevant dimensions of school readiness. For this initial work, we relied on the Québec Longitudinal Study of Child Development (QLSCD).

Second, we wanted to report on the extent to which these school readiness assessments, as well as their predictive associations with later school achievement, were mediated by environmental processes. It is generally assumed that school readiness can be traced back to prior environmental influences, but, as we review below, research also shows that some aspects of school readiness may be heritable and subject to "child effects." In a first step toward disentangling these different possibilities, we used the power of the twin method and turned to the Québec Newborn Twin Study (QNTS).

Finally, given the reported associations between family environment and experiences and school readiness, our final goal was to document further the family processes linking early sociodemographic risk factors, school readiness (as assessed by the EDI and the Lollipop), and later school achievement.

The Predictive Validity of School Readiness Assessment in the QLSCD

The first set of analyses examined the predictive validity of two multidimensional measures of school readiness (the EDI and the Lollipop scales) as predictors of children's trajectories of academic achievement in early elementary school. Data were drawn from the QLSCD, an ongoing prospective longitudinal study of a sample of children, starting at the age of 5 months, representative of the population of infants born in 1998 in the province of Québec, Canada.

Methods

Participants

All singleton infants between 59 and 60 gestational weeks of age in 1998 with mothers living in the province of Québec were targeted, with the exception of (1) infants in the far North administrative region, Cree, or Inuit regions, or living on aboriginal reservations; (2) infants for whom the duration of gestation could not be determined from the birth record; and (3) infants born at less than 24 weeks' gestation, and infants born at greater than 42 weeks' gestation. Infants and their families were selected through a region-based stratified sampling design. More than 2,000 families participated in the study when the infant was age 5 months in 1998 (*N* = 2,120). When the children were 5 months of age, 8.5% of families were headed by a single parent; 31.4% reported an income lower than CAD$ 30,000, and 28.1% reported higher than CAD$ 60,000; and 19.1% of mothers and 20.2% of fathers had not completed high school, while 25.5% of mothers and 24.6% of fathers held a university degree. These children and their families were assessed at home, and their parents were interviewed annually when children were from about 5 months to 8 years of age, and then biannually up to the age of 12 when they finished elementary school. Specifically, follow-up assessments occurred at 17 (*N* = 2,045), 29 (*N* = 1,997), and 41 months (*N* = 1,950), and then in the spring of the following years (50 months, *N* = 1,944, and 61 months, *N* = 1,759). The children all entered grade school in 2003 and were assessed in the spring of 2004 (kindergarten, 74 months, *N* = 1,492), 2005 (grade 1), 2006 (grade 2), 2008 (grade 4), and 2010 (grade 6). These children are now being followed into secondary school (2011–2015). In this report, we focus on the data collected from preschool up to grade 4.

Measures

The QLSCD includes multivariate measures of child developmental outcomes assessed longitudinally, as well as extended and detailed multilevel assessments of environmental factors. Participants were assessed on a broad range of characteristics through computerized, face-to-face interviews of the person most knowledgeable (PMK) about the child (usually the mother). Regular assessments also included questionnaires completed by the mother, the father, and the interviewer, and direct and multifaceted assessments of cognitive development, with a strong emphasis on school readiness at 41, 50, and 61 months (e.g., literacy, vocabulary, numeracy, general IQ), and school achievement at each time point of grade school. Several school readiness measures have been used, beginning at the age of 42 months. In addition to the Lollipop Test and the EDI, these included the Block Design subtest of the Wechsler Preschool and Primary Scale of Intelligence—Revised (WPPSI-R), a measure of visual–spatial organization and a central component of nonverbal intelligence (Wechsler, 1989); the Peabody Picture Vocabulary Test—Revised (PPVT-R), a measure of receptive vocabulary (Dunn, Thériault-Whalen, & Dunn, 1993); the Visually Cued Recall (VCR) test, a measure of short-term visual memory (Zelazo, Jacques, Burack, & Frye, 2002); and the Number Knowledge Test (NKT), a measure of basic knowledge and understanding of number concepts (Okamoto & Case, 1996). Teachers also regularly rated the children's school achievement. These scales, along with the Lollipop Test and the EDI were administered in kindergarten, when the children were about 6 years old.

The Lollipop Test

The French or English version of the Lollipop Test was individually administered to the child in the class setting (i.e., the Diagnostic Screening Test of School Readiness—Revised [Chew, 1987] and as validated by Venet, Normandeau, Letarte, & Bigras, 2003, for the French version). The test takes about 15 minutes, is easy to administer (e.g., by a teacher), and uses stimuli (e.g., suckers, cats) that are familiar to most children. The Lollipop is individually administered using a set of seven stimulus cards and one form on which the child's results are recorded. It comprises four subtests, measuring (1) identification of *colors and shapes*, copying of shapes (14 questions); (2) *spatial recognition* (10 questions); (3) identification of *numbers and counting* (14 questions); and (4) identification of *letters and writing* (14 questions). A total school readiness score may be calculated by adding the scores of the four subtests. During the test, the child is asked questions presented in different forms. First, the interviewer asks the child to identify certain specific stimuli (e.g., a green sucker or the letter *P*), then to name a stimulus that he or she identifies (e.g., a triangle or the number 3), and finally, the child is asked to carry out certain actions (e.g., counting the orange suckers, writing his or her name, or copying a square). The number of points assigned to each question varies from 1 to 5, for a maximum score of 69. In prior research, the Lollipop has shown strong convergent validity with other measures of school readiness and predicts children's school achievement throughout primary school (Chew & Lang, 1990; Chew & Morris, 1984, 1989; Venet et al., 2003).

The EDI

The EDI (Janus & Offord, 2007), a teacher-rated questionnaire of 104 items, is a good example of a holistic, multidimensional approach to the construct of school readiness that can be used in the context of a populationwide coverage. In the QLSCD, an abridged 94-item version was used. The EDI measures five broad domains of school readiness: (1) physical health and well-being, including gross and fine motor skills, physical readiness for the school day, and physical independence; (2) social competence, including responsibility and respect, approaches to learning, overall social competence, and readiness to explore new things; (3) emotional maturity, including prosocial behavior, hyperactivity and inattention, anxious and fearful behavior, and aggressive behavior; (4) language and cognitive development, including basic numeracy, basic literacy, advanced literacy, interest in literacy–numeracy, and capacity to memorize; and (5) communication skills and general knowledge, including the child's ability to tell a story, to communicate needs to an adult or to peers, and to use the native language effectively. The EDI items are coded on various scales, some using a yes–no format, others using 3- or 5-point Likert-type scales. Following the recommendations of Janus and Offord (2007), the items were then recoded on a scale of 0 to 10, to allow the calculation of scores in the five domains, a well as in the 16 dimensions within those domains. The original EDI was translated into French through an inverse-translation procedure (Vallerand, 1989).

School Achievement Trajectories

School achievement was assessed in grades 1 and 2 through teacher ratings of children's performance in three domains (reading, writing, and mathematics), and in the same domains plus science in grade 4. For each of these domains, teachers had to indicate on a 5-point Likert scale to what extent the child's level of achievement was (5) "Near the top of the class," (4) "Above the middle of the class, but not at the top," (3) "In the middle of the class," (2) "Below the middle of the class, but above the bottom," or (1) "Near the bottom of the class." A total school performance score was used in the analyses by averaging the scores in the three (or four) domains. This method of school performance evaluation has been found to be valid and highly correlated with other types of school performance measures, such as report cards (Mattanah, Pratt, Cowan, & Cowan, 2005; Vitaro, Larocque, Janosz, & Tremblay, 2001; Walker, Petrill, Spinath, & Plomin, 2004). Here the resulting scores were found to be highly reliable (Cronbach alphas were all above 0.80).

To describe the school achievement trajectories from grade 1 to grade 4, we used a semiparametric, group-based clustering approach, the ProcTraj procedure in SAS (Jones, Nagin, & Roeder, 2001). This procedure typically identifies prototypical developmental trajectories on the basis of repeated measures of the same characteristic, and allow for the identification of homogeneous subgroups with respect to the shape of their trajectory over time (Nagin, 1999). This approach offers several advantages. First, it considers various individual trajectories to determine the optimal number of groups needed to describe typical patterns of change over time. Second, it does not make strong assumptions about the population distribution of the developmental trajectories, including the assumption that individual trajectories are normally distributed. Third, the procedure assigns each participant to a trajectory based on a probability estimate, calculates the proportion of participants in each trajectory group, and, for each participant, estimates a probability of membership in each trajectory group. As in cluster analysis, a key step is the choice of the optimal number of trajectories to ensure the best fit to the data. The choice of the optimal model is based on the value of the Bayesian Information Criterion (BIC; Jones, Nagin, & Roeder, 2001), which reflects the fit and the parsimony of the competing models. The choice of the optimal model is also based on theoretical likelihood.

Here, models with two to six trajectory groups of teacher-rated school achievement were first estimated on a sample that comprised children with no more than one missing data point on teacher-rated school achievement between grades 1 and 4 (N = 1,276). The BIC improved as the number of groups increased. However, with four groups and more, both high and low stable groups were consistently found, and adding groups only resulted in splitting midlevel groups. Therefore, the four-group solution was retained where children were classified into their most probable achievement trajectory group by the use of posterior probabilities. The same analyses were then conducted, this time using longitudinal sample weights scores to correct for possible biases associated with attrition over time.

Figure 3.1 presents the final model based on un-weighted scores. The 95% confidence intervals around trajectories did not overlap. The *Low* group (estimated at 13.7% of the sample, 56% boys) followed a linear, slightly increasing trajectory that clearly lay lower than all others in terms of school achievement. An *Average* group, clearly the most numerous (38% of the sample; 53% boys), followed a straight trajectory (no change over time) around the mean point of the scale. An *Above average* group was also identified (28% of the sample; 43% boys) also followed a straight above the mean trajectory over time. Finally, the *High* group (20% of the sample; 37% boys) followed a linear, slightly decreasing trajectory near the top of the scale.

The use of sample weights revealed very similar trajectories to that based of unweighted data, with a higher proportion of children in the *Average* group (44.6 vs. 38%) and a lower proportion in the *High* group (12.8 vs. 20%) (data not shown), reflecting a small selection bias toward higher school achievement due to attrition. Given that bias did not affect the trajectories and the proportion of children in the *Low* group, and that sample weights may be complicated to apply given the large number of

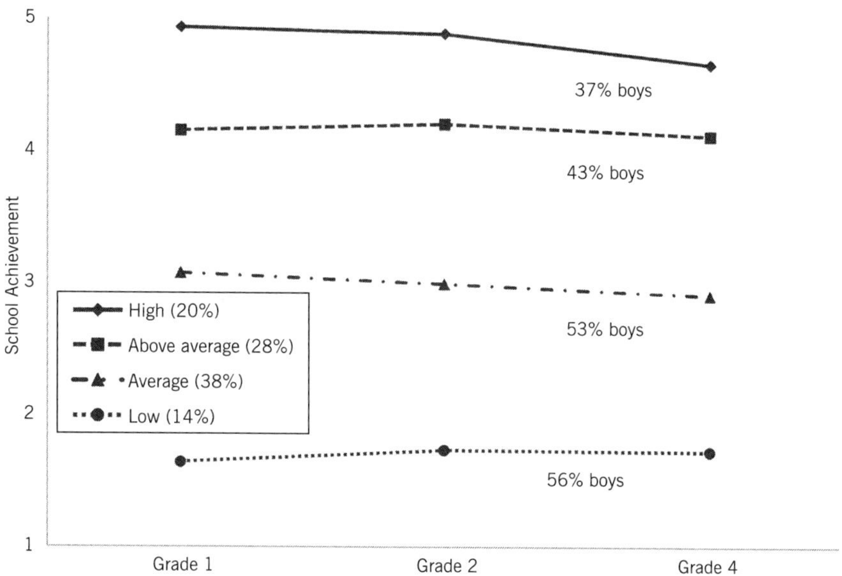

FIGURE 3.1. School achievement trajectories in the early years of school (QLSCD).

variables taken into account, we used unweighted data in the following analysis.

To cross-validate these teacher-based school achievement trajectories, we examined their associations with relevant tests of receptive vocabulary (the PPVT-R) and mathematics (the Canadian Achievement Test, Second Edition [CAT/2]), as well as with the use of speech therapy or special need services, in grade 4. All four trajectory groups differed significantly from each other (all *p*s $< .001$) in the expected direction on measured receptive vocabulary (from the *Low* group to the *High* group, the mean PPVT-R scores were 106.7, 110.2, 115.1, and 118.1, respectively) and mathematic achievement (the mean CAT/2 scores were 11.3, 14.5, 15.7, and 16.8, respectively). Furthermore, of the 161 children (17% of the available sample) who, according to their teacher, had received speech therapy or special needs teacher services in grade 4, 93 were in the *Low* group (58%) and 67 were in the *Average* group (41%), compared to only one in the *Above average* group and none in the *High* group.

These highly convergent results clearly indicate that the teacher ratings provided a valid description of the school achievement trajectories in the early grades of schools for children under study. The validity of these school trajectories being established, we can now turn to the main questions of interest.

Results

Predicting School Achievement from the EDI and the Lollipop

We first wanted to document the predictive validity of both the Lollipop Test and the EDI, both assessed in kindergarten, with respect to early school achievement from grade 1 to grade 4. In an initial prediction attempt, we chose a "shotgun" approach aimed at achieving the best prediction using an extensive battery of various school readiness measures. To do so, we used multiple measures collected in kindergarten, including the Lollipop and the EDI, to predict the achievement trajectories. As indicated previously, the trajectory analysis generates for each individual a probability of belonging to each trajectory. Here, given our interest in achievement difficulties, we aimed at predicting the individual probability associated with the *Low* trajectory. For this initial attempt we used the Block Design, the PPVT-R, the VCR, the NKT, the Lollipop Test, and the EDI. This first regression analysis showed that 41% of the variance of the *Low* achievement trajectory could be predicted from this entire set of predictors.

How does the prediction based on the EDI and the Lollipop compared to this 41%? To answer this question, we then ran a series of regression analyses that considered (1) the Lollipop subscales only, (2) the EDI subscales only, and (3) the Lollipop and EDI subscales combined. For each group of predictors (i.e., 1, 2, and 3), we also ran a series of discriminant function analyses (DFAs) to evaluate more generally the capacity of these different sets of predictors to correctly classify the children in the different trajectory groups. DFA is a statistical procedure that determines whether a set of variables is effective in predicting category membership. As its name implies, DFA defines one or more factors (i.e., a linear combination of predictors, such as school readiness subscores), or "functions" that optimize the prediction of a known membership (i.e., membership in one of the four achievement trajectories).

In a first series of regression and DFA analyses, the four subscales of the Lollipop accounted for 28% of the variance, with the Letters (beta = –0.33, $p < .001$), Numbers (beta = –0.23, $p < .001$), and Colors/Forms (beta = –0.09, $p < .05$), but not Spatial (beta = –0.03, nonsignificant [ns]) subscales, having a significant contribution. When only these four dimensions of the Lollipop were considered in the DFA, 41% of the children were correctly classified in the different trajectory groups. Most interestingly, a greater precision was achieved in the case of the more extreme groups; 68% of the *High* group and 58% of the *Low* groups were correctly classified, versus 29% for both the *Average* and *Above Average* groups.

In a second series of regression and DFA analyses, this time considering only the 16 subscales of the EDI, the prediction was 32%, with Communication Skills and General Knowledge (beta = –0.26, $p < .001$), Basic Numeracy (beta = –0.27, $p < .001$), Overall Social Competence (beta = –0.17, $p < .001$), and Physical Independence (beta = –0.10, p < .05) making unique contributions. The DFA revealed that 47% of the children were correctly classified, again with higher precision for the more extreme groups; 61% of the *High* group and 62% of the *Low* group were correctly classified, versus 44% of *Average* group and 33% of the *Above Average* group.

Finally, in a third series of regression and DFA analyses, when both the Lollipop and the EDI subscales were considered as predictors, the prediction accounted for 40% of the variance (i.e., a level of explanation almost equal to that found earlier with the more extensive battery). The significant predictors were, for the EDI, Communication Skills and General Knowledge (beta = –0.17, $p < .001$), Overall Social Competence (beta = –0.16, $p < .001$), Basic Numeracy (beta = –0.15, $p < .001$), and Physical Independence (beta = –0.09, $p < .01$); and for the Lollipop battery, Letters (beta = –0.19, $p < .001$), Numbers (beta = –0.10, $p < .05$), and Colors/Forms (beta = –0.07, $p < .05$). The corresponding DFA revealed that 51% of the children were correctly classified in the four achievement trajectories, again with higher precision found for the more extreme groups: 66% of the *High* group and 68% of the *Low* group were correctly classified, versus 47% of *Average* group and 37% of *Above Average* group.

Thus, both the EDI and the Lollipop performed very well in predicting early school achievement, especially when the two instruments were used in conjunction, and when predicting children at the top and bottom of the class. School achievement was predicted by a variety of cognitive and social components, including knowledge and basic skills regarding literacy and numeracy, as well as interpersonal skills and behaviors, thus lending support to the multidimensional approach to school readiness.

Because of the logistical constraints associated with assessing populations, preschool and school systems may be hesitant to assess school readiness directly, even with easy-to-use instruments such as the Lollipop. It is therefore important to understand the unique contributions of these two instruments in predicting school achievement difficulties. Accordingly, we ran additional hierarchical regression analyses in which the EDI and the Lollipop subscales were considered in sequence in predicting the probability of being on the *Low* trajectory of school achievement. In a first hierarchical regression, all Lollipop subtests were entered in the first step and all EDI subscales were entered in a second step. We did the reverse in a second regression analysis. As documented earlier, all subscales accounted for 40% of the variance in school achievement difficulties. In these new hierarchical analyses, the EDI added 12%, and the Lollipop, 10% of the variance, respectively, after the other instrument was considered.

The fact that many subtests of the Lollipop and of the EDI uniquely contributed to school achievement difficulties suggests that despite a significant overlap between the two instruments, there is a significant gain in precision in using both. In other words, redundancy was only moderate and important aspects of school readiness, literacy, and numeracy in particular are best covered when the two measures are used.

Given that these two measures of school readiness quite successfully predicted early school achievement, an important ensuing question concerns the nature of the processes underlying the emergence of school readiness skills and their predictive associations with later school achievement. In particular, the relative contributions of genetic versus environmental factors are of interest as potential predictors of school readiness and early learning.

Environmental and Genetic Contributions to School Readiness

As indicated earlier, there is evidence that the development of school readiness is environmentally mediated. A great deal of research has documented the association between school readiness and both proximal and distal facets of the child environment, including family income and maternal employment status (Brooks-Gunn, Han, & Waldfogel, 2002; Dearing, McCartney, & Taylor, 2001); specific favorable home environments, such as sensitive care, verbal stimulation, and access to educational material in the home; and specific parental practices, such as reading with the child (Belsky & Fearon, 2002; Bradley & Caldwell, 1984; Britto, Brooks-Gunn, & Griffin, 2006; Connell & Prinz, 2002; McLoyd, 1998; Melhuish et al., 2008; NICHD Early Child Care Research Network, 2003; see also Welsh, Bierman, & Mathis, Chapter 11, this volume); as well as quality of child care (Connell & Prinz, 2002; Côté, Geoffroy, & Pingault, Chapter 6, this volume).

On the other hand, there is also solid empirical ground for the view that genetically mediated child characteristics may also play a role in school readiness. School readiness has been linked to IQ (Butz, Pulsifer, Leppert, Rimrodt, & Belcher, 2003), an aspect of children's development known to be heritable (see Plomin, DeFries, McClearn, & McGuffin, 2001, for a review). Similarly, the crystallized cognitive components predictive of later school achievement (e.g., the ability to *use* letter and number knowledge) could also stem from fluid cognitive skills (i.e., the capacity to logically *solve* problems independent of acquired knowledge) underlying their learning (Blair, 2006), and these skills could be partly under genetic influence. School readiness has also been linked to infant temperamental features, such as self-regulation through effortful control, that is, the capacity to voluntarily manage attention and to inhibit or activate behavior (Belsky, 2001; Blair & Razza, 2007; Rothbart & Bates, 2006). As for IQ, temperament reflects individual differences in behavioral characteristics that are, at least in part, heritable (Goldsmith, Lemery, Buss, & Campos, 1999). These findings point to possible genetic child "effects" on school readiness. In a first step toward disentangling these different possibilities, we used the power of the twin method and turned to the Québec Newborn Twin Study (QNTS).

The QNTS

A major challenge of developmental research is to infer causal process within a developmental framework. Studies based on correlations, even when they are longitudinal, do not establish cause. As natural experiments, twin studies are the next best thing to an experimental design for investigating developmental pathways. They are uniquely suited to the investigation of child and family contributions to developmental outcomes, and because they provide estimates of both genetic and environmental sources of variance, they can serve as quasi-experimental tests of environmental theories (Rutter, 2007). The twin method uses pairs of identical (monozygotic; MZ) and fraternal (dizygotic; DZ) twins who are raised in their original/biological families. It allows for a statistical estimation of genetic versus shared and nonshared environmental sources of variation for a given phenotype (i.e., an observable characteristic or trait) by comparing the phenotypic similarity among identical-MZ twins, who share 100% of their genes, to that of fraternal-DZ twins, who share on average 50% of their genotype. Higher phenotypic similarity favoring identical-MZ versus fraternal-DZ twins is assumed to reflect genetic sources of variance (i.e., heritability), whereas equivalent or low phenotypic similarity across levels of genetic relatedness (i.e., identical vs. fraternal) represents shared and nonshared environmental sources of variance.

Participants

The QNTS was initiated in 1995 as a parallel study to QLSCD (Boivin et al., 2013). It is an ongoing longitudinal study: More than 1,200 twin children and their parents from the greater Montréal region were assessed when they were 5, 20, 32, 50, and 63 months old, then again in kindergarten, and grades 1, 3, 4, and 6. A follow-up in secondary school is ongoing.

Methods

As in the QLCSD, participants were assessed, through multi-informant and multimethod approaches, on a broad range of characteristics, including school readiness and school achievement. The Lollipop Test was administered in a laboratory setting the summer before the children entered kindergarten when they were age 62 months (i.e., 1 year earlier than in the QLSCD), and school achievement was assessed through teacher ratings as in the QLSCD.

Results

Predicting School Achievement

In a first report, we documented how well the Lollipop Test could predict school achievement in grade 1, examined the genetic and environmental contributions to cognitive school readiness, as assessed by the Lollipop Test, and also extended this analysis to the predictive association between school readiness and school achievement (Lemelin et al., 2007). This series of analyses showed that the Lollipop Test substantially predicted school achievement in grade 1 (20% of the variance) over and above nonverbal intelligence, as measured by the Block Design subtest of the WPPSI-R (Wechsler, 1989). Three of the four subscales, Numbers (beta = 0.29, $p < .001$), Spatial (beta = 0.16, $p < .001$), and Letters (beta = 0.14, $p < .001$) significantly contributed to the prediction. In other words, as in the QLSCD, the Lollipop battery showed an appreciable capacity to predict early school achievement. Furthermore, the prediction was from an earlier time (before entry in kindergarten), and it was found to be substantial and in addition to the prediction by fluid cognitive skills central to nonverbal IQ.

Estimating Genetic and Environmental Contributions

We then turned our attention to estimating, through the twin method, the genetic and environmental contributions to school readiness. We first computed intraclass correlations (ICCs) for MZ and DZ twins. ICCs may vary from –1 to +1, and reflect the degree of association among co-twins (i.e., twins of the same family) on a specific dimension/measure, with a high positive correlation indicating high similarity among twins of the same family. As Figure 3.2 illustrates, these ICCs were uniformly high across subscales, and most importantly, of similar magnitude for both MZ and DZ twins. The values ranged from .54 (MZ) and .55 (DZ) for the Spatial subtest to .89 (MZ) and .79 (DZ) for the Letters subtests (all highly significant *p*s < .0001). Note that the ICCs for the Letter subtest were as high as values generally accepted for test–retest reliability. This

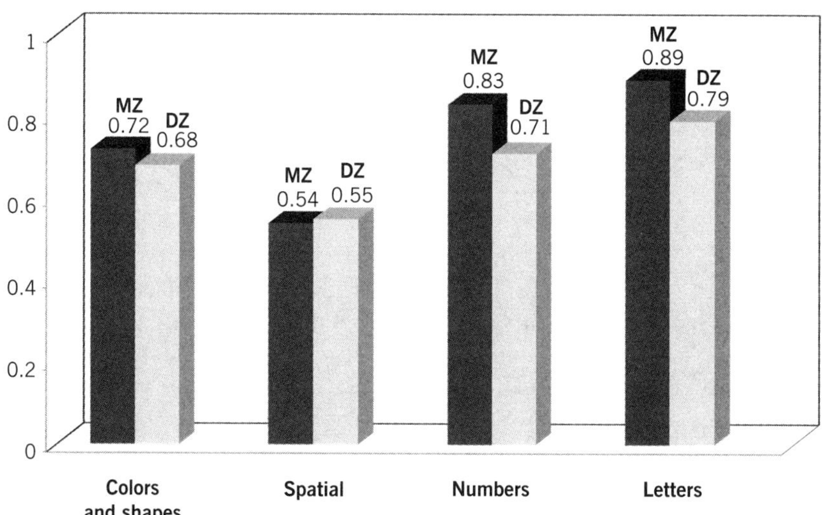

FIGURE 3.2. Intraclass correlation between co-twins' prekindergarten school readiness scores (Lollipop Test) as a function of zygosity.

pattern of family aggregation strongly suggests that there are familywide factors accounting for these various cognitive school readiness skills, and that shared environmental rather than genetic factors (i.e., heritability) mostly account for this family aggregation (i.e., as reflected by the low differential in MZ vs. DZ ICCs). The further modeling of the data for each subscale confirmed this initial view, with moderate heritability only found for Numbers (see Lemelin et al., 2007, for details about the modeling procedure).

A more qualified, yet similar picture emerged when we used a multivariate approach to assessing the genetic and environmental contributions to the Lollipop Test. Here, the four school readiness components were examined simultaneously in an integrated *longitudinal common pathway model* extending to the prediction of school achievement in grade 1 (see Figure 3.3). This model assumed (1) that general cognitive school readiness derives from the convergence of the four Lollipop subscales, and (2) that general school achievement in grade 1 derives from the four teacher assessments of specific school achievement (i.e., in reading, writing, mathematics, and general). The model was designed to disentangle the genetic and environmental sources of variance for (1) general school readiness, (2) general school achievement in grade 1, and (3) their association.

The resulting complex model is illustrated in Figure 3.3. Providing the minutiae is beyond the scope of this chapter but, by and large, three important features should be emphasized (see Lemelin et al., 2007, for details). First, the (latent) school readiness factor resulting from the convergent information provided by the four subtests was only moderately accounted for by genetic factors (29% of the variance), and environmental sources of variance, especially environment shared by twins of the same family (54% of the variance), were the dominant source of variance. The fact that genetic factors seemed more important here than when examining each subtest separately could be due to the fact that the school readiness factor reflects fluid cognitive skills partly under genetic influence.

Second, school achievement was more heritable (41% accounted for by genetic factors), but with the environment still playing an important role (32 and 27% of the variance, respectively). The significant heritability found for school achievement could be due to possible interplay of behavior tendencies, such as aggressive and hyperactive behaviors, known to be heritable, in school achievement difficulties.

Third, the predictive association, that is, the putative contribution of school readiness to school achievement, was also mediated by common shared and nonshared environmental factors, in addition to common genetic factors, as indicated by the corresponding correlations at the top of Figure 3.3. All correlations were high, which indicates that, in

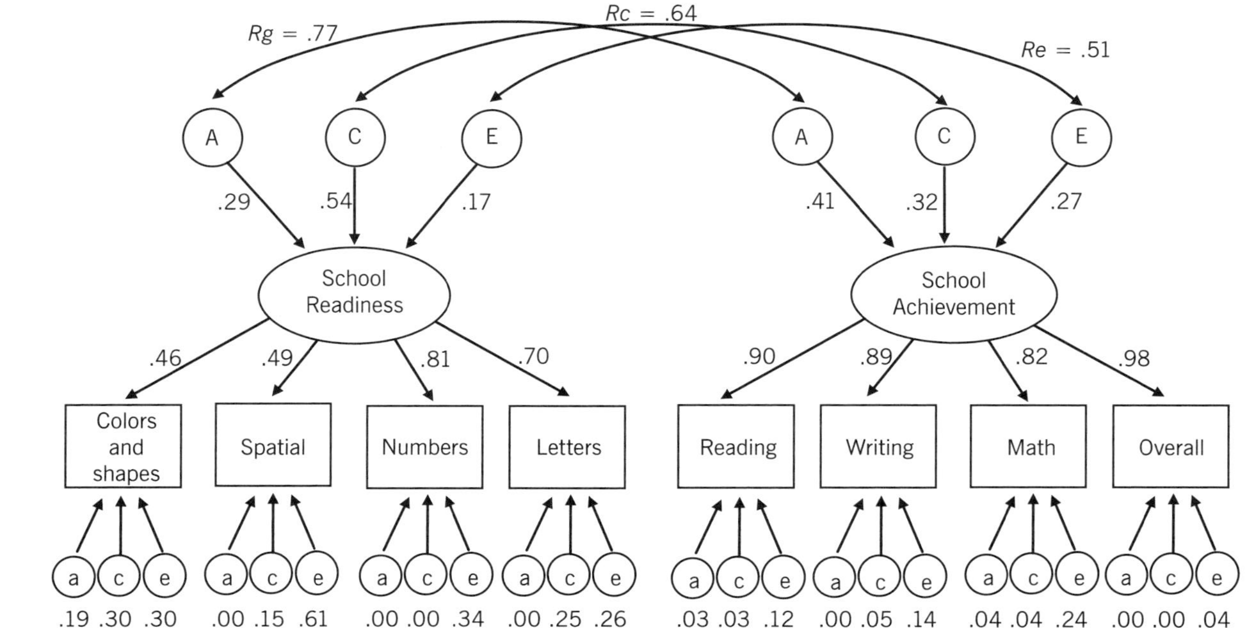

FIGURE 3.3. Bivariate common pathway model linking school readiness and school achievement. *Note.* A and a stand for additive genetic variance, C and c for shared (or common) environmental variance, E and e for unique environmental variance.

large part, the same genetic and shared environmental factors influenced school readiness and school achievement. In other words, not only were shared environmental factors important for general school readiness but to a large extent, the same factors also played a role as predictors of school achievement 2 years later.

The implications of these results are clear; although some genetic factors contributed to general school readiness and predicted early school achievement, environmental factors, especially those fostering similarities among members of the same family (and thus differences between families) accounted for most of the prediction. These results point to the importance of the home environment and experiences for school readiness, and to the need to document further the family processes involved in the emergence of school readiness. We conclude our chapter by presenting two pieces of evidence that speak to this issue.

FAMILY RISK, SCHOOL READINESS, AND SCHOOL ACHIEVEMENT

The association between school achievement difficulties and sociodemographic risk factors, such as low socioeconomic status (SES), teenage parenting, and early single parenthood is well documented (Foster, Lambert, Abbott-Shim, McCarty, & Franze, 2005; McLoyd, 2008). A final goal of this chapter was to use data from the QLSCD and the QNTS to address the question of how well the EDI and the Lollipop measures of school readiness account for the association between early family sociodemographic risk factors and the child's later school achievement.

In the QLSCD, we examined the contribution of early sociodemographic risk factors, including components of low SES assessed when the child was age 5 months, to early school achievement difficulties (e.g., the probability of membership in the *Low* achievement trajectory as presented in Figure 3.1). Specifically, we distinguished single parenthood, insufficient income (below the low-income cutoff before taxes (LICO) defined by *Statistics Canada,* which take into account the size of the household and the size of the region of residence), young parenthood for both mother and father (i.e., age 20 or less at the birth of the child), and low education (not having completed high school) for both mother and father. Globally, these early sociodemographic risk factors at 5 months were significantly, but only moderately associated with later school difficulties, accounting for 9% of the variance in early school achievement difficulties. Interestingly, the only unique contributions were made by mother's low education level (beta = 0.20, $p < .001$), father's low education level (beta = 0.15, $p < .001$), and young motherhood (beta = 0.10, $p < .05$).

We then looked at the contribution of the EDI and the Lollipop to the prediction of early school achievement, after taking into account the early sociodemographic risk factors. The EDI and the Lollipop not only accounted for an additional 39% of the variance in early school achievement, but most interestingly, they also explained most of the prediction of school achievement difficulties by early sociodemographic risk factors. Specifically, the amount of explained variance by the sociodemographic risk factors dropped from 9 to 2.6%, a 6.4% reduction, or 71% of the original association.

These results are interesting on two accounts. First, they clearly show that low levels of school readiness are far from being entirely accounted for by the sociodemographic factors associated with low SES. It is not clear at this point what mediates this unaccounted-for prediction by early sociodemographic risk factors (likely family processes independent of these early risks, see below), but there is an added value (i.e., as shown by a quite impressive 39% of additional variance) to assessing school readiness at the end of preschool. Second, most of the predictive association between early sociodemographic risk factors and later school difficulties (i.e., mainly due to low education background of both parents) was explained by the fact that the child was less prepared for school (as assessed by these two instruments). Thus, the two instruments successfully "accounted" for the predictive association, which points to possible family processes. Given the results of gene–environment contributions to cognitive school readiness, the most likely "learning assumption" is that these associations reflect differences between families in creating a nurturing setting for learning, possibly due to parental practices.

Data from the QNTS were used to start addressing this question by looking at early language development (Forget-Dubois et al., 2009). In this study, the Lollipop Test (i.e., total score combining the four subscales) was considered the outcome measure. SES was estimated on the basis of household income and parent education when the child was 6 and 19 months old. Child language was measured at 19 and 32 months using the parent-reported assessment of expressive vocabulary (the MacArthur–Bates Communicative Development Inventory; Fenson et al., 1995). Exposure to reading was assessed though parent report at 19 months. General cognitive abilities were assessed by the Block Design, and as with sex and age, were used as controls. First, using the twin method, the study showed that the association between early language and later school readiness was essentially accounted for by shared and unique environmental sources of variance (i.e., no genetic contribution). Forget-Dubois et al. (2009) then proceeded to examine the extent to which the association between early SES and later school readiness was mediated by (1) exposure to reading

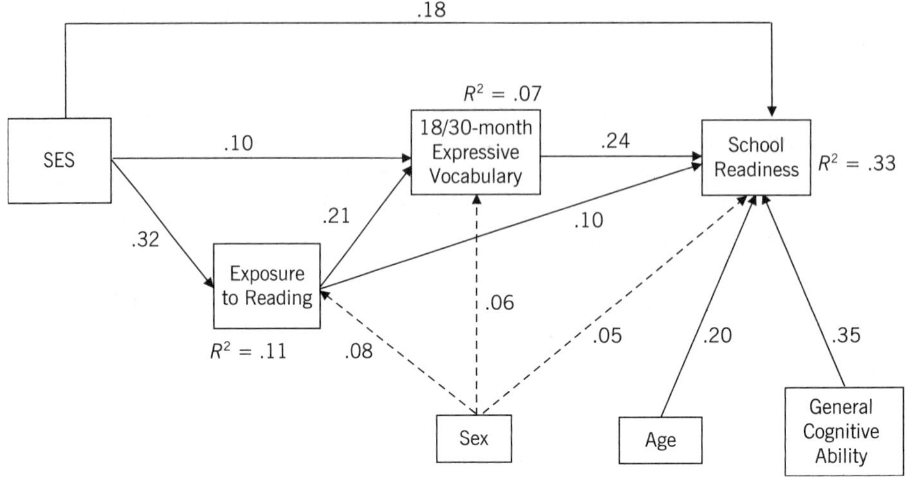

FIGURE 3.4. Direct and indirect paths linking SES to on school readiness. *Note.* $\chi^2 = 10.18$ ($df = 7$), $p = .18$; RMSEA = .03 (90% CI: .00–.06); CFI = .99; AIC = 66.18. Nonsignificant ($p > .05$) paths are indicated by a dashed line. Relevant correlations between exogenous variables are omitted for simplicity.

resulting in (2) stronger expressive vocabulary. The resulting model with corresponding estimates, presented in Figure 3.4, showed that the link between SES and school readiness was partly accounted for by parent–child reading, which predicted child vocabulary.

Summary and Implications for Policy and Practice

This chapter presents a strong case for the utility of the EDI and the Lollipop for assessing school readiness in the context of a populationwide approach. The reported analyses and review of previous research clearly indicate that the two instruments predict early school achievement in a significant way, especially when they are used in conjunction, and particularly when predicting at the extreme of the distribution (i.e., children experiencing school achievement difficulties, as well as those who achieve well). These composite measures of school readiness also significantly accounted for the contribution of a variety of early ECD risk indicators (i.e., child, parental, and family factors) to early school achievement difficulties, suggesting that they can document quite effectively and in a multidimensional way the nature of the difficulties awaiting children at risk in the early years of school. Finally, the cognitive facets of school readiness, as well as their (substantial) contribution to later school achievement were mainly accounted for by environmental factors and processes shared and uniquely experienced by children of the same family (in contrast to genetic factors and processes).

This work is ongoing, but this initial series of analyses illustrates that reliable and valid assessment tools are available to monitor preschool school readiness in populations. It also suggests that the level of school readiness is accounted for by specific early risk indicators that could become the target of early preventive interventions aimed at improving school readiness and, by way of consequence, early school achievement.

There are, however, caveats to the actual research and remaining challenges for future work in this field. For instance, replication will be necessary to ensure that the estimates and patterns revealed through the trajectory analysis apply not only to the population from which it has been drawn (i.e., using appropriate population weights and accounting for the sampling design), but also in other population contexts where the social inequalities and social services available to families and young children differ substantially. Given the biases toward "normalization" possibly leading to a restriction in the sample variance through attrition, it is likely that the reported figures are conservative estimates. However, this is an empirical question that should be put to test in future work.

It will be important to document whether the combined use of these two instruments will reveal a significant level of prediction of school achievement beyond the early years of school (i.e., for late primary and secondary school). A variety of social (i.e., social competence) and cognitive (i.e., literacy, numeracy) dimensions predicted early school achievement, which speaks to the value of a multidimensional approach to school readiness. However, it will be interesting to see whether these specific predictions will be maintained over time, and to what extent they will extend to school-related outcomes that are likely to play a more decisive role in early to late adolescence (e.g., peer relationships, quality of the relation with the teacher, school motivation). Finally, we will also need to more specifically examine the family factors and practices accounting for the various aspects of school readiness. These questions will be examined in a near future as these two longitudinal studies unfold.

The finding that important school readiness components, especially language-related aspects and numeracy, are mainly associated with shared and unique environment is supportive of efforts to improve the quality of the environments in which at-risk children are developing in order to enhance their school readiness skills, and set them on a more promising trajectory in school. It should be seen as a further incentive for continued implementation and evaluation of preventive intervention programs and services aimed at improving the level of school readiness in children from at-risk families. It should also encourage us to forge ahead in building a comprehensive early childhood policy agenda (Boivin & Hertzman, 2012).

Acknowledgments

We are grateful to the children and parents of the Québec Longitudinal Study of Child Development and the Québec Newborn Twin Study (QNTS), and the participating teachers and schools. We thank the Québec Institute of Statistics, Mireille Jetté, Bertrand Perron, Jocelyn Malo, and the GRIP staff for data collection and management, as well as Bei Feng, Alain Girard, and Hélène Paradis for assistance with statistical analyses. This research was supported by grants from the Québec Ministries of Health and Families, the Fondation Lucie et André Chagnon, the Fonds Québécois de la Recherche sur la Société et la Culture (FQRSC), the Fonds de la Recherche en Santé du Québec, the Social Science and Humanities Research Council of Canada (SSHRC), the National Health Research Development Program, the Canadian Institutes for Health Research (CIHR), and Ste. Justine Hospital's Research Center. Michel Boivin was supported by the Canada Research Chair Program.

References

Battin-Pearson, S., Newcomb, M. D., Abbott, R. D., Hill, K. G., Catalano, R. F., & Hawkins, J. D. (2000). Predictors of early high school dropout: A test of five theories. *Journal of Educational Psychology, 92*, 568–582.

Belsky J. (2001). Developmental risks (still) associated with early child care. *Journal of Child Psychology and Psychiatry, 42*, 845–859.

Belsky, J., & Fearon, R. M. P. (2002). Infant–mother attachment security, contextual risk, and early development: A moderational analysis. *Development and Psychopathology, 14*, 293–310.

Bierman, K. L., Nix, R. L., Greenberg, M. T., Blair, C., & Domitrovich, C. E. (2008). Executive functions and school readiness intervention: Impact, moderation, and mediation in the Head Start REDI Program. *Development and Psychopathology, 20*, 821–843.

Bierman, K. L., Torres, M. M., Domitrovich, C. E., Welsh, J. A., & Gest, S. D. (2009). Behavioral and cognitive readiness for school: Cross-domain associations for children attending Head Start. *Social Development, 18*, 305–323.

Blair, C. (2002). School readiness: Integrating cognition and emotion in a neurobiological conceptualization of children's functioning at school entry. *American Psychologist, 57*, 111–127.

Blair, C. (2006). How similar are fluid cognition and general intelligence?: A developmental neuroscience perspective on fluid cognition as an aspect of human cognitive ability. *Behavioral and Brain Sciences, 29*, 109–125.

Blair, C., & Diamond, A. (2008). Biological processes in prevention and intervention: Promotion of self-regulation and the prevention of early school failure. *Development and Psychopathology, 20*, 899–911.

Blair, C., & Razza, R. P. (2007). Relating effortful control, executive function, and false-belief understanding to emerging math and literacy ability in kindergarten. *Child Development, 78*, 647–663.

Boivin, M., Brendgen, M., Dionne, G., Dubois, L., Pérusse, D., Robaey, P., et al. (2013). The Québec Newborn Twin Study into adolescence: 15 years later. *Twin Research and Human Genetics, 16*(1), 64–69.

Boivin, M., & Hertzman, C. (Eds.). (2012). *Early childhood development: Adverse experiences and developmental health.* Royal Society of Canada, Canadian Academy of Health Sciences Expert Panel (with Ronald Barr, Thomas Boyce, Alison Fleming, Harriet MacMillan, Candice Odgers, Marla Sokolowski, & Nico Trocmé). Ottawa, ON: Royal Society of Canada. Available from *https://rsc- src.ca/sites/default/files/pdf/ ecd%20report_0.pdf.*

Bradley, R. H., & Caldwell, B. M. (1984). The relation of infants' home environments to achievement test performance in first grade: A follow-up study. *Child Development, 55*, 803–809.

Britto, P. R., Brooks-Gunn, J., & Griffin, T. (2006). Story readers and story tellers: Stylistic differences in low income, young, African-American mothers' reading styles. *Reading Research Quarterly, 41*, 68–89.

Brooks-Gunn, J., Han, W.-J., & Waldfogel, J. (2002). Maternal employment and child cognitive outcomes in the first three years of Life: The NICHD Study of Early Child Care. *Child Development, 73*, 1052–1072.

Butz, A. M., Pulsifer, M. B., Leppert, M., Rimrodt, S., & Belcher, H. (2003). Comparison of intelligence, school readiness skills, and attention in in-utero drug-exposed and nonexposed preschool children. *Clinical Pediatrics, 42*, 727–739.

Chew, A. L. (1987). *Developmental and interpretive manual for the Lollipop Test: A Diagnostic Screening Test of School Readiness–Revised.* Atlanta, GA: Humanics.

Chew, A. L., & Lang, W. S. (1990). Predicting academic achievement in kindergarten and first grade from Prekindergarten scores on the Lollipop Test and DIAL. *Educational and Psychological Measurement, 50*, 431–437.

Chew, A. L., & Morris, J. D. (1984). Validation of the Lollipop Test: A Diagnostic Screening Test of School Readiness. *Educational and Psychological Measurement, 44*, 987–991.

Chew, A. L., & Morris, J. D. (1989). Predicting later academic achievement from kindergarten scores on the Metropolitan Readiness Tests and the Lollipop Test. *Educational and Psychological Measurement, 49*, 461–465.

Christenson, S. L., Sinclair, M. F., Lehr, C. A., & Godber, Y. (2001). Promoting successful school completion: Critical conceptual and methodological guidelines. *School Psychology Quarterly, 16*, 468–484.

Connell, C. M., & Prinz, R. J. (2002). The impact of childcare and parent–child interactions on school readiness and social skills development for low-income African American children. *Journal of School Psychology, 40*, 177–193.

Dearing, E., McCartney, K., & Taylor, B. A. (2001). Change in family income-to-needs matters more for children with less. *Child Development, 72*, 1779–1793.

Duncan, G. J., Dowsett, C. J., Claessens, A., Magnuson, K., Huston, A. C., Klebanov, P., et al. (2007). School readiness and later achievement. *Developmental Psychology, 43*, 1428–1446.

Dunn, L. M., Thériault-Whalen, C. M., & Dunn, L. M. (1993). *Échelle de vocabulaire en images Peabody (EVIP), Adaptation française du Peabody Picture Vocabulary Test–Revised. Manuel pour les formes A et B* [French Adaptation of The Peabody Picture Vocabulary Test—Revised (PPVT). Manual for Forms A and B]. Toronto: Psycan.

Ensminger, M. E., & Slusarcick, A. L. (1992). Paths to high school graduation or dropout: A longitudinal study of a first-grade cohort. *Sociology of Education, 65*, 95–113.

Fenson, L., Dale, P. S., Bates, E., Reznick, J. S., Thal, D. J., Pethick, S. J., et al. (1994). Variability in early communicative development. *Monograph of the Society for Research in Child Development, 59*(5, Serial No. 242), 1–185.

Forget-Dubois, N., Dionne, G., Lemelin, J. P., Pérusse, D., Tremblay R. E., Boivin, M. (2009). Early child language mediates the relation between home environment and school readiness. *Child Development, 80*(3), 736–749.

Foster, M. A., Lambert, R., Abbott-Shim, M., McCarty, F., & Franze, S. (2005). A model of home learning environment and social risk factors in relation to children's emergent literacy and social outcomes. *Early Childhood Research Quarterly, 20*, 13–36.

Galéra, C., Côté, S. M., Bouvard, M.-P., Pingault, J.-B., Melchior, M., Michel, G., et al. (2011). Early risk factors of hyperactivity–impulsivity and inattention trajectories from 17 months to 8 years. *Archives of General Psychiatry, 68*(12), 1267–1275.

Garnier, H. E., Stein, J. A., & Jacobs, J. K. (1997). The process of dropping out of school: A 19 year perspective. *American Educational Research Journal, 34*, 395–419.

Goldsmith, H. H., Lemery, K. S., Buss, K. A., & Campos, J. J. (1999). Genetic analyses of focal aspects of infant temperament. *Developmental Psychology, 35*, 972–985.

Janus, M., & Offord, D. R. (2007). Development and psychometric properties of the Early Development Instrument (EDI): A measure of children's school readiness. *Canadian Journal of Behavioral Science, 39*(1), 1–22.

Jones, B. L., Nagin, D. S., & Roeder, K. (2001). A SAS procedure based on mixture models for estimating developmental trajectories. *Sociological Methods and Research, 29*, 374–393.

Kurdek, L. A., & Sinclair, R. J. (2000). Psychological, family, and peer predictors of academic outcomes in first through fifth-grade children. *Journal of Educational Psychology, 92*, 449–457.

Ladd, G. W., Herald, S. L., & Kochel, K. P. (2006). School readiness: Are there social prerequisites? *Early Education and Development, 17*, 115–150.

LaParo, K., & Pianta, R. C. (2000). Predicting children's competence in the early school years: A meta-analytic review. *Review of Educational Research, 70*, 443–484.

Lemelin, J.-P., Boivin, M., Forget-Dubois, N., Dionne, G., Séguin, J. R., Brendgen, M., et al. (2007). The genetic–environmental etiology of cognitive school readiness in early childhood. *Child Development, 78*(6), 1855–1869.

Mattanah, J. F., Pratt, M. W., Cowan, P. A., & Cowan, C. P. (2005). Authoritative parenting, parental scaffolding of long-division mathematics, and children's academic competence in fourth grade. *Journal of Applied Developmental Psychology, 26*, 85–106.

McLoyd, V. C. (1998). Socioeconomic disadvantage and child development. *American Psychologist, 53*, 185–204.

Melhuish, E. C., Phan, M. B., Sylva, K., Sammons, P., Siraj-Blatchford, I., & Taggart, B. (2008). Effects of the home learning environment and preschool center experience upon literacy and numeracy development in early primary school. *Journal of Social Issues, 64*, 95–114.

Moffitt, T. E., Arseneault, L., Belsky, D., Dickson, N., Hancox, R. J., Harrington, H., et al. (2011). A gradient of childhood self-control predicts health, wealth, and public safety. *Proceedings of the National Academy of Science, 108*, 2693–2698.

Nagin, D.S. (1999). Analyzing developmental trajectories: A semiparametric, group-based approach. *Psychological Methods, 4*, 139–157.

NICHD Early Child Care Research Network. (2003). Do children's attention processes mediate the link between family predictors and school readiness? *Developmental Psychology, 39*, 581–593.

Normandeau, S., & Guay, F. (1998). Preschool behavior and first-grade school achievement: The mediational role of cognitive self-control. *Journal of Educational Psychology, 90*, 111–121.

Okamoto, Y., & Case, R. (1996). Exploring the microstructure of children's central conceptual structures in the domain of number. *Monographs of the Society for Research in Child Development, 61*, 27–59.

Pingault, J.-B., Tremblay, R. E., Vitaro, F., Carbonneau, R., Genolini, C., Falissard, B., et al. (2012). Childhood trajectories of inattention and hyperactivity and prediction of educational attainment in early adulthood: A 16-year longitudinal population-based study. *American Journal of Psychiatry, 168*(11), 1164–1170.

Plomin, R., DeFries, J. C., McClearn, G. E., & McGuffin, P. (2001). *Behavioral genetics* (4th ed.). New York: Worth.

Rothbart, M. K., & Bates, J. E. (2006). Temperament. In W. Damon & N. Eisenberg (Eds.), *Social, emotional, and personality development* (5th ed., Vol. 3, pp. 105–176). New York: Wiley.

Rutter, M. (2007). Proceeding from observed correlation to causal inference: The use of natural experiments. *Perspectives on Psychological Science, 2*(4), 377–395.

Tramontana, M. G., Hooper, S. R., & Selzer, S. C. (1988). Research on the preschool prediction of later academic achievement: A review. *Developmental Review, 8*, 89–146.

Vallerand, R. J. (1989). Vers une méthodologie de validation trans-culturelle de questionnaires psychologiques: Implication pour la recherche en langue française [Toward a methodology of cross-cultural validation of psychological questionnaires: Implications for research in French]. *Psychologie Canadienne, 30*, 662–680.

Venet, M., Normandeau, S., Letarte, M.-J., & Bigras, M. (2003). Les propriétés psychométriques du Lollipop [The psychometric properties of the Lollipop]. *Revue de Psychoeducation, 32*, 165–176.

Vitaro, F., Larocque, D., Janosz, M., & Tremblay, R. E. (2001). Negative social experiences and dropping out of school. *Educational Psychology, 21,* 401–415.

Walker, S. O., Petrill, S. A., Spinath, F. M., & Plomin, R. (2004). Nature, nurture and academic achievement: A twin study of teacher assessments of 7-year-olds. *British Journal of Educational Psychology, 74,* 323–342.

Wechsler, D. (1989). *Manual for the Wechsler Preschool and Primary Scale of Intelligence–Revised.* San Antonio, TX: Psychological Corporation.

Worrell, F. C. (1997). Predicting successful or non-successful at risk status using demographic risk factors. *High School Journal, 81*(1), 46–53.

Zelazo, P. D., Jacques, S., Burack, J., & Frye, D. (2002). The relation between theory of mind and rule use: Evidence from persons with autism-spectrum disorders. *Infant and Child Development, 11,* 171–195.

PART II

Determinants of School Readiness

CHAPTER 4

A Multilevel Approach to the Examination of Cognitive Skills in School Readiness

MARK WADE, HEATHER PRIME, DILLON BROWNE, and JENNIFER M. JENKINS

Most definitions of school readiness cover a broad range of skills involving cognition, social skills, and emotion regulation. In this chapter we concentrate on two cognitive skills—language and early print recognition—that have a well-established impact on children's academic trajectories (see Snow, Burns, & Griffin, 1998). For example, Kurdek and Sinclair (2001) have shown that fourth graders' reading achievement is predicted by verbal abilities measured in kindergarten. Likewise, Walker, Greenwood, Hart, and Carta (1994) have shown that early language assessed between 7 and 36 months is predictive of receptive and spoken language, as well as reading and spelling achievement, up to 7 years later. Using data from six longitudinal studies, Duncan et al. (2007) demonstrated that school-entry reading and math skills were the strongest predictors of later academic outcomes. Thus, owing to the predictive power of early language and reading on later academic competencies, it is important to identify the multilevel factors that predate these skills prior to school entry. Such an approach has the potential to enhance a range of childhood outcomes through policy and practice.

Bronfenbrenner (1979) and others (e.g., Lerner, 2006) have suggested that development occurs within embedded "layers" of context. The most proximal layer involves relationships in which the child takes part: relationships with parents, siblings, and peers. In turn, these relationships are nested within more distal circumstances that also have a bearing on the proximal influences. For instance, social disadvantage is associated with more negative parenting practices (Dodge, Pettit, & Bates, 1994; Jenkins, Rasbash, & O'Connor, 2003; McLoyd, 1990), as well as with more negative sibling relationships (Dunn, Slomkowski, & Beardsall, 1994). Broader contextual factors such as the economic state of the community may also be associated with the functioning of children through influences on child care, school, and family structures (e.g., Conger, Ge, Elder, Lorenz, & Simons, 1994).

The multilevel structure described earlier constitutes a complex mixture of distal and proximal influences in the context of children's ongoing adaptations to their environment. Despite our knowledge about the various factors associated with children's developmental outcomes, the relative contributions of these various types of influence and the ways that they combine together in the prediction of children's early language and reading skills have been underinvestigated. In this chapter we describe findings from the Kids, Families and Places, a longitudinal study of an ethnically diverse sample of 501 parents, a newborn, and an older child, living in two cities in Southern Ontario, who are being followed up until the youngest child is school age. This study focuses on distal and proximal processes that predict the youngest child's reading and language at age 3. Four categories of distal and proximal influence were considered: (1) sociodemographic characteristics of parents; (2) neighborhoods; (3) parenting behaviors; and (4) earlier child adaptations.

Furthermore, research has consistently shown that development must be understood in terms of moderating influences (e.g., Luthar, Cicchetti, & Becker, 2000; Jenkins, 2008). Contingencies operate across these different types of risk. Thus, we cannot simply examine main effects on school readiness; instead, we must also consider how factors combine to explain child outcomes. That is, even if children are exposed to a contextual influence that is normally associated with low achievement, in the presence of another factor, they may perform well (Bierman, Nix, Greenberg, Blair, & Domitrovich, 2008). For example, higher parental acceptance and lower parental hostility is associated with better prereading scores among kindergartners from low-income families (Hill, 2001). This study was designed to examine the relative influence of categories of risk, as well as the ways in which risks combine, in understanding early reading and language.

Sociodemographic Characteristics of Parents

Sociodemographic characteristics of parents (e.g., income and education) have consistently shown associations with children's language and reading achievement. Children who grow up in low- income families have less advanced language skills in terms of vocabulary acquisition (Hart & Risley, 1995; Hoff, 2003), onset of combinatorial speech, and language complexity (Arriaga, Fenson, Cronan, & Pethick, 1998) compared to children from middle-income homes. Similarly, Dollaghan et al. (1999) showed that maternal education was related to 3-year-olds' receptive vocabulary, length of utterances, and vocabulary size. Indeed, maternal education was a significant predictor of children's receptive vocabulary upon entry to kindergarten (Christian, Morrison, & Bryant, 1998). The relationship between socioeconomic status [SES] and reading abilities is also well established, with SES accounting for about 5% of the variance in school achievement (see White, 1982). Moreover, maternal education is longitudinally predictive of preacademic reading skills such as letter and word recognition (Hirsh-Pasek & Burchinal, 2006). Finally, in some samples, ethnicity has been shown to have associations with children's receptive vocabulary, reading recognition, math skills, and letter recognition at kindergarten entry (e.g., Christian et al., 1998), and it also predicts preacademic skills such as expressive language and letter–word identification (e.g., Hirsh-Pasek & Burchinal, 2006). Importantly, the data for the current study were drawn from an ethnically heterogeneous population with a large proportion of immigrant families. Immigrant parents earn less money, accept lower paying jobs, and receive more offers of employment that do not match their educational attainment than do their nonimmigrant counterparts (Leyendecker, Harwood, Comparini, & Yalcinkaya, 2005). This diversity necessitated the uncoupling of income, education, and ethnicity in the present analysis. Thus, we examined the independent effects of these sociodemographic variables on children's language and reading outcomes.

One criterion for entry into the current study was that the mothers be fluent in English. However, some mothers used their heritage language in the home. Since all target children had lived in Canada for 3 years at the time of testing and had older siblings (most of whom were in school), all children were exposed to some level of English. We formed a variable of low versus high English exposure to reflect this. We expected children with little exposure to English to show lower print recognition and vocabulary at 3 years than children with higher exposure. However, we also expected that this effect would be moderated by family size, based on research documenting lower achievement among children who have more siblings. This association may reflect the dilution of parental resources, given that parental time and energy are finite resources that become less available as more children require them (Blake, 1981). Consequently, we were interested in whether sibship size in families interacted with English exposure to explain children's early language/literacy.

Neighborhood Factors

Neighborhood characteristics can be classified along two different dimensions: *structural characteristics*, which entail aspects such as poverty and employment rates, and *social organizational* factors, which include measures of informal social control and social cohesion. This chapter focuses on social organizational factors because their relation to school readiness has been relatively understudied. Two key social processes fall under the banner of "social organization": (1) social control, reflecting the extent to which youth are monitored by the collective community; and (2) social cohesion, a measure of mutual trust and shared values (Silk, Sessa, Morris, Steinberg, & Avenevoli, 2004). Together, these processes comprise the concept of *collective efficacy*, which represents a community-level influence on child outcomes (Sampson, Raudenbush, & Earls, 1997). There is evidence that social control and social cohesion are associated with higher levels of prosociality and fewer behavior problems in adolescent populations (Elliott et al., 1996), as well as with lower levels of psychopathology in both adolescents (Aneshensel & Sucoff, 1996) and young children (Xue, Leventhal, Brooks-Gunn, & Earls; 2005). With regard to school readiness outcomes, Kohen, Brooks-Gunn, Leventhal, and Hertzman (2002) showed that higher ratings of neighborhood disorder were associated with lower receptive vocabulary scores in a sample of Canadian preschoolers, whereas higher ratings of social cohesion were related to higher verbal scores. Here, we attempt to replicate this finding and extend it to early reading.

Parenting

The sensitivity that mothers show toward their children has been found to be an important predictor of language and reading outcomes, and it is easy to understand why. From a young age children engage in a variety of activities that elicit both verbal and nonverbal responses from caregivers, who in turn vary in the type and quality of their reactions. Mothers who respond rapidly and sensitively evoke a sense of security and accomplishment in their children (Ainsworth, 1973), while also scaffolding language development by providing labels and expressions that match the object(s) of their children's attention. It turns out that both *what mothers say* and *what mothers do* is related to their children's readiness. Tamis-LeMonda, Bornstein, and Baumwell (2001; Tamis-LeMonda, Bornstein, Kahana-Kalman, Baumwell, & Cyphers, 1998) have shown that contingent verbal responsiveness at 13 months predicts children's mastery of fundamental language abilities in the second year, including an accelerated acquisition of vocabulary and combinatorial speech. Likewise, sensitive parenting behavior has been shown to predict language ability at 15 to 36 months (National Institute of Child and Human Development Early Child Care Research Network [NICHD-ECCRN], 1999), and is also predictive of teacher-reported readiness skills, social skills, communication skills, and receptive communication (Connell & Prinz, 2002). Others have broadened the construct of sensitivity to include maternal behaviors that provide cognitive challenge and scaffolding. Thus, Pianta and Harbers (1996) have shown that, in addition to sensitivity-type behaviors (encouragement, warmth, and emotional support), behaviors that challenge the child cognitively (quality instructions and respect for their autonomy) are also important predictors of academic achievement during the first few years of school. In general, these kinds of parenting behaviors are longitudinally associated with reading skills, language skills, and phonemic knowledge at school entry (Bradley, Corwyn, Burchinal, McAdoo, & Garcia Coll, 2001; Poe, Burchinal, & Roberts, 2004).

Another parenting behavior that may influence child outcomes is *reflective functioning*. This process refers to parents' ability to interpret and understand their child's behavior by reflecting on their own (and their child's) internal mental experience (Fonagy, Steele, Moran, Steele, & Higgitt, 1991). Such a capacity is crucial to one's management of affective and behavioral responses, as well as basic social functioning (Slade, 2005). Perhaps unsurprisingly, deficits in maternal reflective functioning are associated with poorer dyadic affective communication, which has been shown to mediate the relationship between reflective functioning and unfavorable attachment outcomes (Kelly, Slade, & Grienenberger, 2005). Thus, reflective functioning represents another characteristic that may have a bearing on the way parents interact with their children and, in turn, influences school readiness. This study examined the joint role of both parental responsivity (including sensitivity, mutuality, and cognitive challenge) and reflective functioning on children's early language and reading skills, and extends previous findings by contrasting the roles of different types of risk, including their interactions, in the prediction of these skills. One factor that might be expected to interact with parenting behaviors in the prediction of language and literacy is children's previous level of language adaptation.

Previous Adaptation

In the current study, language and literacy outcomes at 3 years were the target of investigation. One of the best predictors of future functioning is earlier levels of that behavior. Thus, previous adaptation—operationalized as language functioning at 18 months—was hypothesized to relate to these later language-based competencies. Support for this claim comes from research showing that children who have poor expressive language abilities at 24 to 31 months are at risk for continued language delays approximately 2 years later (Rescorla & Schwartz, 1990); and these same children are more likely to demonstrate language and reading deficits at age 9 compared to control children (Rescorla, 2002). Similarly, Dale, Price, Bishop, and Plomin (2003) showed that over 40% of children showing language delays at 2 years showed persistent delays at 3 and 4 years. Scarborough (1990) showed that spoken language at 30 months is predictive of receptive vocabulary 1 year later, and that poor language was a risk factor for the development of reading disabilities at age 5. In a meta-analytic review of 61 studies, Scarborough (2001) demonstrated that the strongest predictors of reading ability in grade 1 were print processing skills, oral language skills, and phonological awareness (in that order) during kindergarten. Regardless of the pathway through which language operates, there is a common theme across these studies: Early oral language lays the foundation upon which reading faculties develop.

Risk and Resilience in School Readiness

Risk and resilience models of development (Luthar et al., 2000; Jenkins, 2008) have demonstrated that there is large variation in the degree to which psychosocial adversity compromises child outcomes. Whether children show negative outcomes when exposed to adversity is dependent on factors in themselves and their environments that combine (i.e., interact) with risk exposure to exacerbate or attenuate those effects (Rutter, 2012). In this chapter we examine the contribution of person and environmental risks to children's language and reading ability at 3 years. Recall the types of risk included in this study: neighborhood (i.e., social cohesion and social control), sociodemographic (SES, exposure to English, sibship size), parental (maternal responsivity and reflective functioning), and child (previous adaptation; language). Operating within a risk-resiliency framework, we examined contingencies that operated within and across types of risk. That is, we examined how the effect of one type of risk factor (e.g., exposure to English; *sociodemographic*) was contingent on the presence of the same type of risk (e.g., number of siblings in the home;

sociodemographic), as well as how one type of risk (e.g., previous language skills; *child previous adaptation*) was contingent on another type of risk (e.g., maternal responsivity; *family process*).

The moderation (or interaction) models just described can be further differentiated on the basis of patterns of contingent influences. For example, Luthar et al. (2000) describe one of these patterns as "protective-stabilizing," which refers to a pattern in which an individual is exposed to a particular risk, yet functions well due to the presence of a positive factor that helps him or her to cope. For instance, Gass, Jenkins, and Dunn (2007) reported that although exposure to adverse life events is usually associated with more mood disorders in children, the existence of close sibling relationships seems to protect against these negative effects. In this study, we predicted that children with poor language at 18 months (the risk) would be protected from language and literacy problems at 3 years when they received high levels of positive parenting behaviors (the protective factor). This hypothesized interaction was based on the finding that maternal sensitivity is protective to children in the development of cooperation when the children show poor joint attention skills (Frampton, Moore, Astington, Perlman, & Jenkins, 2012). We also hypothesized that children exposed to low levels of English by their mothers would show worse language and reading outcomes when they had large sibships, whereas there would be less negative developmental consequences for children in small sibships. This is based on the resource dilution hypothesis described earlier (Downey, 1995, 2001). For literacy in English, both large sibships (Downey, 1995) and mothers not talking to children in English constitute risks prior to school entry, with the idea that these two risks will potentiate one another. Moderation hypotheses, in which the presence of certain risks potentiate or attenuate the impact of other risks, are not only critical to our understanding of development (Rutter et al., 2008) but also inform our thinking about social policy and the implementation of targeted and universal intervention programs that promote school readiness.

Research Questions

This study addressed four major research questions to shed light on the various multilevel influences on children's language and reading ability at 3 years: (1) how much of the variance in language and reading at age 3 is attributable to the sociodemographic characteristics of parents; (2) after accounting for sociodemographic influences, how much parenting behaviors, characteristics of neighborhoods, and earlier child adaptations account for language and reading when children are 3 years old; (3) how much unique variance each of these categories of risk explains; and (4) whether there is evidence of protective effects. In examining protective influences, we explored a variety of interactions, including those in which parenting behaviors protected against sociodemographic disadvantage. We hypothesized that children with poor language at 18 months would be protected from poor reading and language at 3 years if their mothers showed high sensitivity. Furthermore, we hypothesized that children would be protected from a lack of English input from mothers if they had fewer siblings, because more available resources would provide other avenues to facilitate language and reading competencies. In turn, questions (1), (2), and (3) could provide valuable information regarding the most important targets for social policy and intervention based on the relative influence of certain risks on reading and language development, while question (4) would speak to the contingent processes that operate in development.

METHOD

Participants

All women giving birth to infants in the cities of Toronto and Hamilton between February 2006 and February 2008 were considered for participation. Families were recruited through a program called Healthy Babies Healthy Children, run by Toronto and Hamilton Public Health Units. Inclusion criteria for participation in the *Intensive* sample of the Kids, Families and Places (IKFP) study included an English-speaking mother, a newborn weighing more than 1,500 grams, and two or more children in the family who were less than 4 years old. At Time 1 (when infants were about 2 months old), 501 families took part in the *Intensive* sample data collection, and these families were followed up at Time 2 (about 18 months) and Time 3 (about 3 years). We compared the IKFP sample with the general population of Toronto and Hamilton using 2006 Canada Census Data. The IKFP sample was similar to the general population in terms of number of persons in the household and personal income but had had a lower proportion of nonintact (step- or lone-parent) families (5%), fewer immigrants (47%), and more educated mothers (53% had a Bachelor's degree) than the total population from which the sample was drawn. Only the youngest sibling was included in the current study, as the developmental progression toward school entry was of particular interest.

At the time of writing this chapter, Time 3 data collection (including the language and reading outcome measures) was still ongoing. Thus, we report on a subset of families for whom data collection was complete (N =

230 families). Of participating mothers, 59% were born in Canada, 90% were from intact families at the beginning of the study, and the average age was 33.3 years (*SD* = 4.7). The majority of participants were of European descent, though 12.4% identified themselves as East Asian, 12% as South Asian, and 6% as black. The average number of persons in each household was 4.55 (*SD* = 1.07), and the average number of children was 2.40 (*SD* = 0.62). Children were initially seen when they were 2 months old, and 42% of the current sample were female.

Measures

Covariates

Child gender (female = 1; male = 0) and age (in years and months) at Time 3 were included as covariates. We also included birthweight as a covariate, since this perinatal factor has been shown to be associated with children's cognitive and academic outcomes (e.g., Saigal, Szatmari, Rosenbaum, Campbell, & King, 1991), including children in the normal birthweight range (Richards, Hardy, Kuh, & Wadsworth, 2001). Mothers reported on their child's birthweight using either pounds and ounces or kilograms and grams. All scores were converted to kilograms and grams. In order to adjust for normative variation in birthweight curves as a function of maternal ethnic ancestry (*www.stmichaelshospital.com/birthweights.php*), each child's score was expressed as a standardized deviation from their ethnic average birthweight. In the KFP study, the ethnic categories were European, African/black, East Asian, and Southeast Asian. The resultant scores were combined into a single standardized, ethnicity-adjusted birthweight.

Sociodemographics

Immigrant status was evaluated by asking the mother whether or not she was born in Canada (1 = yes; 0 = no). Another dummy variable was created to indicate whether or not mothers spoke to their children in English during observed mother–child interaction. Mothers were asked to speak in English but some chose to speak in their heritage language. We coded 1 = low exposure to English. To assess SES, maternal education was measured as the number of years of formal study the mother received, excluding kindergarten. Mothers also reported on their partners' education level. To assess material wealth, mothers reported their best estimate of annual household income on a scale ranging from 1 (*No income*) to 16 (*$105,000 or more*). This score was standardized.

Maternal Responsivity

Responsivity was coded using a combination of three domains from the Parent–Child Interaction System of global ratings (PARCHISY; Deater-Deckard, 2000; Deater-Deckard, Pylas, & Petrill, 1997) and the Coding of Attachment-Related Parenting (CARP; Matias, Scott, & O'Connor, 2006): (1) *Sensitivity* (CARP) was the degree to which the parent displayed awareness of the child's needs and showed sensitivity to his or her signals, supported autonomy, and demonstrated an ability to see things from the child's point of view; (2) *Mutuality* (CARP) indexed reciprocity in conversation, affect sharing, joint engagement in a task, and open body posture; and (3) *Positive control* (PARCHISY) captured the parents' positive means of securing child cooperation, using praise, open-ended questions, rewards, and explanations. All three codes were *z*-scored within each task and summed (alpha = 0.85).

Maternal Reflective Parenting

Mothers were asked "How have your experiences in your childhood affected you as a parent?" The scoring was based on the mothers' ability to talk about her early experience, current parenting, and her attention to thoughts and feelings. We were guided in our coding categories by the work of Fonagy and Target (1997). A 5-point scale was used, from *no reflective parenting* (0) to *high reflective parenting* (5). Two coders were trained to criterion and then reliability was checked throughout the coding period on 10% of narratives. Interrater reliability for children's reflective parenting was alpha = 0.80.

Neighborhood Quality

This was assessed using questionnaire and observation data. First, mothers reported on (1) *social cohesion and trust,* which refers to the degree of closeness and camaraderie among members of the neighborhood (e.g., "This is a close-knit neighborhood"; "People in this neighborhood can be trusted"). Items were rated on a 5-point Likert scale ranging from 1 (*strongly agree*) to 5 (*strongly disagree*); (2) *social control* refers to the extent to which neighbors have control over events in the community, in addition to their ability to prevent harm and trouble (e.g., "If some children were spray-painting graffiti on a local building, how likely is it that your neighbors would do something about it?"). Items were rated on a 5-point Likert scale, from 1 (*very unlikely*) to 5 (*very likely*). These two areas were combined to form a score of neighborhood quality (alpha = 0.83).

Early Child Language

The MacArthur–Bates Communicative Development Inventories (CDI) assessed expressive language at 18 months. Mothers reported on children's vocabulary (in English and in their heritage language). The CDI has proven to be a valid and reliable measure of expressive language for typically developing children (Dale, 1991; Dale, Bates, Reznick, & Morisset, 1989) and children with language delays (Heilmann, Weismer, Evans, & Hollar, 2005; Thal & Bates, 1988).

Cognitive School Readiness

Two components of cognitive school readiness were assessed when children were 3-years-old. *Language (*i.e., *receptive vocabulary)* was assessed using the Peabody Picture Vocabulary Test—Fourth Edition (PPVT-4). Children listen to a set of words, and identify each meaning by pointing to one of four pictures. *Prereading skills (i.e., print recognition)* were evaluated using the Get Ready to Read (GRTR) screening tool, designed to predict future reading success among preschool children (Whitehurst, 2003). GRTR consists of 20 items assessing book, letter, and word identification abilities, as well as early phonological skills. GRTR converges with measures of receptive vocabulary, letter knowledge, and phonological ability (rs = .44–.67).

Data Presentation

First, variables were evaluated for univariate normality. Second, descriptive analyses were conducted, examining means and standard deviations for continuous variables, and frequencies and percentages for categorical variables. Then, hierarchical linear regressions were conducted to examine associations with school readiness outcomes (receptive vocabulary and print recognition). A seven-step hierarchical regression was used to test whether new variables entered into the model predicted language and print recognition over and above the covariates and other predictors already in the model. Interactions that were deemed to be significant were entered last, following entry of the main effects. Variables were entered in the following steps: (1) covariates (child gender, age, and birthweight); (2) sociodemographic variables (maternal/partner education, household income, number of siblings in household, and low exposure to English); (3) child language at 18 months; (4) parenting behavior (maternal responsivity and reflective functioning); (5) neighborhood quality; (6) the interaction between child language and parenting behavior; and (7) the interaction between low exposure to English and sibship size. Variables were entered in blocks to determine the amount of additional variance explained by each new level entered in the analysis. In a final analysis, we entered the variables from each level after the variables from every other level in order to determine the unique variance explained by each level of influence, over and above the effects of all other levels.

RESULTS

As we had several ethnicity and immigration variables that were strongly related to one another (born in Canada, low exposure to English, and ethnicity), we carried out preliminary analyses to determine whether some immigration and ethnicity variables could be excluded from the model to reduce the risk of *multicollinearity*. Results showed that only "low English exposure" remained a significant predictor of language when other variables were in the model. Consequently, immigration status and ethnicity were excluded from all models. Prior to conducting the main analysis we investigated two other plausible interactions: that the effects of neighborhood and parental education would be contingent on parental sensitivity. These were not found to be significant and are not reported in the following analyses.

Descriptive statistics are presented in Table 4.1. The hierarchical regression predicting early reading skills (print recognition) is presented

TABLE 4.1. Descriptive Statistics for Continuous Study Variables

	Min.	Max.	*M*	*SD*
PPVT score	50.00	137.00	92.10	16.62
GRTR score	0.00	19.00	8.60	3.42
Sensitive responding (18 months)	1.33	5.78	3.54	0.81
Reflective functioning (18 months)	–1.00	7.00	2.64	1.61
Language (18 months)	–1.98	3.54	0.01	1.03
Household income	–2.73	1.04	0.12	0.90
Maternal education in years	10.00	22.00	15.36	2.56
Partner education in years	7.00	22.00	15.30	2.36
Neighborhood quality	1.00	5.00	3.74	0.67
Child age	2.50	3.58	3.58	0.14
Ethnicity-adjusted birthweight	–3.22	5.35	0.09	1.01

Note. PPVT, Peabody Picture Vocabulary Test; GRTR, Get Ready to Read.

in Table 4.2. In this regression, the block of sociodemographic variables accounted for 4.3% of the variance in print recognition. None of the variables made significant unique contributions, although having three or more children in the household showed a trend toward significance, with more siblings associated with lower print recognition scores. Adding child language ability at 18 months accounted for an additional 8.8% of the variance in print recognition, with better language ability at 18 months associated with higher print recognition at 3 years after we controlled for demographics. Adding parenting behavior (maternal responsivity and reflective functioning) accounted for an additional 7.1% of the variance in print recognition. Higher levels of maternal responsivity, but not reflective functioning, were associated with significantly higher print recognition after we controlled for demographic characteristics and children's

TABLE 4.2. Hierarchical Regression Summary for Predictors of Prereading (Print Recognition) at Age 3

	Print recognition	B	SE_B	ΔR^2	R
Step 1	Child age	.172	.100	.030	
	Male	–.118	.179		
	Birthweight	.062	.091		
Step 2	Maternal education	–.100	.116	.043	
	Partner education	.020	.109		
	Household income	.182	.137		
	Three or more children	–.352	.201		
	Low English exposure	–.163	.222		
Step 3	Child language (18 months)	$.311^{***}$	.085	$.088^{***}$	
Step 4	Sensitive responding (18 months)	$.293^{**}$	.095	$.071^{**}$	
	Reflective functioning (18 months)	.123	.087		
Step 5	Neighborhood quality	.157	.097	.016	
Step 6	Sensitive responding (18 months)* Child language (18 months)	.049	.074	.003	
Step 7	Low English exposure* Three or more children	-1.387^{**}	.488	$.046^{**}$	.545

$^{*}p < .05$; $^{**}p < .01$; $^{***}p < .001$.

earlier language ability. Neighborhood quality, added in step 5, did not account for a significant amount of additional variance, after we controlled for demographic variables, early language, and parenting behavior, nor did the inclusion of the interaction term (maternal responsivity by child language). However, the inclusion of the other retained interaction term (low English exposure by sibship size) accounted for an additional 4.6% of the variance in children's print recognition after we controlled for all previous variables (including main effects of interaction variables). The final model accounted for 30% of the variance in children's print recognition skills at age 3. Regarding the interactions, the hypothesis was confirmed that the effect of low exposure to English was strongest for children in larger families. Indeed, there was evidence of a protective effect for children in small families (see Figure 4.1; interactions are plotted one standard deviation above and below the mean). On the other hand, we did not find support for the protective influence of parenting on children's reading at 3 years when they demonstrated low language ability at 18 months.

We examined the role of each level of risk after controlling for all other levels. Child language at 18 months accounted for the most unique variance (6.7%), followed by parenting behavior (5.5%). Neighborhood and sociodemographic characteristics did not predict a significant amount of unique variance in children's print recognition at 3 years.

Results for the hierarchical regression predicting children's receptive vocabulary are presented in Table 4.3. In the first step, neither child

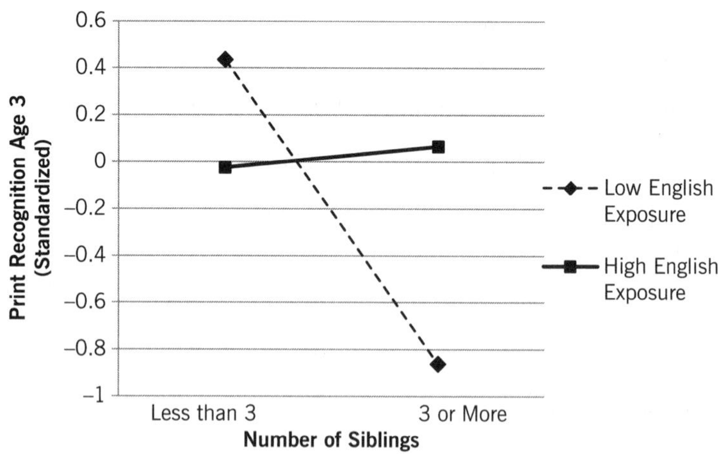

FIGURE 4.1. The effect of sibship size on print recognition is moderated by exposure to English.

TABLE 4.3. Hierarchical Regression Summary for Predictors of Language (Receptive Vocabulary) at Age 3

	Receptive vocabulary	B	SE_B	ΔR^2	R
Step 1	Child age	.096	.096	.060*	
	Child gender	–.202	.170		
	Birthweight	.218*	.087		
Step 2	Maternal education	.111	.096	.264***	
	Partner education	–.064	.090		
	Household income	.377**	.113		
	Three or more children	–.241	.166		
	Low English exposure	–.706***	.184		
Step 3	Child language (18 months)	.203**	.071	.040**	
Step 4	Sensitive responding (18 months)	.229**	.080	.044*	
	Reflective functioning (18 months)	.079	.074		
Step 5	Neighborhood quality	.251**	.080	.043**	
Step 6	Sensitive responding (18 months)* Child language (18 months)	.122*	.060	.018*	
Step 7	Low English exposure* Three or more children	–1.124**	.398	.032**	.707

* $p < .05$; ** $p < .01$; *** $p < .001$.

age nor gender made unique predictions to vocabulary scores, but higher birthweight was associated with significantly higher language ability at 3 years. At step 2, the family sociodemographic variables explained an additional 26% of the variance in child vocabulary at age 3, with household income and low exposure to English each making significant unique contributions. At step 3, child language at 18 months predicted an additional 4% of the variance in age 3 vocabulary, after we controlled for demographics, with higher expressive language at 18 months associated with significantly higher receptive language at 3 years. In step 4, parenting behavior was entered into the model, predicting an additional 4.4% of the variance, or 34% overall. As with print recognition, only maternal responsivity (not reflective functioning) was associated with significantly higher language ability at 3 years. It is notable that when parenting behavior was entered into the equation, the effects of income and exposure to English that were significant in step 2 remained significant, suggesting that the effects of these risks on receptive vocabulary cannot be fully explained by parenting behaviors. In step 5, neighborhood quality was entered and found to be a significant predictor of receptive vocabulary, explaining an additional 4% of the variance (or 38% overall) after we accounted for sociodemographic influences, early child language, and parenting behavior. Children who lived in higher-quality neighborhoods had significantly higher receptive vocabulary scores. In the final step, the hypothesized interactions were entered, revealing a significant interaction between maternal responsivity and early child expressive language on receptive vocabulary at 3 years. Children who displayed both good early language skills *and* received high levels of maternal responsivity at 18 months demonstrated the highest receptive language at 3 years (see Figure 4.2). This interaction explained 2% of the variance in receptive language. The pattern of this interaction was different from our hypothesis, however, which we discuss below. Second, there was a significant interaction between exposure to English and size of the sibship. Children who showed the lowest receptive vocabulary had low exposure to English and lived in large families (see Figure 4.3). Exposure to just one of these risks was not associated with lower vocabulary scores. This interaction explained 3.2% of the variance in children's language. In summary, about 50% of the variance in children's vocabulary scores at age 3 was explained by factors evident between birth and 18 months.

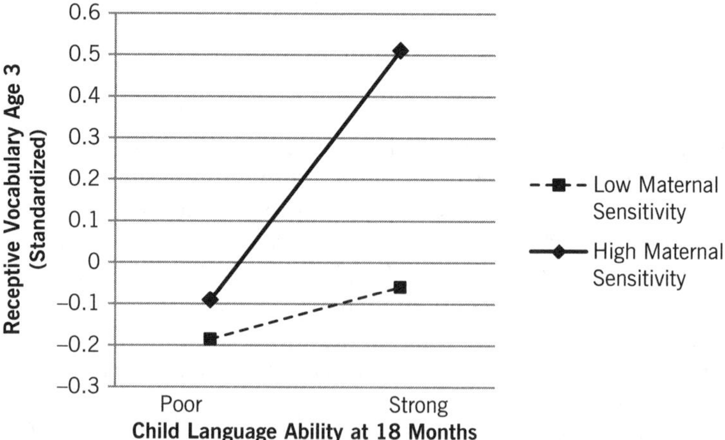

FIGURE 4.2. The effect of early child language on later receptive vocabulary is moderated by maternal sensitivity.

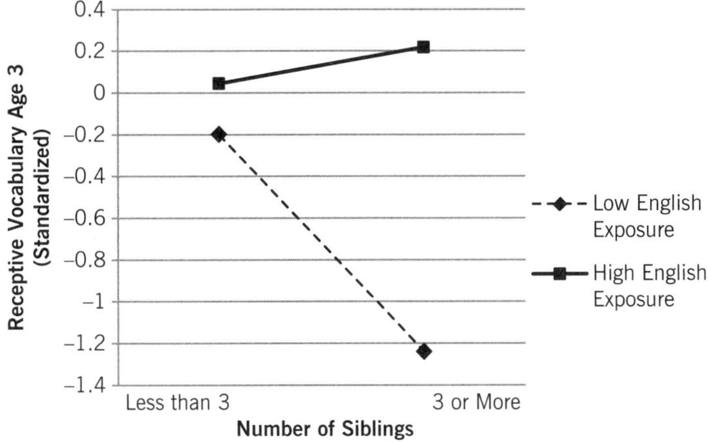

FIGURE 4.3. The effect of sibship size on receptive vocabulary is moderated by exposure to English.

We examined the role of each of our levels, controlling for all other levels. Sociodemographic influences explained the most unique variance (11.8%), followed by parenting factors (4.8%), neighborhood efficacy (4.6%) and child language at 18 months (2.7%).

Discussion

Types of Risk and Contingent Effects

This study provided support for multilevel predictors of children's language and early literacy prior to school entry. With respect to sociodemographic risk, family income and a lack of exposure to English in the household were significant predictors of children's language at 3 years, whereas ethnicity, immigration status, parental education, and size of the sibship were less strongly associated with either language or reading. Within this type of risk, only exposure to English predicted more variance in literacy than family SES. These results suggest that socioeconomically disadvantaged children, and children receiving low levels of English exposure at home, are at risk for poor literacy outcomes, especially in the area of language development. These results are consistent with the noted achievement gap that exists between low- and middle-income children at school entry—a difference that widens over time and predicts later learning difficulties (Ryan, Fauth, & Brooks-Gunn, 2006). Indeed, enriched early learning programs that aim to foster these preacademic skills may prove effective in reducing the purported gap in cognitive school readiness that is associated with socioeconomic disadvantage (Lonigan, Burgess, & Anthony, 2000; Welsh, Nix, Blair, Bierman, & Nelson, 2010).

We also found evidence for the importance of previous adaptation—in the form of children's language at 18 months—on subsequent language and reading at 3 years, over and above the effects of family sociodemographics. Coupled with the finding that educational interventions provided in preschool are more effective at fostering long-term achievement than those administered later in development (Campbell & Ramey, 1995), these results suggest programs that build language skills and offer other supports (Ramey et al., 2000) from a young age may have the benefit of improving children's cognitive school readiness. These findings have been replicated in many projects, including the Infant Health and Development Project, wherein early educational treatment at or prior to 12 months was associated with more advanced cognitive and linguistic competence by 3 years (Gross, Spiker, & Haynes, 1997).

When problematic trajectories become established, there is evidence for continuities over the life course (Hart & Risley, 1995), with many arguing that experience becomes embedded in the biology of the individual (Hertzman & Boyce, 2010). Thus, preventive techniques that address child difficulties before they worsen may be more beneficial than intervention programs once problems are evident. For example, children in early preschool programs that build linguistic competencies are less likely to experience grade retention or placements in special education (Campbell & Ramey, 1995). As the cost of special education is over two times that of regular classroom placements (Ramey & Ramey, 2007), and grade retention imposes school-level economic costs, early programming that targets children at risk of experiencing language difficulties may prove more cost-effective than remedial programs that serve children with problems that have already emerged over time. Indeed, participation in early intervention programs that target cognitive and linguistic skills produce a return-on-investment rate of 7%, factoring in elements such as forecasted participant earnings and maternal monetary gains due to workforce participation (Masse & Barnett, 2002).

Parenting behavior also accounted for a significant portion of the variance in both language and reading at 3 years. However, only maternal responsivity, and not maternal reflective functioning, was associated with these outcomes. In our study, maternal responsivity comprised elements of the mother–child relationship that may be considered important predictors of language and literacy. These included the mother's responsiveness to the child's verbal and nonverbal help-seeking behavior, as well as autonomy promotion and the ability to facilitate activities. Mutuality, on the other hand, measured the interactive style of the dyad, including positive shared attention, affect matching, imitation of verbalizations, and fluid conversation. Positive control comprised the mother's ability to control her child's behavior through praise, explanation, and open-ended questions. That these maternal behaviors were associated with language and reading ability at 3 years is consistent with the notion that specific dimensions of parenting may be particularly important for children's literacy development, such as the mother's responsiveness to her child's vocalizations, vocal imitations, and questions (Tamis-LeMonda et al., 2001). These results support models wherein maternal responsiveness and verbal sensitivity (Baumwell, Tamis-LeMonda, & Bornstein, 1997) promote children's language development. Importantly, the precise elements of parenting that contribute to language and reading cannot be elucidated from this study as our responsivity measure comprised multiple maternal behaviors. However, the finding that maternal reflective functioning was not related to later language or reading suggests that this element of parenting may not be particularly important to children's cognitive school readiness at age 3. Although this cognitive-reflective style seems important in promoting other areas of children's psychosocial health such as attachment security (Kelly et al., 2005), it appears that behaviors specifically related to responsiveness—sensitivity, mutuality, and positive control—represent more pertinent targets for policy efforts geared toward enhancing children's readiness via improvements in parenting behavior.

Evaluations of several randomized control trials reveal promising effects for the impact of parenting interventions on children's health and development (see Olds, Sadler, & Kitzman, 2007, for a review). Communitywide programs that aim to improve parenting have been shown to reduce problems in early development (e.g., Sanders et al., 2008; Jones, Daley, Hutchings, Bywater, & Eames, 2007). Moreover, there is growing evidence for the efficacy of attachment-based interventions that target parental sensitivity (Bakermans-Kranenburg, van IJzendoorn, & Juffer, 2003). These programs may assist parents in becoming more accurate perceivers of their children's signals and/or developing adequate ways of responding to those signals. The finding that parental responsivity is a significant predictor of children's cognitive school readiness points to the parent–child relationship as a potential target for intervention to help alleviate the risks associated with poor reading and language.

In line with past studies, the current study also demonstrated a link between neighborhood efficacy and children's language (Kohen et al., 2002; Leventhal & Brooks-Gunn, 2000). Controlling for family demographic and parenting variables, as well as previous levels of adaptation, we showed that lower social cohesion and social control (i.e., collective efficacy) within neighborhoods was associated with poorer language at 3 years. The concept of collective efficacy is related to the notion of social capital, which reflects the degree of civic engagement and the establishment of social networks and norms that foster community cooperation. From this perspective, neighborhoods higher in collective efficacy may provide more access to peers, nonparental adults, and activities and events within the community (Sampson et al., 1997). A mother who perceives her community as safe and unified may be more motivated to take her child to community sites such as parks, libraries, and recreation centers than a mother who feels the neighborhood is dangerous. This exposure to novel and changing contexts may afford her child enriched opportunities to communicate and interact with other children and adults, in turn facilitating cognitive school readiness. Thus, social programs that aim to increase community cohesiveness through the establishment of recreation centers, parks, and neighborhood events may prove effective in fostering children's healthy development. Results of studies examining change in functioning as a result of neighborhood influences are mixed, with some suggesting improved outcomes when neighborhoods change or when families move out of disadvantaged neighborhoods (Dalgard & Tambs, 1997; Leventhal & Brooks-Gunn, 2004). However, the benefits of these changes to neighborhoods may not be long-lasting (Leventhal, Fauth, & Brooks-Gunn, 2005). Furthermore, because there is some evidence that the effect of neighborhoods on 3-year-olds' school readiness is mediated by learning experiences within the family (Klebanov, Brooks-Gunn, McCarton, & McCormick, 1998) it may be more direct and efficient to target learning experiences within the family through programs situated in high-risk neighborhoods (Welsh et al., 2010).

We also found evidence for contingencies operating across types of risk. The adverse effect of mothers not talking to children in English was attenuated when children lived in small families. Thus, even though opportunities for learning English are lower when mothers speak mainly in their heritage language, when the family is small there are compensatory processes operating. These compensatory processes were seen both for vocabulary and early reading. These might be processes such as maternal word explanations, father or sibling talk to children, and more time engaged with books or other literary materials. For example, parents who are not overcome by the demands of caring for multiple children may have more time to engage in book reading with their child, a process that facilitates both language (Wasik & Bond, 2001) and reading (Bus, van IJzendoorn, & Pellegrini, 1995). It is important to note that when children lived in small families and their mothers spoke in their heritage language, their English vocabulary and reading was at a similar level to that of children whose mothers spoke to them in English. In contrast, the pattern of combined effects of maternal responsivity and child language on later receptive vocabulary was unexpected. Instead of the compensatory effect that was hypothesized (i.e., children low in language would benefit more from maternal responsivity), effects of maternal responsivity on later receptive language were strongest when children also showed relatively high expressive language at 18 months. Thus, we saw children "advantaged" by having both good early language *and* sensitive mothers. These findings on contingent processes in children explained between 2.0 to 4.6% of the variance in vocabulary and early reading outcomes.

Program and Policy Implications

Having identified *where* resources and intervention efforts should be directed to improve children's readiness for school, we are in a position to consider *how* those efforts should be implemented. Generally speaking, intervention efforts can be universal or targeted. *Universal* interventions are directed at the whole population–both those in need and those not in need. *Targeted* programs, on the other hand, are aimed at assisting specific individuals or families. Compared to targeted programs, universal programs have the advantage of not relying on screening tools to determine "need," nonstigmatization, and program maintenance (Offord, Kraemer, Kazdin, Jensen, & Harrington, 1998). However, they have the disadvantage of expense and resource dilution.

One model that combines both universal and targeted program delivery is Triple P (Sanders, Markie-Dadds, & Turner, 2003). This model has been shown to be effective in the treatment of parenting and behavioral problems in children (Sanders et al., 2008), but to our knowledge a staged universal to targeted program has not been evaluated for the promotion of child language and literacy skills. Under this model, intervention is provided along a tiered continuum of increasing intensity and specificity. At the broadest level, the entire population receives services, perhaps in the form of print and electronic media such as tip sheets about parent–child interactions or developmental problems in children, with information about where parents can seek additional support. This kind of program increases in strength across levels, with more targeted services offered to at-risk children/families. For example, the results of our study suggest that children with little English exposure who also live in large families are likely to show language and reading difficulties at age 3. Thus, it may not be efficient to provide services to all children who are not exposed to English, but rather to those experiencing multiple risks (large families and low exposure to English). The overall idea of the Triple P model is to provide the *minimally sufficient level* of support to parents and children to optimize developmental outcomes. The results of our present study suggest that an investigation of contingent processes may help to identify children most at risk.

In accordance with the wealth of literature examining the adverse effects of poor early language on later reading ability (see Scarborough, 2001), our results also support the implementation of early diagnostic and preventative programs that target the development of expressive language skills as early as 18 months (also see Dionne, Mimeau, & Mathieu, Chapter 5, this volume). Hammer, Lawrence, and Miccio (2007) have shown that English and Spanish children involved in Head Start programs showed increased language abilities over a 2-year period, and that language growth was associated with end-of-preschool reading skills. These researchers argue that changing children's language trajectories will have a positive impact on early reading abilities, thus setting into motion a vehicle for later achievement.

The number and types of intervention studies that seek to improve early language skills are widespread. Efforts to support language development via curriculum-based or programmatic interventions with teacher coaching and professional development have been shown to be effective at facilitating language growth (Ashe, Reed, Dickinson, & Wilson, 2009; Assel, Landry, Swank, & Gunnewig, 2007). However, these programs are most relevant for older children who are already attending funded educational programs. On the other hand, small-scale parent book reading interventions (e.g., *diologic reading*), which involve strategies such as questioning, repeated reading, attention to vocabulary, supportive discussion, and feedback, have been shown to yield significant effects on young children's expressive language, with effect sizes as large as $d = 0.59$ (Mol, Bus, & de Jong, 2008). These parent-driven reading approaches offer one means of fostering positive language and reading outcomes in children. Moreover, extending these reading programs to the school system may actually prove more effective than having parents implement them in the home (Lonigan & Whitehurst, 1998; Mol, Bus, & de Jong, 2009).

The challenge of screening and treating young children who may be falsely identified or who undergo a spontaneous remission of language difficulties highlights the importance of also developing communitywide language programs. One such program, Reach Out and Read (ROR), is a clinic-based program wherein pediatricians incorporate literacy development into standard health care routines. During each regular child health checkup from 6 months through 4 years, parents are provided with individualized guidance about reading techniques and are given developmentally sensitive books that are used to facilitate children's language and reading skills. In addition, clinics are equipped with volunteers who read to children in the waiting room in order to scaffold for parents the appropriate way to read to their children (see Needlman, Klass, & Zuckerman, 2006, for an overview). The effectiveness of this program is well-documented. In a cross-sectional, between-clinics comparison, Mendelsohn et al. (2001) showed that children in the ROR intervention group had higher receptive and expressive vocabulary than children in the comparison site after 3 years of exposure to the program. Likewise, using a prospective, quasi-randomized control design, High, LaGasse, Becker, Ahlgren, and Gardner (2000) demonstrated increases in receptive and expressive vocabulary in the intervention group compared to the control group, and this effect was mediated by the amount of parent–child book reading that took place at home. These results provide evidence for the effectiveness of inexpensive, communitywide literacy programs that can be integrated into regular public health services. A more reasonable approach may be a combination of both universal and targeted interventions. For example, children who partake in basic literacy development programs (e.g., ROR) but fail to show age-appropriate growth in language skills can then be referred for more specialized programs, such as phonological training interventions (e.g., Bus & van IJzendoorn, 1999) and syntactic interventions (e.g., Fey, Cleave, Long, & Hughes, 1993), which effectively improve particular aspects of language and reading. This integrated method ensures that children with minor difficulties receive the basic support they need for literacy development, whereas those with pronounced deficits can be targeted for more intensive levels of intervention.

This study has provided evidence for individual, family, and contextual risks that operate both independently and in combination to explain variation in the development of language and literacy in young children. Working within an ecological framework of development, and drawing upon research into the effectiveness of specific prevention and remedial programs, we have outlined programs and program models that have been found to improve the language and literacy outcomes of children. Owing to the complex manner in which various types of risk impact children's school readiness, it is suggested that social policies and programs consider how to incorporate multilevel components into their agenda.

References

Ainsworth, M. (1973) The development of infant–mother attachment. In B. Caldwell & H. Ricciuti (Eds.), *Review of child development research* (Vol. 3, pp. 1–95). Chicago: University of Chicago Press.

Aneshensel, C. S., & Sucoff, C. A. (1996). The neighborhood context of adolescent mental health. *Journal of Health and Social Behavior, 37*, 293–310.

Arriaga, R. I., Fenson, L., Cronan, T., & Pethick, S. J. (1998). Scores on the MacArthur Communicative Development Inventory of children from low and middle-income families. *Applied Psycholinguistics, 19*, 209–223.

Ashe, M. K., Reed, S., Dickinson, D. K., & Wilson, S. J. (2009). Cross-site effectiveness of Opening the World of Learning and site-specific strategies for supporting implementation. *Early Childhood Services, 3*, 179–191.

Assel, M. A., Landry, S. H., Swank, P. R., & Gunnewig, S. (2007). An evaluation of curriculum, setting, and mentoring on the performance of children enrolled in pre-kindergarten. *Reading and Writing, 20*, 463–494.

Bakermans-Kranenburg, M. J., van IJzendoorn, M. H., & Juffer, F. (2003). Less is more: Meta-analyses of sensitivity and attachment interventions in early childhood. *Psychological Bulletin, 129*, 195–215.

Baumwell, L., Tamis-LeMonda, C. S., & Bornstein, M. H. (1997). Maternal verbal sensitivity and child language comprehension. *Infant Behavior and Development, 20*(2), 247–258.

Bierman, K. L., Nix, R. L., Greenberg, M. T., Blair, C., & Domitrovich, C. E. (2008). Executive functions and school readiness intervention: Impact, moderation, and mediation in the head start REDI program. *Development and Psychopathology, 20*, 821–843.

Blake, J. (1981). Family size and the quality of children. *Demography, 18*(4), 421–442.

Bradley, R. H., Corwyn, R. F., Burchinal, M., McAdoo, H. P., & Garcia Coll, C. G. (2001). The home environments of children in the United States: Part II. Relations with behavioral development through age thirteen. *Child Development, 72*, 1868–1886.

Bronfenbrenner, U. (1979). Contexts of child rearing: Problems and prospects. *American Psychologist, 34*, 844–850.

Bus, A. G., & van IJzendoorn, M. H. (1999). Phonological awareness and early reading: A meta-analysis of experimental training studies. *Journal of Educational Psychology, 91*, 403–414.

Bus, A. G., van IJzendoorn, M. H., & Pellegrini, A. D. (1995). Joint book reading makes for success in learning to read: A meta-analysis on intergenerational transmission of literacy. *Review of Educational Research, 65*(1), 1–21.

Campbell, F. A., & Ramey, C. T. (1995). Cognitive and school outcomes for high-risk African-American students at middle adolescence: Positive effects of early intervention. *American Educational Research Journal, 32*, 743–772.

Christian, K., Morrison, F., & Bryant, F. (1998). Predicting kindergarten academic skills: Interactions among child care, maternal education, and family literacy environments. *Early Childhood Research Quarterly, 13*, 501–521.

Conger, R. D., Ge, X., Elder, G. H., Lorenz, F. O., & Simons, R. L. (1994). Economic stress, coercive family process, and developmental problems of adolescents. *Child Development, 65*, 541–561.

Connell, C. M., & Prinz, R. J. (2002). The impact of childcare and parent–child interactions on school readiness and social skills development for low-income African American children. *Journal of School Psychology, 40*, 177–193.

Dale, P. (1991). The validity of a parent report measure of vocabulary and syntax at 24 months. *Journal of Speech and Hearing Research, 34*, 565–571.

Dale, P. S., Bates, E., Reznick, J. S., & Morisset, C. (1989). The validity of a parent report instrument of child language at twenty months. *Journal of Child Language, 16*, 239–249.

Dale, P. S., Price, T. S., Bishop, D. V. M., & Plomin, R. (2003). Outcomes of early language delay: I. Predicting persistent and transient delay at 3 and 4 years. *Journal of Speech, Language, and Hearing Research, 46*, 544–560.

Dalgard, O. S., & Tambs, K. (1997). Urban environment and mental health. A longitudinal study. *British Journal of Psychiatry, 171*(6), 530–536.

Deater-Deckard, K. (2000). Parenting and child behavioral adjustment in early childhood: A quantitative genetic approach to studying family processes and child development. *Child Development, 71*, 468–484.

Deater-Deckard, K., Pylas, M. V., & Petrill, S. A. (1997). *Parent–Child Interaction System (PARCHISY)*. Unpublished manuscript, Institute of Psychiatry, London, UK.

Dodge, K. A., Pettit, G. S., & Bates, J. E. (1994). Socialization mediators of the relation between socioeconomic status and child conduct problems. *Child Development, 65*, 649–665.

Dollaghan, C. A., Campbell, T. F., Paradise, J. L., Feldman, H. M., Janosky, J. E., Pitcairn, D. N., et al. (1999). Maternal education and measures of early speech and language. *Journal of Speech, Language, and Hearing Research, 42*, 1432–1443.

Downey, D. B. (1995). When bigger is not better: Family size, parental resources, and children's educational performance. *American Sociological Review, 60*, 746–761.

Downey, D. B. (2001). Number of siblings and intellectual development: The resource dilution explanation. *American Psychologist, 56*, 497–504.

Duncan, G. J., Dowsett, C. J., Claessens, A., Magnuson, K., Huston, A. C., Klebanov, P., et al. (2007). School readiness and later achievement. *Developmental Psychology, 43*, 1428–1446.

Dunn, J., Slomkowski, C. L., & Beardsall, L. (1994). Sibling relationships from the preschool period through middle childhood and adolescence. *Developmental Psychology, 30*, 315–324.

Elliott, D., Wilson, W. J., Huizinga, D., Sampson, R., Elliott, A., & Rankin, B. (1996). The effects of neighborhood disadvantage on adolescent development. *Journal of Research in Crime and Delinquency, 33*, 389–426.

Fey, M., Cleave, P., Long, S., & Hughes, D. (1993). Two approaches to the facilitation of grammar in children with language impairment–an experimental evaluation. *Journal of Speech and Hearing Research, 36*, 141–157.

Fonagy, P., Steele, M., Steele, H., Moran, G. S., & Higgitt, A. C. (1991). The capacity for understanding mental states: The reflective self in parent and child and its significance for security of attachment. *Infant Mental Health Journal, 12*(3), 201–218.

Fonagy, P., & Target, M. (1997). Attachment and reflective function: Their role in self-organization. *Development and Psychopathology, 9*(4), 679–700.

Frampton, K., Moore, C., Astington, J.W., Perlman, M., & Jenkins, J. M. (2012). *The combined influence of maternal sensitivity and children's joint attention in the development of children's cooperation*. Manuscript submitted for publication.

Gass, K., Jenkins, J., & Dunn, J. (2007). Are sibling relationships protective?: A longitudinal study. *Journal of Child Psychology and Psychiatry and Allied Disciplines, 48*, 167–175.

Gross, R. T., Spiker, D., & Haynes, C. W. (1997). *Helping low birth weight, premature babies: The Infant Health and Development Program*. Stanford, CA: Stanford University Press.

Hammer, C. S., Lawrence, F. R., & Miccio, A. W. (2007). Bilingual children's language abilities and early reading outcomes in head start and kindergarten. *Language, Speech, and Hearing Services in Schools, 38*, 237–248.

Hart, B., & Risley, T. R. (1995). *Meaningful differences in the everyday experience of young American children*. Baltimore: Brookes.

Heilmann, J., Weismer, S. E., Evans, J., & Hollar, C. (2005). Utility of the MacArthur–Bates Communicative Development Inventory in identifying language abilities of late-talking and typically developing toddlers. *American Journal of Speech–Language Pathology, 14*, 40–51.

Hertzman, C., & Boyce, T. (2010). How experience gets under the skin to create gradients in developmental health. *Annual Review of Public Health, 31*, 329–347.

High, P. C., LaGasse, L., Becker, S., Ahlgren, I., & Gardner, A. (2000). Literacy promotion in primary care pediatrics: Can we make a difference? *Pediatrics, 105*, 927–934.

Hill, N. E. (2001). Parenting and academic socialization as they relate to school readiness: The roles of ethnicity and family income. *Journal of Educational Psychology, 93*(4), 686–697.

Hirsh-Pasek, K., & Burchinal, M. (2006). Mother and caregiver sensitivity over time: Predicting language and academic outcomes with variable- and person-centered approaches. *Merrill–Palmer Quarterly, 52*, 449–485.

Hoff, E. (2003). The specificity of environmental influence: Socioeconomic status affects early vocabulary development via maternal speech. *Child Development, 74*, 1368–1378.

Jenkins, J. M. (2008). Psychosocial adversity and resilience. In M. Rutter, D. Bishop, D. Pine, S. Scott, J. Stevenson, E. A. Taylor, & A. Thapar (Eds.), *Rutter's handbook of child and adolescent psychiatry* (pp. 377–391). Oxford, UK: Blackwell.

Jenkins, J. M., Rasbash, J., & O'Connor, T. G. (2003). The role of the shared family context in differential parenting. *Developmental Psychology, 39*, 99–113.

Jones, K., Daley, D., Hutchings, J., Bywater, T., & Eames, C. (2007). Efficacy of The Incredible Years Basic Parent Training Programme as an early intervention for children with conduct problems and ADHD. *Child Care Health and Development, 33*, 749–756.

Kelly, K., Slade, A., & Grienenberger, J. F. (2005). Maternal reflective functioning, mother–infant affective communication, and infant attachment: Exploring the link between mental states and observed caregiving behavior in the intergenerational transmission of attachment. *Attachment and Human Development, 7*(3), 299–311.

Klebanov, P. K., Brooks-Gunn, J., McCarton, C., & McCormick, M. C. (1998). The contribution of neighborhood and family income to developmental test scores over the first three years of life. *Child Development, 69*(5), 1420–1436.

Kohen, D. E., Brooks-Gunn, J., Leventhal, T., & Hertzman, C. (2002). Neighborhood income and physical and social disorder in Canada: Associations with young children's competencies. *Child Development, 73*, 1844–1860.

Kurdek, L. A., & Sinclair, R. J. (2001). Predicting reading and mathematics achievement in fourth-grade children from kindergarten readiness scores. *Journal of Educational Psychology, 93*, 451–455.

Lerner, R. M. (2006). Developmental science, developmental systems, and contemporary theories of human development. In R. M. Lerner & W. Damon (Eds.), *Handbook of child psychology: Vol. 1. Theoretical models of human development* (6th ed., pp. 1–17). New York: Wiley.

Leventhal, T., & Brooks-Gunn, J. (2000). The neighborhoods they live in: The effects of neighborhood residence upon child and adolescent outcomes. *Psychological Bulletin, 126*, 309–337.

Leventhal, T., & Brooks-Gunn, J. (2004). A randomized study of neighborhood effects on low-income children's educational outcomes. *Developmental Psychology, 40*(4), 488–507.

Leventhal, T., Fauth, R., & Brooks-Gunn, J. (2005) Neighborhood poverty and public policy: A 5-year follow-up of children's educational outcomes in the New York City moving to opportunity demonstration. *Developmental Psychology, 41*, 933–952.

Leyendecker, B., Harwood, R. L., Comparini, L., & Yalcinkaya, A. (2005). Socioeconomic status, ethnicity, and parenting. In T. Luster & L. Okagaki (Eds.), *Parenting: An ecological perspective* (2nd ed., pp. 319–341). Mahwah, NJ: Erlbaum.

Lonigan, C. J., Burgess, S. R., & Anthony, J. L. (2000). Development of emergent literacy and early reading skills in preschool children: Evidence from a latent-variable longitudinal study. *Developmental Psychology, 36*(5), 596–613.

Lonigan, C. J., & Whitehurst, G. J. (1998). Relative efficacy of parent and teacher involvement in a shared-reading intervention for preschool children from low-income backgrounds. *Early Childhood Research Quarterly, 13*(2), 263–290.

Luthar, S. S., Cicchetti, D., & Becker, B. (2000). The construct of resilience: A critical evaluation and guidelines for future work. *Child Development, 71*, 543–562.

Masse, L. N., & Barnett, W. S. (2002). A benefit–cost analysis of the Abecedarian early childhood intervention. In *Cost-Effectiveness and Educational Policy* (pp. 157–173). Larchmont, NY: Eye on Education, Inc.

Matias, C., Scott, S., & O'Connor, T. G. (2006). *Coding of Attachment-Related Parenting (CARP)*. Unpublished manuscript, Institute of Psychiatry, King's College, London, UK.

McLoyd, V. C. (1990). The impact of economic hardship on black families and children: Psychological distress, parenting, and socioemotional development. *Child Development, 62*, 311–346.

Mendelsohn, A. L., Mogilner, L. N., Dreyer, B. P., Forman, J. A., Weinstein, S. C., Broderick, M., et al. (2001). The impact of a clinic-based literacy intervention on language development in inner-city preschool children. *Pediatrics, 107,* 130–134.

Mol, S. E., Bus, A. G., & de Jong, M. T. (2009). Interactive book reading in early education: A tool to stimulate print knowledge as well as oral language. *Review of Educational Research, 79,* 979–1007.

Mol, S., Bus, A., de Jong, M., & Smeets, D. (2008). Added value of dialogic parent-child book readings: A meta-analysis. *Early Education And Development, 19,* 7-26.

National Institute of Child and Human Development Early Child Care Research Network (NICHD-ECCRN). (1999). Chronicity of maternal depressive symptoms, maternal sensitivity and child functioning at 36 months. *Developmental Psychology, 35,* 1297–1310.

Needlman, R., Klass, P., & Zuckerman, B. (2006). A pediatric approahc to early literacy. In D.K. Dickinson & S. B. Neuman (Eds.), *Handbook of early literacy research* (Vol. 2, pp. 333–346). New York: Guilford Press.

Offord, D. R., Kraemer, H. C., Kazdin, A. E., Jensen, P. S., & Harrington, R. (1998). Lowering the burden of suffering from child psychiatric disorder: Trade-offs among clinical, targeted, and universal interventions. *Journal of the American Academy of Child and Adolescent Psychiatry, 37,* 686–694.

Olds, D. L., Sadler, L., & Kitzman, H. (2007). Programs for parents of infants and toddlers: Recent evidence from randomized trials. *Journal of Child Psychology and Psychiatry, 48*(34), 355–391.

Pianta, R., & Harbers, K. (1996). Observing mother and child behavior in a problem-solving situation at school entry: Relations with academic achievement. *Journal of School Psychology, 34,* 307–322.

Poe, M. D., Burchinal, M. R., & Roberts, J. E. (2004). Early language and the development of children's reading skills. *Journal of School Psychology, 42*(4), 315–332.

Ramey, C. T., Campbell, F. A., Burchinal, M., Skinner, M. L., Gardner, D. M., & Ramey, S. L. (2000). Persistent effects of early childhood education on high-risk children and their mothers. *Applied Developmental Science, 4*(1), 2–14.

Ramey, C. T., & Ramey, S. L. (2007). Early learning and school readiness: Can early intervention make a difference? *Merrill–Palmer Quarterly, 50,* 471–491.

Rescorla, L. (2002). Language and reading outcomes to age 9 in late-talking toddlers. *Journal of Speech, Language, and Hearing Research, 45*(2), 360–371.

Rescorla, L., & Schwartz, E. (1990). Outcome of toddlers with specific expressive language delay. *Applied Psycholinguistics, 11,* 393–407.

Richards, M., Hardy, R., Kuh, D., & Wadsworth, M. E. J. (2001). Birth weight and cognitive function in the British 1946 birth cohort: Longitudinal population based study. *British Medical Journal, 322*(7280), 199–203.

Rutter, M. (2002). Nature, nurture, and development: From evangelism through science toward policy and practice *Child Development,* 73(1), 1–21.

Rutter, M., Bishop, D., Pine, D., Scott, S., Stevenson, J., Taylor, E., et al. (2008). *Rutter's child and adolescent psychiatry.* Oxford, UK: Blackwell.

Ryan, R. M., Fauth, R. C., & Brooks-Gunn, J. (2006). Childhood poverty: Implications for school readiness and early childhood education. In B. Spodek

& O. Saracho (Eds.), *Handbook of research on the education of young children* (pp. 323–346). Mahwah, NJ: Erlbaum.

Saigal, S., Szatmari, P., Rosenbaum, P., Campbell, D., & King, S. (1991). Cognitive abilities and school performance of extremely low birth weight children and matched term control children at age 8 years: A regional study. *Journal of Pediatrics, 118*(5), 751–760.

Sampson, R., Raudenbush, S., & Earls, F. (1997). Neighborhoods and violent crime: A multilevel study of collective efficacy. *Science, 277,* 918–924.

Sanders, M. R., Markie-Dadds, C., & Turner, K. M. T. (2003). Theoretical, scientific and clinical foundations of the Triple P—Positive Parenting Program: A population approach to the promotion of parenting competence. *Parenting Research and Practice Monograph, 1,* 1–21.

Sanders, M. R., Ralph, A., Sofronoff, K., Gardiner, P., Thompson, R., Dwyer, S., et al. (2008). Every family: A population approach to reducing behavioral and emotional problems in children making the transition to school. *Journal of Primary Prevention, 29,* 197–222.

Scarborough, H. S. (1990). Very early language deficits in dyslexic children. *Child Development, 61,* 1728–1743.

Scarborough, H. (2001). Connecting early language and literacy to later reading (dis)abilities: Evidence, theory, and practice. In S. B. Neuman & D. K. Dickinson (Eds.), *Handbook of early literacy research* (pp. 97–110). New York: Guilford Press.

Silk, J., Sessa, F., Morris, A., Steinberg, L., & Avenevoli, S. (2004). Neighborhood cohesion as a buffer against hostile maternal parenting. *Journal of Family Psychology, 18,* 135–146.

Slade, A. (2005). Parental reflective functioning: An introduction. *Attachment and Human Development, 7*(3), 269–281.

Snow, C. E., Burns, M. S., & Griffin, P. (1998). *Preventing reading difficulties in young children.* Washington, DC: National Academy Press.

Tamis-LeMonda, C. S., Bornstein, M. H., & Baumwell, L. (2001). Maternal responsiveness and children's achievement of language milestones. *Child Development, 72,* 748–748.

Tamis-Lemonda, C. S., Bornstein, M. H., Kahana-Kalman, R., Baumwell, L., & Cyphers, L. (1998). Predicting variation in the timing of language milestones in the second year: An events history approach. *Journal of Child Language, 25,* 675–700.

Thal, D., & Bates, E. (1988). Language and gesture in late talkers. *Journal of Speech and Hearing Research, 31,* 115–123.

Walker, D., Greenwood, C., Hart, B., & Carta, J. (1994). Prediction of school outcomes based on early language production and socioeconomic factors. *Child Development, 65,* 606–621.

Wasik, B. A., & Bond, M. A. (2001). Beyond the pages of a book: Interactive book reading and language development in preschool classrooms. *Journal of Educational Psychology, 93*(2), 243–250.

Welsh, J. A., Nix, R. L., Blair, C., Bierman, K. L., & Nelson, K. E. (2010). The development of cognitive skills and gains in academic school readiness for children from low-income families. *Journal of Educational Psychology, 102*(1), 43–53.

White, K. R. (1982). The relation between socioeconomic status and academic achievement. *Psychological Bulletin, 91*, 461–481.

Whitehurst, G. J. (2003). The NCLD Get Ready to Read!: Screening tool technical report. Retrieved from *www.stage.pearsoned.com/resrpts_for_posting/reading_research_studies/r13*.

Xue, Y., Leventhal, T., Brooks-Gunn, J., & Earls, F. (2005). Neigborhood residence and mental health problems of 5- to 11-year-olds. *Archives of General Psychiatry, 62*, 554–563.

CHAPTER 5

The Role of Oral Language Development in Promoting School Readiness

GINETTE DIONNE, CATHERINE MIMEAU, and EMYLIE MATHIEU

A substantial portion of the research on school readiness and early school achievement has focused on the readiness to read and the early determinants of reading ability. This focus appears justified as learning to read is the first major milestone of primary school, and reading ability is astonishingly stable throughout the school years (Scarborough, 2009), with long-term associations with school achievement (Gabrieli, 2009), educational attainment (Challen, King, Knapp, & McNally, 2008), and individual and social economic success (Organization for Economic Cooperation and Development [OECD], 2010).

Given the crucial role reading plays in the foundation of human capital, a wealth of cross-linguistic data has been gathered on the predictors of reading ability in normal and at-risk populations. Most of this research targets a specific developmental period that spans the late preschool years to the early primary grades, and addresses reading readiness.

Reading readiness can be defined as a time point in development when the *skills* and the *knowledge* a child requires to commence reading instruction are in place. Most agree that early language development provides the foundation for this endeavor (National Institute of Child Health and Human Development [NICHD] Early Child Care Research Network, 2005). However, whereas the readiness for oral language is inborn and develops through natural social interactions, learning to read requires explicit instruction for most children. This instruction taps onto a set of fluid cognitive skills that develop through maturation and experience and onto basic knowledge most children acquire through simple exposure during the preschool years. The *skill* basis of reading readiness refers to processing strategies, such as being able to establish the letter–sound correspondence rapidly and to extract meaning from a succession of decoded words. The *knowledge* basis refers to information stored in memory, such as the conventions of the written code and the meaning of words.

The prerequisites of learning to read have been fairly well established in both typical and atypical development (see Scarborough, 2009, for a review); they have been shown to be the product of both brain maturation and individual cognitive predispositions, and explicit instructions and prior experiences with the written and oral forms of language. Nonetheless, the question of continuities versus discontinuities in the links between early oral language development and reading continue to baffle researchers and educators, as we are just beginning to understand how the developmental story unfolds.

The focus of this chapter is the developmental story of how reading readiness emerges from birth onward, with an emphasis on the putative processes that account for continuities and discontinuities between language development and learning to read. Drawing from two longitudinal epidemiological studies of over 2,000 children followed prospectively from birth in the Québec Longitudinal Study of Child Development (QLSCD), a representative cohort of children born in the province of Québec, Canada in the mid 1990s, and the Québec Newborn Twin Study (QNTS), a population-based cohort of twins born during the same period in the greater Montréal area, we propose a conceptual model that describes the mechanisms linking predictors of reading readiness over time. In particular, we consider what roles early literacy practices in the home and genetic liabilities play in these processes and how empirical results can inform prevention and intervention efforts.

Building a Conceptual Model: The Theoretical Framework

The general consensus among researchers and experts is that oral language development lays the general foundation for learning to read (Catts, Bridges, Little, & Tomblin, 2008; Flax, Realpe-Bonilla, Roesler, Choudhury, & Benasich, 2009; Lervåg, Bråten, & Hulme, 2009; Liu et al., 2010; NICHD Early Child Care Research Network, 2005; Scarborough, 2009; Silvén, Poskiparta, Niemi, & Voeten, 2007). Accordingly, reading can be viewed as one component of language development, with significant continuities and common underlying processes linking the oral and written, as well as the expressive and receptive forms of language (Silvén et al., 2007; St-Pierre, Dalpé, Lefebvre, & Giroux, 2010), and form-specific determinants, such as the motor components of expressive language or the visual–spatial tracking involved in reading. Individual differences in the rate at which this development occurs stem from both genetic predispositions and the degree of exposure to facilitating environments (Harlaar, Hayiou-Thomas, Dale, & Plomin, 2008). Within this theoretical framework, reading is the receptive and written form of language.

Continuities in language development can occur through bootstrapping processes. *Bootstrapping* refers to the use of a mastered skill to build new knowledge. In language development, skills such as the perception of the distinctive sounds of a language (i.e., phonemes), the accumulated vocabulary in one's lexicon, the knowledge and control of the rules governing word combinations and inflections (i.e., syntax and morphology), and the meaning of it all (i.e., semantics) build upon each other from birth onward (MacWhinney, 2010). For example, from birth, the process through which babies' inborn ability to discriminate and segment speech sounds helps them identify words (Kuhl, 1993) can be termed *phonological bootstrapping*. Around their first birthday, children begin using words in a referential manner and once they have the necessary vocabulary, usually around 18 months, they move on to combining words through *lexical bootstrapping* (Bates, Dale, & Thal, 1995). Indeed, as they learn about words, they also learn something about their grammatical properties (e.g., that *throw* is an action and a *ball* is a possible object of that action) that facilitates word order. Then, once word combinations begin, *syntactical bootstrapping* helps children expand their vocabulary with the morphological and grammatical elements needed to accommodate the demands of the adult-like sentences they usually produce by age 4–5 years. This is the time when written language development begins for most children as they are taught about letters, what they represent, and how they make up words, sentences, and books.

According to this view, reading readiness can be explained by bootstrapping processes involving previously mastered language skills and knowledge. Most theorists consider two distinctive sets of skills needed to read efficiently: those required for word decoding and those required for comprehension (Nation, Cocksey, Taylor, & Bishop, 2010). The puzzle of the converging language-general and form-specific skills and knowledge that make reading possible has been best illustrated by Scarborough (2009, p. 24). She describes it as the coming together of multiple strands leading to the increasingly strategic and automatic nature of skillful reading. Each strand represents a specific skill/knowledge essential to decoding or to comprehension. For decoding, these include phonological awareness, that is, the understanding that words are made up of sounds and syllables, letter knowledge, letter–sound (sometimes letter–syllable/idea) correspondences, and visual tracking/sight recognition. Skills/knowledge essential to comprehension include vocabulary, grammar, background knowledge, and verbal reasoning/working memory. The relative mastery of these skills and the brain's capacity to consolidate them into an automatic process determine reading ability. How children get there is the developmental story we want to unearth.

Continuities from Oral Language to Reading

A substantial portion of the research on the predictors of reading has focused on early reading, the period starting with the introduction of formal instruction, usually in first grade, up until the reading process is automatized, that is, when children no longer need to decode individual letters and sounds and can read fluently. This usually occurs within 1 to 3 years after formal instruction begins, but the duration varies across individuals and languages.

In a meta-analysis of kindergarten predictors of reading in the early school grades (Scarborough, 1998), knowledge of *print conventions* and of letters and what they stand for best predicted early word decoding (21 to 33% of the variance). One could argue, however, that print knowledge is itself an early measure of written language. Oral language measures were a close second, explaining from 16 to 24% of word decoding and comprehension in various samples of typically developing children, language-impaired children, and children at risk for dyslexia. Although dyslexia constitutes a major learning disability, empirical evidence suggests it is one extreme of the reading ability continuum (Boscardin, Muthén, Francis, & Baker, 2008; Shaywitz, Escobar, Shaywitz, Fletcher, & Makuch, 1992) with similar predictors to those of typical reading. Phonological awareness has been deemed the best single oral language predictor of reading, explaining on average 22% of the variance of word decoding, more so in phonetically transparent languages in which letter–sound correspondences are more straightforward (Silvén et al., 2007). Yet, surprisingly, taken together, general receptive and expressive oral language indices of vocabulary and grammar predict reading ability as well as phonological awareness (Nation & Snowling, 2004; Roth, Speece, & Cooper, 2002), with expressive vocabulary as the best single predictor among them. Finally, verbal memory, verbal IQ, *rapid naming* (i.e., the ability to rapidly identify sequences of colors, objects, letters, or numbers), and speech production/perception, as well as nonverbal abilities, including performance IQ, are all significant predictors of early reading but predict less than 10% of individual differences.

Typically, proximal measures (i.e., measures that are closer in time) predict more variance in a given outcome. For example, phonological awareness in kindergarten predicts reading in the early school grades better than later in schooling. The prediction of reading from oral language, however, spans well beyond kindergarten measures. As early as age 2 years, expressive and receptive vocabularies (Lyytinen et al., 2004; Silvén et al., 2007) and grammar (Scarborough, 1990) predict up to 9% of individual differences in early reading. By age 3, expressive and receptive language predicts up to 21% of the variance in early reading (Lyytinen et al., 2004; NICHD Early Child Care Research Network, 2005; Scarborough, 1990; Snowling, Gallagher, & Frith, 2003; Walker, Greenwood, Hart, & Carta, 1994). This is well before phonological awareness is consolidated (Dodd & Gillon, 2001), which indicates that the rate of language development in the early preschool years is already indicative of reading readiness.

The Québec-based longitudinal studies replicate these general findings. Briefly, the QLSCD is a demographically and geographically representative cohort of 2,133 singletons recruited from birth records to constitute a sample of families in which there was a birth between October 1997 and July 1998 and assessed annually on a host of developmental indices. The QNTS conducted comparable assessments on a population-based sample of 1,430 twins from all twin births recruited at delivery in the greater Montréal area between November 1995 and July 1998. Both studies assessed preschool language development using state-of-the-art expressive and receptive vocabulary and grammar measures at three time points between ages 18 months and 5 years (30, 42, and 60 months in the QLSCD, and 18, 30, and 60 months in the QNTS). These measures and other study details are described in Dionne, Boivin, Séguin, Pérusse, and Tremblay (2008). In grade 2, children were assessed on reading achievement using the Word Decoding subtest of the Kaufman Assessment Battery for Children (K-ABC; Kaufman & Kaufman, 1983) Word Decoding subtest for 1,459 French- or English-speaking children in the QLSCD, and the computerized Reading Comprehension subtest of the *Test d'Habiletés en Lecture* (Reading Skills Test; THAL; Pépin & Loranger, 1999) for 520 French-speaking twins only in the QNTS.

Figure 5.1 shows the association between average preschool oral language (vocabulary and grammar) between 18 months and 5 years and grade 2 decoding in the QLSCD (left panel) and comprehension in the QNTS (right panel). For ease of illustration, the language scores are expressed in quartiles and the reading scores have been *Z*-standardized with a sample mean of 0, shown as a dashed line, and a standard deviation of 1.

The similarity in slopes across samples is striking: the correlation between language and reading was $r = .43$, $p < .001$ in the QLSCD and $r = .39$, $p < .001$ in the QNTS. Differences between average reading in the

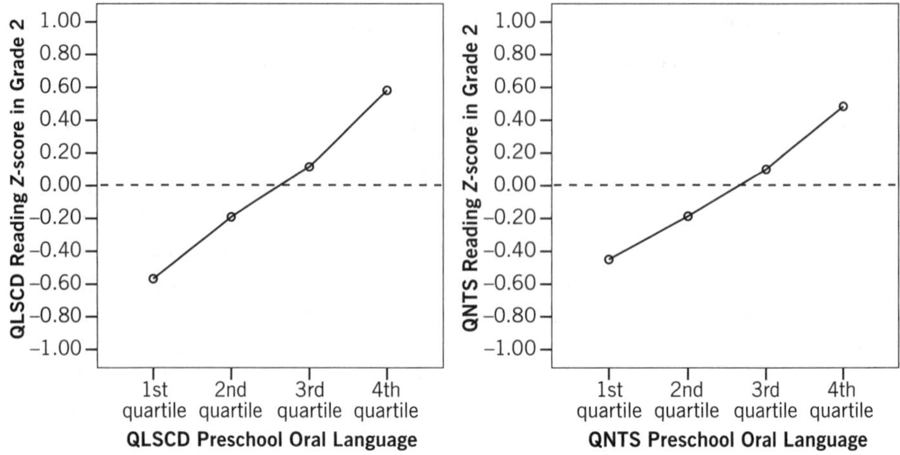

FIGURE 5.1. Associations between quartiles of longitudinal preschool oral language and *Z*-standardized reading score in grade 2 in the QLSCD (left panel) and the QNTS (right panel). The dashed lines indicate sample means.

first and fourth quartiles reached 1.15 *SD* in the QLSCD (standard score $M = -0.57$ vs. $M = 0.58$ for the bottom and top 25%, respectively) and 0.99 *SD* in the QNTS ($M = -0.49$ vs. $M = 0.50$ for the bottom and top 25%, respectively) with different reading measures. This is strikingly similar to what Harlaar and colleagues (2008) observed in their U.K. sample; specifically, using a teacher-assessed qualitative measure of reading, they found a correlation of $r = .40$ between a latent factor of vocabulary and grammar assessed at ages 2, 3, and 4 years, and a latent factor of reading at ages 7, 9, and 10 years. Moreover, the correlations in both the QNTS and QLSCD were not due simply to measures being proximal in time. Expressive vocabulary, as early as 18 months in the QNTS, predicted 7% of the variance in grade 2 reading comprehension, with early talkers (fourth quartile expressive vocabulary) having a 0.59 *SD* advantage over children with no expressive vocabulary at 18 months (first quartile). In the QLSCD, those in the first and fourth quartiles of expressive vocabulary at 30 months differed by 0.93 *SD* in word decoding in grade 2 (for 11% of the variance explained). By 42 months, receptive vocabulary accounted for 13% of the variance in grade 2 decoding.

Therefore, the continuity from preschool oral language to early reading appears early, is strikingly robust across language/reading measures and samples, and can be observed across languages with differing orthographic systems.

THE DEVELOPMENTAL STORY: WHY IS THERE CONTINUITY FROM ORAL LANGUAGE TO READING?

Observing continuity from oral language to reading is only one piece of the puzzle. The more important question is why preschool language, as early as age 18 months, predicts reading more than 6 years later. To answer this question, we draw from two prevalent but not mutually exclusive positions (see Cain, Oakhill, & Lemmon, 2004; Harlaar et al., 2008). Each proposal involves different bootstrapping mechanisms: The first view posits a *direct* contribution of oral language to reading, and the second, a series of *indirect* contributions. Figure 5.2 illustrates the direct and indirect processes that may account for how the developmental story unfolds.

A *direct* contribution of oral language to reading is supported by studies showing that children use their oral language skills in a top-down fashion to understand what they read. In top-down processes, *lexical, semantic,* and *syntactic bootstrapping,* such as using one's vocabulary and knowledge of sentence structure, provide cues to reading comprehension (see Snowling, 2000, for a review).

Indirect pathways lead to the association between early oral language and reading through bottom-up processes, where decoding depends on

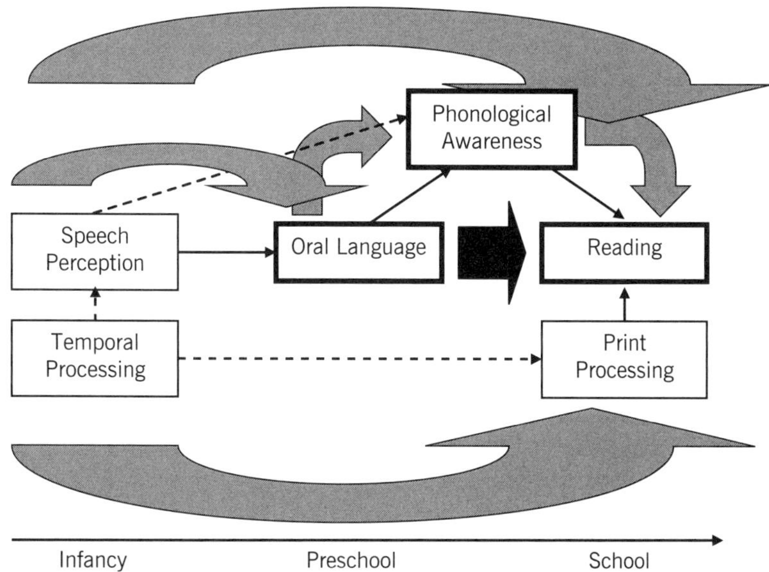

FIGURE 5.2. The developmental model of continuity from oral language to reading through direct and indirect pathways from infancy to the early school years.

phonological bootstrapping (i.e., using the sounds of letters to decode words) and *print processing* (i.e., identifying letters and the orthography of groups of letters; see Walker, Hall, Klein, & Phillips, 2006, for a description of this dual pathway to reading).

In the most documented indirect process, phonological awareness mediates the association between oral language and reading (Silvén et al., 2007; Storch & Whitehurst, 2002). When encoding new vocabulary words, children encode their phonological properties (i.e., the sounds that make up words). As vocabulary increases, children gain an implicit understanding of how the sounds are organized in their language, and this understanding is what facilitates the letter–sound association needed for decoding written words. This is the prevailing view of how oral language and reading are linked, and the reason why reading readiness focuses on developing early language and reading instruction targets letter–sound correspondences as the main decoding strategy.

A second indirect process also involves phonological bootstrapping, but the developmental story starts unfolding much earlier, with speech perception from birth onward. In this process, the rate of oral language development is partly determined by early speech processing capabilities. Presumably, these are the very early phonological processes that serve to fine-tune the phonological awareness skills central to learning to read. Accordingly, oral language and reading may become associated because of the shared influences from early speech processing. Coherent with this developmental story, many studies have shown that early speech processing is crucial to oral language development (Benasich & Tallal, 2002; Kuhl, Conboy, Padden, Nelson, & Pruitt, 2005; Tsao, Liu, & Kuhl, 2004), and at least one Finnish study has shown that speech processing at birth and at 6 months of age predicts both preschool language and reading (Lyytinen et al., 2006).

Other indirect processes that may explain the language–reading association have also been identified as key features of learning to read. These include, but are not restricted to, processing speed and *automatization* (i.e., the fluid and effortless sequencing of the complex cognitive processes involved in reading), the role of verbal memory and procedural learning, as well as low-level perceptual skills involved in the processing of rapidly occurring stimuli, also called *temporal processing*. These low-level skills are thought to play a role in speech perception (Tallal, Miller, Jenkins, & Merzenich, 1997) and have been linked to both early oral language (Choudhury, Leppanen, Leevers, & Benasich, 2007) and reading (Tallal, 2004; Walker et al., 2006; Zhang & McBride-Chang, 2010). Using data from the QNTS, we have recently shown that temporal processing of nonverbal auditory and visual stimuli predicts reading through both a phonological and a possible visual path linked to the processing of print (Malenfant et al., 2012).

Thus, there are many developmental reasons explaining why oral language is central to reading readiness. It not only serves as the foundation for *reading comprehension* (i.e., understanding what one reads), but it also provides the clues to the phonological structure that links spoken and written words in *decoding*. However, from a developmental perspective, oral language may be more important to reading readiness in that it may indicate how efficient the brain has been at speech/signal processing and learning. Because early language milestones are easily monitored, many suggest that they should be used to identify at-risk children who could potentially benefit from reading readiness interventions. However, before we conclude that at-large interventions to promote language development may be the key to prevent reading difficulties, we need to consider discontinuities from oral language to reading.

Discontinuities from Oral Language to Reading

So far, the empirical evidence strongly suggests that children with delays in early oral language skills are more likely to experience difficulties in learning to read, whereas those with good oral language skills should do well. However, this is not always the case. Consider, in Figure 5.3, the scatterplot of reading in grade 2 in the QLSCD as a function of average preschool oral language (expressed as *Z*-standardized scores).

The correlation depicted earlier in Figure 5.1 ($r = .43$, $p < .001$) is still apparent, but we can now see the variations around this correlation. Dividing up the plot into four quadrants, based on having scores above or below the mean reading and oral language, shows that two-thirds of the sample have results consistent with the expected continuity from oral language to reading (i.e., at or above the mean for both reading and oral language or at or below the mean for both). However, one-third of the members of the sample do not read at the level expected for their preschool oral language. Half of these children perform above what could be expected based on their preschool oral language (upper-left quadrant), and half perform below what could be expected (lower-right quadrant). Given that reading is assessed at a single time point and that performing below or above the mean is an arbitrary cutoff for ability–disability, the proportion of children who show discontinuities from oral language to reading may be overestimated. Nonetheless, the main point here is that the continuity model does not seem to apply to some children, and the reasons for this have baffled educators and researchers alike. Discontinuities in the

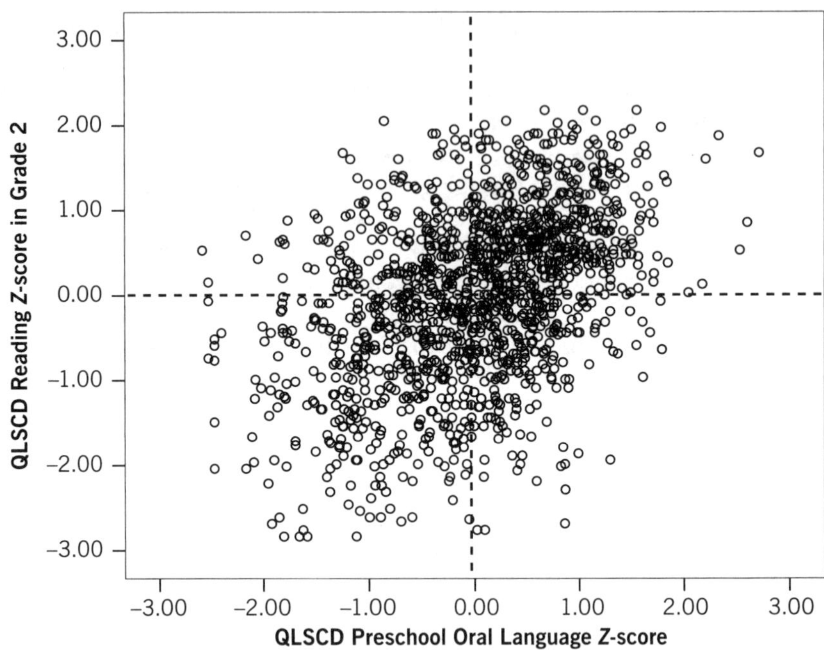

FIGURE 5.3. Scatterplot of QLSCD children's reading as a function of their average preschool oral language expressed in *Z*-standardized scores illustrating discontinuities from oral language to reading. The upper-left quadrant identifies false positives for reading difficulties based on preschool oral language, and the lower-right quadrant identifies false negatives.

longitudinal association between early oral language and later reading suggest that for some children, good oral language skills may not be sufficient for mastering reading and, alternatively, for others, they may not even be necessary.

In the next sections, we explore three possible explanations for the observed discontinuities: (1) the role of other skills in reading readiness; (2) the genetic liability to reading ability–disability; and (3) the role of family literacy in reading readiness.

The Role of Other Reading Readiness Skills/Knowledge

One way to look at the factors underlying discontinuities from oral language to reading is to compare children who have similar preschool oral language but differ in reading outcomes to document other possible reading readiness skills/knowledge that differentiate them. When children were 5 years of age in the QNTS, and 6 years of age (kindergarten) in the QLSCD, letter knowledge was assessed with the Lollipop Test (Chew, 1981), nonverbal IQ was assessed with the Block Design subtest of the Wechsler Preschool and Primary Scale of Intelligence—Revised (WPPSI-R; Wechsler, 1989), and visual memory was assessed with the Visually Cued Recall (VCR) task (Zelazo, Jacques, Burack, & Frye, 2002). Concomitant to reading in grade 2, verbal memory was assessed using the Nonword Repetition subtest of the Neuropsychological Assessment (NEPSY; Korkman, Kirk, & Kemp, 1998), and rapid naming was assessed through the color-naming task of a rapid automatized naming (RAN) test (Denckla & Rudel, 1974). Additionally, in the QNTS, temporal processing was assessed using two temporal order judgment tasks, one an auditory task and the other a bimodal (visual/auditory) task (see Grondin et al., 2007; Malenfant et al., 2012, for a description of tasks), and phonological awareness was assessed with a phoneme deletion task (Cormier, MacDonald, Grandmaison, & Ouellet-Lebel, 1995), again concomitant with reading. All measures were corrected for chronological age and *Z*-standardized.

Dividing up groups along the quadrants in Figure 5.3, we compared the poor and good reading groups of children with poor language (upper-left quadrant, poor language/good reading; lower-left quadrant, poor language and reading) and those with good language (lower-right quadrant, good language/poor reading; upper-right quadrant, good language and reading). Results are summarized in Table 5.1.

In both the QLSCD and the QNTS, children within the same language group, but with poor versus good reading outcomes differed on all reading readiness measures, even after we controlled for small differences in oral language. Children with good reading skills, regardless of their poor oral language skills, had average or above average scores on all measures, with the largest differences compared to their counterparts with poor language and poor reading apparent on letter knowledge (0.61 *SD* difference in the QLSCD and 0.66 *SD* difference in the QNTS) and phonological awareness (0.80 *SD* difference in the QNTS). Phonological awareness also largely differentiated the children with good language skills, with or without poor reading in the QNTS (e.g., 0.91 *SD* difference in the QNTS), as did letter knowledge (0.66 *SD* difference in the QNTS) and temporal processing (0.60 *SD* difference in the QNTS), which may explain why some children with good oral language struggle with learning to read.

For instance, for a small proportion of children, good oral language skills may mask difficulties in other areas (i.e., phonological awareness, letter knowledge, and temporal processing) that may lead to reading difficulties. Conversely, for some children with poor language skills, a good

TABLE 5.1. *t*-Tests Comparing Children with Poor Language Skills, with or without Poor Reading (Top Panel), and Children with Good Language Skills, with or without Poor Reading (Lower Panel)

	QLSCD			QNTS		
	Poor reading			Poor reading		
Measures	No	Yes	*t*	No	Yes	*t*
Children with poor language skills versus low language/reading						
Letters	.13	–.48	6.66***	.18	–.48	5.06***
Rapid naming	.12	–.27	5.34***	.16	–.49	4.66***
Phonological memory	.11	–.47	7.10***	.04	–.47	3.89***
Nonverbal IQ	–.01	–.41	4.63***	.27	–.22	3.64***
Phonological awareness				.29	–.51	5.85***
Temporal processing				.21	–.42	4.59***
Children with good language skills versus high language/reading						
Letters	.37	–.04	5.24***	.45	–.21	5.79***
Rapid naming	.21	–.01	3.56***	.19	–.22	4.05***
Phonological memory	.36	–.07	5.67***	.29	–.07	2.97**
Nonverbal IQ	.30	.07	2.62**	.40	–.18	4.91***
Phonological awareness				.54	–.37	9.02***
Temporal processing				.37	–.23	5.77***

*** $p < .001$; ** $p < .01$.

level on key prereading skills such as letter knowledge and phonological awareness may buffer the negative effects of poor oral skills on learning to read. The discontinuities from oral language to reading therefore highlight the need to consider other skills in addition to oral language in the developmental story of learning to reading.

The results presented here further emphasize the overlapping and cumulative nature of the skills and knowledge basis of reading readiness and explain why a single preschool measure is limited in predicting reading ability. However, Scarborough (2009) argues that from a few reading readiness measures taken together, "the predictability of future reading ability is about as strong from kindergarten onward as it is from grade to grade [around $r = .70$] once formal reading instruction has commenced" (p. 26). In the QLSCD, oral language, letter knowledge, rapid naming, phonological memory, and nonverbal IQ predict over 30% of the variance in grade 2 decoding ($r = .58$). All of the measures except nonverbal IQ make unique contributions to decoding (*p*s < .001) and the strongest unique contribution stems from oral language (beta = 0.28). In the QNTS, the same measures predict 37% of the variance in reading comprehension in grade 2 (r = .61), with unique contributions from all measures (ps < .001) and letter knowledge as the strongest unique predictor (beta = 0.28). When phonological awareness and temporal processing were added to the regression model, the prediction became strikingly similar to the grade-to-grade stability reported by Scarborough (r = .71). The strongest unique contribution stemmed from phonological awareness (beta = 0.35), with reduced contributions from letter knowledge, phonological memory, and rapid naming, and no longer any unique contribution from oral language or nonverbal IQ. This suggests that together, phonological awareness and temporal processing mediate some or all of the contributions of oral language and IQ to reading comprehension.

The Genetic Liability to Reading

Another possible explanation for the observed discontinuity between oral language and reading comes from genetically informative studies: Although early oral language and reading are associated, they have been shown to have very different genetic etiologies. For instance, preschool indices of oral language, particularly vocabulary, have been shown to be highly permeable to the family environment and only slightly heritable (10–20%; Dionne, Dale, Boivin, & Plomin, 2003). By contrast, reading is consistently shown to be one of the most heritable cognitive skills of childhood, with heritability estimates generally around 60–70% (Byrne et al., 2009; Harlaar et al., 2008, 2010; Haworth et al., 2009; Logan et al., 2011; Petrill, Deater-Deckard, Thompson, DeThorne, & Schatschneider, 2006), which means that the cumulative effect of genes explains 60–70% of individual differences over the entire continuum of reading disability–ability.

One way to illustrate the differing genetic etiologies of language and reading is to compare the within-pair similarities across identical and fraternal twins. As identical twins (monozygotic [MZ]) share 100% and fraternal twins (dizygotic [DZ]) share 50% of their genes, the extent to which the MZ similarity exceeds the DZ similarity represents the cumulative effect of genes. Heritability can be grossly estimated by doubling the MZ–DZ correlations differences. Figure 5.4 illustrates the QNTS MZ and DZ correlations for preschool oral language, grade 2 reading comprehension, and the reading readiness skills/knowledge measures just explored.

The large difference in MZ–DZ correlations for reading comprehension replicates previous findings of the high heritability of reading. More importantly, similar differences can be observed for temporal processing, and somewhat for rapid naming, nonverbal IQ, and phonological awareness, which indicates that part of the genetic liability to reading may lie

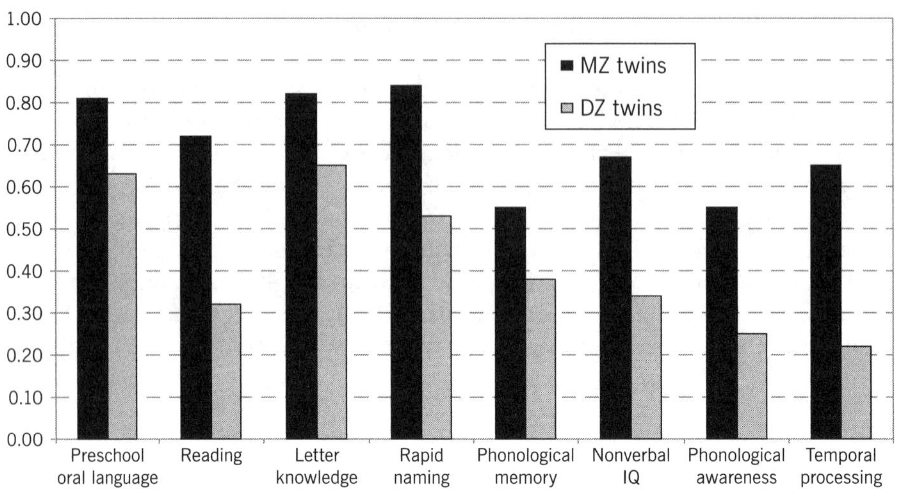

FIGURE 5.4. Within-pair correlations for MZ and DZ twins on preschool oral language, grade 2 reading comprehension, and reading readiness skills/knowledge in the QNTS.

within these reading readiness skills. By contrast, the MZ–DZ correlations differences for oral language, letter knowledge, and, to a lesser extent, phonological memory are small, indicating modest heritability.

Moreover, the overall high within-family correlations for oral language and letter knowledge indicate that experiences shared by children of the same family account for most of the differences on these measures. In other words, if the skills basis of reading readiness appears largely under the influence of one's genetic factors, its knowledge basis rather seems more permeable to environmental influences. This discrepancy indicates that the knowledge basis of reading may be more easily enhanced by familywide interventions and opens one window of opportunity to maximize reading readiness.

The Role of Family Literacy in Reading Readiness

More than 15 years ago, a meta-analysis showed that family- and community-based literacy programs significantly improved emergent literacy and reading (Bus, van IJzendoorn, & Pellegrini, 1995). Part of the contribution of literacy programs came from effects on children's language development, including not only receptive vocabulary (Frijters, Barron, & Brunello, 2000; Sénéchal & Cornell, 1993), expressive vocabulary

(Whitehurst et al., 1994), and oral language (Aram & Levin, 2002; Burgess, Hecht, & Lonigan, 2002), but also effects on print/letter knowledge (Neuman, 1999). By contrast, contributions of literacy programs to phonological awareness were found to be mainly indirect, through their effect on language skills (Sénéchal, 2006). These results are consistent with the genetic–environmental etiology of the reading readiness skill/knowledge measures described earlier: Literacy practices appear to promote the oral language and print knowledge basis of reading readiness.

The effects of literacy programs are usually tested through experimental designs, but the associations with reading can also be assessed in naturally occurring differences in family literacy practices. In the QLSCD and the QNTS, we assessed family literacy practices longitudinally during the preschool years. For illustrative purposes, we report data derived from a single question about literacy assessed at 18, 32, and 42 months in the QLSCD, and at 18, 30, and 48 months in the QNTS. Parents were asked about the frequency with which they read to their child(ren): less than once a month, a few times a month, at least once a week, many times a week, or every day. In both the QLSCD and the QNTS, frequency of parent–child reading from age 18 months onward predicted reading in grade 2 (ps < .001) and was moderately stable (rs = .32–.44 in both samples). Therefore, longitudinal scores were averaged and rounded to the nearest frequency category. The modal longitudinal frequency in both samples was many times/week.

Figure 5.5 shows the associations between early parent–child reading frequency and grade 2 decoding in the QLSCD (left panel), and grade 2 reading comprehension in the QNTS (right panel). In linear regression models, the pooled age 18–42 months (QLSCD) and age 18–48 months (QNTS) parent–child reading frequency predicted 2% of the variance in reading in grade 2 in the QLSCD and 4% in the QNTS, which appears quite modest. However, it amounts to a 0.59 *SD* difference in the QLSCD, and a 0.83 *SD* difference in the QNTS between children who were read to less than once a month and those who were read to every day.

Moreover, as was the case in previous studies, early parent–child reading frequency predicted oral language (8% of the variance in the QLSCD and 9% of the variance in the QNTS) better than it predicted reading. In fact, regression models indicated that preschool oral language completely mediated the association between early parent–child reading frequency and reading in grade 2 in the QLSCD (15% variance explained), and it mediated more than half of this same association in the QNTS. In the QNTS, parent–child reading frequency made a unique contribution to reading comprehension in grade 2 (beta = 0.16, p = .001) even once preschool oral language was taken into account (16% total variance explained). As expected, parent–child reading frequency predicted letter

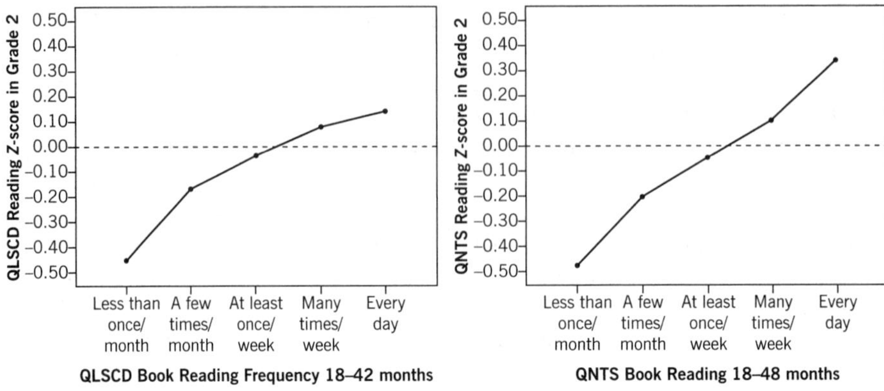

FIGURE 5.5. Associations between parent–child book-reading frequency before age 4 years and reading in grade 2 in the QLSCD (left panel) and the QNTS (right panel). The dashed lines indicate sample means.

knowledge (6% of the variance) better than it did phonological awareness (3% of the variance) or temporal processing (4% of the variance) in the QNTS, both skills that are more heritable.

One problem with data on literacy practices derived from correlations versus experimentation is that associations can be spurious. In this case, the association between early parent–child reading frequency and language/reading outcomes may stem from the fact that more educated parents tend to read more to their children, and as parents and children share their genetic makeup, it could account for the observed associations. However, this is unlikely for several reasons. First, parent–child reading frequency is more strongly associated with oral language, the less heritable component of reading readiness, than with phonological awareness, temporal processing, and reading, which are more heritable. Second, we have shown in a previous study (Forget-Dubois et al., 2009) that the contribution of parents and family socioeconomic characteristics to language development, and to school readiness through language, is an environmental process not mediated by genetic liabilities. Finally, all contributions from parent–child reading frequency to oral language or reading in both the QLSCD and the QNTS remain significant when mothers' education level (no high school diploma, high school or technical diploma, university degree) is taken into account. Thus, the contribution of early parent–child reading frequency to reading level in grade 2 is unlikely to be a simple reflection of shared genetic factors between parents and children.

Parent–child reading frequency assessed with a single question at multiple time points remains a gross measure of family literacy practices. Sénéchal (2006) has shown that different literacy activities can promote different aspects of reading readiness: Reading to a child enhances vocabulary, but it is teaching about literacy and print that predicts letter knowledge. Together, results from previous studies and novel results from our studies presented here are consistent with the hypothesis that family literacy practices have an impact on the knowledge basis of reading readiness, and prepare for learning to read through enhanced language skills and better knowledge of print conventions.

IMPLICATIONS FOR THE PREVENTION OF READING READINESS DELAYS

What the previously reviewed evidence means for children at risk for reading readiness delays and reading difficulties remains unclear. Do they benefit equally from family literacy practices? There is evidence from some studies that children at risk, whether from a socioeconomic standpoint or because of familial antecedents (possibly genetic in nature) of reading or language difficulties, do not benefit as much from at-large family-based literacy interventions (Byrne, Shankweiler, & Hine, 2008; Justice, Skibbe, McGinty, Piasta, & Petrill, 2011). To address this question, we now consider how socioeconomic risk in the QLSCD and genetic risk for reading in the QNTS moderate the contribution of parent–child reading frequency to preschool oral language and grade 2 reading.

In the QLSCD, maternal education was used as a proxy for socioeconomic risk. Figure 5.6 shows the association between parent–child reading frequency and preschool oral language as a function of maternal education separately for children of mothers with no high school diploma, children of mothers with a high school or technical diploma, and children of mothers with a university degree. The corresponding analysis of variance showed that there were main contributions of both maternal education, $F(2, 1{,}915) = 22.75$, $p < .001$, and parent–child reading frequency, $F(4, 1{,}915) = 15.20$, $p < .001$, to preschool oral language in the QLSCD. Although more educated mothers did tend to read more frequently to their children (Spearman's $r = .26$, $p < .001$), regression models tested separately for each maternal education level indicated that frequency of parent–child reading explains barely 2% of the variance in language for children of mothers who did not have a high school diploma, but 4% of the variance for children of mothers with a high school or a technical diploma, and 9% of the variance for children of mothers with a university degree.

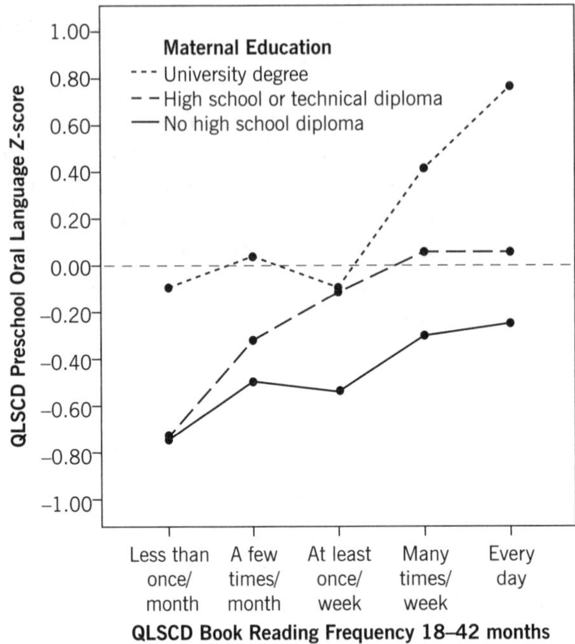

FIGURE 5.6. Association between parent–child reading frequency between 18 and 42 months and preschool oral language in the QLSCD as a function of maternal education level. The dashed line indicates the sample mean.

Clearly, all children gained from being exposed to a higher frequency of parent–child reading. However, the contribution of parent–child reading frequency to children's oral language development does seem to vary as a function of socioeconomic status, as indexed here by maternal education. Children of more educated mothers appear to benefit more from parent–child reading at lesser frequencies. For instance, with a high frequency of parent–child reading, children of mothers with high school or technical diplomas did as well on language as children of more educated mothers who were read to once a week or less. By contrast, children of mothers with no high school diploma had the lowest language scores overall: The average language level of those who were read to every day failed to reach that of children of mothers with a university degree who were read to less than once a week. However, children of mothers with no high school or technical diploma who were read to every day ($N = 44$) had language scores 0.45 *SD* above those who were read to less than once a month ($N = 31$), showing that within this socioeconomic group, a higher frequency of parent–child book reading is associated with a better language outcome.

The gains from parent–child reading frequency are therefore significant, but more modest in children at socioeconomic risk, based on mothers' educational attainment. The main problem, however, is that children at socioeconomic risk were less likely to be read to frequently in this sample: The modal reading frequency of mothers with no high school diploma was less than a few times a month, whereas the modal frequency of the more educated mothers was many times a week (high school or technical diploma) or every day (university degree).

Let us now consider children with a genetic risk for reading difficulties. Do they benefit from a higher frequency of parent–child reading? Genetic risk is not as easily identified as socioeconomic risk. Indeed, some genes have been associated with reading disability, including *DYX1C1* (Taipale et al., 2003), *DCDC2* (Meng et al., 2005), and *KIAA0319* (Paracchini et al., 2008), but they only account for a very small portion of the variance and are not suited for screening. Another way to identify genetic risk is to look at the reading disabilities of close relatives. Many studies on reading readiness have focused on children at familial risk for reading disability based on dyslexic family members (Lyytinen et al., 2001; Puolakanaho et al., 2008; Torppa, Lyytinen, Erskine, Eklund, & Lyytinen, 2010). Similarly, in twin studies, genetic risk can be inferred based on the co-twin and the twins' genetic relatedness (see Jaffee et al., 2005). Using this strategy in the QNTS, we coded genetic risk for reading difficulties based on co-twin's reading being below the mean (high risk) or at or above the mean (low risk).

Figure 5.7 illustrates the association between parent–child reading frequency between 18 and 48 months and reading comprehension in grade 2 in the QNTS as a function of the estimated genetic risk for reading difficulty. The corresponding analysis of variance shows that there were main contributions of both genetic risk, $F(1, 483) = 74.96$, $p < .001$, and parent–child reading frequency, $F(4, 483) = 5.02$, $p = .001$, on reading comprehension in grade 2, as well as a significant interaction between genetic risk and parent–child reading frequency, $F(4, 483) = 5.76$, $p < .001$. Regression analyses conducted separately for each genetic risk category indicate that parent–child reading frequency between 18 and 48 months predicts 5% of the variance in reading comprehension in grade 2 in the low-risk group, but only marginally predicts reading in the high-risk group ($p = .08$). To make matters worse, the high-risk children have less educated mothers (60% of those without a high school diploma) and have been read to less frequently (modal frequency is many times a week for the high-risk group vs. every day for the low-risk group) even when maternal

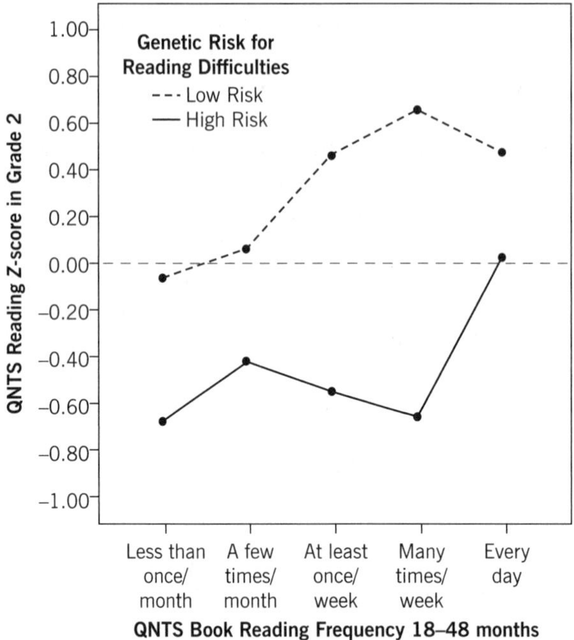

FIGURE 5.7. Association between parent–child reading frequency between 18 and 48 months and reading in grade 2 in the QNTS as a function of the genetic risk for reading difficulties. The dashed line indicates the sample mean.

education is controlled. The genetic risk is thus associated with a higher environmental risk, what is referred to as a gene–environment correlation (GEcor), possibly enhancing the overall risk of reading difficulties. In other words, the bad news is that the genetically at-risk children tended to also be the children who received less environmental stimulation in the form of parent–child reading.

However, the good news is that there were children in the high-genetic-risk group who were exposed to the highest frequency of parent–child reading (i.e., every day). Their reading scores are striking: Reading comprehension in grade 2 was within the mean for these children. Exposure to parent–child reading every day was the only frequency category that showed a gain in reading for the children at genetic risk for reading difficulties. This gain remained significant even after we controlled for maternal education, the severity of the co-twin reading difficulty (M = –0.79), and multiple tests ($p < .05/4$). This suggests that children at genetic (co-twin reading difficulties) and environmental risk (low maternal education) for reading difficulties can achieve average reading levels under intensive environmental stimulation. A parent-report measure of reading frequency is a gross measure of environmental stimulation but it may be that significant gains are *only* achieved with very intensive stimulation for children genetically at risk of reading difficulties. This stimulation can be implemented not only in the family but also in community-based programs and even in a clinical setting when risk is detected early.

Closing the gap on reading achievement between at-risk children and their more advantaged peers is an ongoing challenge. Along with more targeted interventions, namely, to develop phonological awareness in preschool settings, family-based literacy practices may play a significant role toward reaching that goal with the proper intensity level. Indeed, they can translate into significant gains even from something as informal as being read to every day from an early age. In a sample of 41 2-year-olds, DeBaryshe (1993) observed that age of onset of parent–child reading was a better predictor of gains in oral language than reading frequency. Given the wealth of information on the benefits of early literacy, even for genetically and socially at-risk children, one challenge for policymakers to tackle is how to foster literacy stimulation in the home, especially in households where parents may not believe it can have a significant impact on their child's outcome.

Mothers of children at high genetic risk for reading difficulties in the QNTS and mothers without a high school diploma in the QLSCD reported significantly lower perceived parental impact (i.e., a measure of how much parents believe they can affect their child's general development by their actions; see Boivin et al., 2005, for a description of this measure) than other mothers when their infants were 5 and 18 months of age ($ps < .001$). This result points to attitudes and beliefs that may limit educational opportunities in the home and call for creative ways to bring less educated parents to reconsider the value of their contributions. Additionally, given the challenges of promoting family literacy in disadvantaged geographical areas and the overwhelming demands social disadvantage already creates for families, community-based services meant to close the gap created by social and biological risk should be fostered. Among these, quality formal child care services are one venue that has been shown to have a normalizing effect on disadvantaged children's early language milestones (Geoffroy et al., 2007).

CONCLUSION

For most children, the developmental story from early language skills to reading is straightforward and promoting early language development is likely to have benefits down the line when they learn to read. For a smaller proportion of children, the developmental story is more complex: Genetic and environmental liabilities in particular call for creative, tailored, and evidence-based intervention strategies.

In this chapter, we have focused on the central role of early language skills in the emergence of reading readiness by looking at the putative processes that account for continuities and discontinuities in the language–reading association. On the one hand, we have exposed how reading, as the receptive and written form of language, relies on previously mastered oral language skills through bootstrapping processes and have illustrated a developmental model depicting the direct and indirect pathways linking early oral language development to later reading. We also have shown that the consistent finding of continuity between early oral language and reading can be replicated in our samples comprising over 2,000 children followed prospectively.

On the other hand, we also have illustrated discontinuities between oral language and reading in these samples and explored possible explanations for them. First, we showed that other reading readiness skills, including phonological awareness, letter knowledge, rapid naming, phonological memory, temporal processing, and nonverbal IQ are also part of the developmental story. They can buffer the effect of poor language skills on learning to read or, by contrast, lead to poor reading skills in some children with otherwise good language skills. Second, we showed that there is a strong underlying genetic predisposition to reading and other reading readiness skills such as temporal processing and phonological awareness, whereas oral language and letter knowledge appear to be shaped by environmental experiences, namely, those shared by children of the same family. The differing genetic etiology of oral language and reading therefore partly explains why early oral language alone may not be the best indicator of future reading ability in some children. Finally, we showed that even a gross measure of family literacy practices, namely, early parent–child reading frequency, is associated with meaningful differences in reading ability by grade 2. Along with results from intervention studies, these results imply that the knowledge basis of reading readiness, including oral language skills and print knowledge, can be enhanced through early stimulation. Therefore, evidence-based and creative interventions can modify how the developmental story unfolds.

We conclude this chapter with an empirical note of caution regarding the possible contribution of such interventions. We showed that gains, in language skills or reading, from family-based literacy practices were more modest in children at genetic or socioeconomic risk. However, we found that genetically at-risk children for reading difficulties who were read to every day in early childhood had reading comprehension scores within the mean in grade 2. Part of the problem appears to be that the vulnerable children tend to be exposed to lesser levels of literacy stimulation and have parents who seem unaware of the benefits their child could gain from it. Enhancing reading readiness stimulation in the home and the community, as well as informing parents of more at-risk children of the value of their educational input, is luckily something that can be tackled through targeted intervention strategies. The challenge resides in how to inform and support the parents and communities of the more vulnerable children in their efforts to promote reading readiness. With all we have learned about promoting the readiness to read, the central role of early language skills and how early the developmental story unfolds, parents, educators, and communities should be urged to maximize early literacy exposure.

References

Aram, D., & Levin, I. (2002). Mother–child joint writing and storybook reading: Relations with literacy among low SES kindergartners. *Merrill–Palmer Quarterly, 48*, 202–224.

Bates, E., Dale, P. S., & Thal, D. (1995). Individual differences and their implications for theories of language development. In P. Fletcher & B. MacWhinney (Eds.), *Handbook of child language* (pp. 96–151). Oxford, UK: Blackwell.

Benasich, A. A., & Tallal, P. (2002). Infant discrimination of rapid auditory cues predicts later language impairment. *Behavioural Brain Research, 136*, 31–49.

Boivin, M., Pérusse, D., Dionne, G., Saysset, V., Zoccolillo, M., Tarabulsy, G. M., et al. (2005). The genetic–environmental etiology of parents' perceptions and self-assessed behaviours toward their 5-month-old infants in a large twin and singleton sample. *Journal of Child Psychology and Psychiatry, 46*, 612–630.

Boscardin, C. K., Muthén, B., Francis, D. J., & Baker, E. L. (2008). Early identification of reading difficulties using heterogeneous developmental trajectories. *Journal of Educational Psychology, 100*, 192–208.

Burgess, S., Hecht, S., & Lonigan, C. (2002). Relations of the home literacy environment (HLE) to the development of reading-related abilities: A one-year longitudinal study. *Reading Research Quarterly, 37*, 408–426.

Bus, A., van IJzendoorn, M., & Pellegrini, A. (1995). Joint book reading makes for success in learning to read: A meta-analysis on intergenerational transmission of literacy. *Review of Educational Research, 65*, 1–21.

Byrne, B., Coventry, W. L., Olson, R. K., Samuelsson, S., Corley, R., Willcutt, E. G., et al. (2009). Genetic and environmental influences on aspects of literacy and language in early childhood: Continuity and change from preschool to Grade 2. *Journal of Neurolinguistics, 22*, 219–236.

Byrne, B., Shankweiler, D. P., & Hine, D. W. (2008). Reading development in children at risk of dyslexia. In M. Mody & E. R. Silliman (Eds.), *Brain, behavior, and learning in language and reading disorders* (pp. 240–270). New York: Guilford Press.

Cain, K., Oakhill, J., & Lemmon, K. (2004). Individual differences in the inference of word meanings from context: The influence of reading comprehension, vocabulary knowledge, and memory capacity. *Journal of Educational Psychology, 96,* 671–681.

Catts, H. W., Bridges, M. S., Little, T. D., & Tomblin, J. B. (2008). Reading achievement growth in children with language impairments. *Journal of Speech, Language, and Hearing Research, 51,* 1569–1579.

Challen, A., King, D., Knapp, M., & McNally, S. (2008). *Foresight Mental Capital and Wellbeing Project: The economic consequences of specific learning difficulties and the cost-effectiveness of prevention strategies.* London: Government Office for Science.

Chew, A. L. (1981). *The Lollipop Test: A diagnostic screening test of school readiness.* Atlanta, GA: Humanics.

Choudhury, N., Leppanen, P. H. T., Leevers, H. J., & Benasich, A. A. (2007). Infant information processing and family history of specific language impairment: Converging evidence for RAP deficits from two paradigms. *Developmental Science, 10,* 213–236.

Cormier, P., MacDonald, G. W., Grandmaison, É., & Ouellette-Lebel, D. (1995). Développement d'un test d'analyse auditive en français: Normes et validation de construit [Development of an auditory analysis test in French: Norms and construct validation]. *Revue des Sciences de l'Éducation, 21,* 223–240.

DeBaryshe, B. D. (1993). Joint picture-book reading correlates with early oral language skill. *Journal of Child Language, 20,* 455–461.

Denckla, M. B., & Rudel, R. (1974). Rapid "automatized" naming of pictured objects, colors, letters and numbers by normal children. *Cortex, 10,* 186–202.

Dionne, G., Boivin, M., Séguin, J. R., Pérusse, D., & Tremblay, R. E. (2008). Gestational diabetes hinders language development in offspring. *Pediatrics, 122,* e1073–e1079.

Dionne, G., Dale, P. S., Boivin, M., & Plomin, R. (2003). Genetic evidence for bidirectional effects of early lexical and grammatical development. *Child Development, 74,* 394–412.

Dodd, B., & Gillon, G. (2001). Exploring the relationship between phonological awareness, speech impairment, and literacy. *Advances in Speech–Language Pathology, 3,* 139–147.

Flax, J. F., Realpe-Bonilla, T., Roesler, C., Choudhury, N., & Benasich, A. (2009). Using early standardized language measures to predict later language and early reading outcomes in children at high risk for language-learning impairments. *Journal of Learning Disabilities, 42,* 61–75.

Forget-Dubois, N., Dionne, G., Lemelin, J.-P., Pérusse, D., Tremblay, R. E., & Boivin, M. (2009). Early child language mediates the relation between home environment and school readiness. *Child Development, 80,* 736–749.

Frijters, J. C., Barron, R. W., & Brunello, M. (2000). Direct and mediated influences of home literacy and literacy interest on prereaders' oral vocabulary and early written language skill. *Journal of Educational Psychology, 92,* 466–477.

Gabrieli, J. D. E. (2009). Dyslexia: A new synergy between education and cognitive neuroscience. *Science, 325,* 280–283.

Geoffroy, M.-C., Côté, S. M., Borge, A. I. H., Larouche, F., Séguin, J. R., & Rutter, M. (2007). Association between nonmaternal care in the first year of life and children's receptive language skills prior to school entry: The moderating role of socioeconomic status. *Journal of Child Psychology and Psychiatry, 48,* 490–497.

Grondin, S., Dionne, G., Malenfant, N., Plourde, M., Cloutier, M., & Jean, C. (2007). Temporal processing skills of children with and without specific language impairment. *Canadian Journal of Speech–Language Pathology and Audiology, 31,* 38–46.

Harlaar, N., Cutting, L., Deater-Deckard, K., DeThorne, L. S., Justice, L. M., Schatschneider, C., et al. (2010). Predicting individual differences in reading comprehension: A twin study. *Annals of Dyslexia, 60,* 265–288.

Harlaar, N., Hayiou-Thomas, M. E., Dale, P. S., & Plomin, R. (2008). Why do preschool language abilities correlate with later reading? A twin study. *Journal of Speech, Language, and Hearing Research, 51,* 688–705.

Haworth, C. M. A., Kovas, Y., Harlaar, N., Hayiou-Thomas, M. E., Petrill, S. A., Dale, P. S., et al. (2009). Generalist genes and learning disabilities: A multivariate genetic analysis of low performance in reading, mathematics, language and general cognitive ability in a sample of 8,000 12-year-old twins. *Journal of Child Psychology and Psychiatry, 50,* 1318–1325.

Jaffee, S. R., Caspi, A., Moffitt, T. E., Dodge, K. A., Rutter, M., Taylor, A., et al. (2005). Nature × nurture: Genetic vulnerabilities interact with physical maltreatment to promote conduct problems. *Development and Psychopathology, 17,* 67–84.

Justice, L. M., Skibbe, L. E., McGinty, A. S., Piasta, S. B., & Petrill, S. (2011). Feasibility, efficacy, and social validity of home-based storybook reading intervention for children with language impairment. *Journal of Speech, Language, and Hearing Research, 54,* 523–538.

Kaufman, A. S., & Kaufman, N. L. (1983). *Kaufman Assessment Battery for Children.* Circle Pines, MN: American Guidance Service.

Korkman, M., Kirk, U., & Kemp, S. I. (1998). *NEPSY: A developmental neuropsychological assessment.* San Antonio, TX: Psychological Corporation.

Kuhl, P. K. (1993). Developmental speech perception: Implications for models of language impairment. *Annals of the New York Academy of Sciences, 682,* 248–263.

Kuhl, P. K., Conboy, B. T., Padden, D., Nelson, T., & Pruitt, J. (2005). Early speech perception and later language development: Implications for the "critical period." *Language Learning and Development, 1,* 237–264.

Lervåg, A., Bråten, I., & Hulme, C. (2009). The cognitive and linguistic foundations of early reading development: A Norwegian latent variable longitudinal study. *Developmental Psychology, 45,* 764–781.

Liu, P. D., McBride-Chang, C., Wong, A. M.-Y., Tardif, T., Stokes, S. F., Fletcher, P., et al. (2010). Early oral language markers of poor reading performance in Hong Kong Chinese children. *Journal of Learning Disabilities, 43,* 322–331.

Logan, J., Petrill, S. A., Flax, J., Justice, L. M., Hou, L., Bassett, A. S., et al. (2011). Genetic covariation underlying reading, language and related measures in a sample selected for specific language impairment. *Behavior Genetics, 41,* 651–659.

Lyytinen, H., Ahonen, T., Eklund, K., Guttorm, T., Laakso, M.-L., Leinonen, S., et al. (2001). Developmental pathways of children with and without familial risk for dyslexia during the first years of life. *Developmental Neuropsychology, 20,* 535–554.

Lyytinen, H., Aro, M., Eklund, K., Erskinel, J., Guttorm, T., Laakso, M.-L., et al. (2004). The development of children at familial risk for dyslexia: Birth to early school age. *Annals of Dyslexia, 54,* 184–220.

Lyytinen, H., Erskine, J., Tolvanen, A., Torppa, M., Poikkeus, A.-M., & Lyytinen, P. (2006). Trajectories of reading development: A follow-up from birth to school age of children with and without risk for dyslexia. *Merrill–Palmer Quarterly, 52,* 514–546.

MacWhinney, B. (2010). A tail of two paradigms. In M. Kail & M. Hickmann (Eds.), *Language acquisition across linguistic and cognitive systems* (pp. 17–32). Amsterdam, Netherlands: Benjamins.

Malenfant, N., Grondin, S., Boivin, M., Forget-Dubois, N., Robaey, P., & Dionne, G. (2012). Contribution of temporal processing skills to reading comprehension in 8-year-olds: Evidence for a mediation effect of phonological awareness. *Child Development, 83,* 1332–1346.

Meng, H., Smith, S. D., Hager, K., Held, M., Liu, J., Olson, R. K., et al. (2005). DCDC2 is associated with reading disability and modulates neuronal development in the brain. *Proceedings of the National Academy of Sciences, 102,* 17053–17058.

Nation, K., Cocksey, J., Taylor, J. S. H., & Bishop, D. V. M. (2010). A longitudinal investigation of early reading and language skills in children with poor reading comprehension. *Journal of Child Psychology and Psychiatry, 51,* 1031–1039.

Nation, K., & Snowling, M. J. (2004). Beyond phonological skills: Broader language skills contribute to the development of reading. *Journal of Research in Reading, 27,* 342–356.

National Institute of Child Health and Human Development [NICHD] Early Child Care Research Network. (2005). Early child care and children's development in the primary grades: Follow-up results from the NICHD Study of Early Child Care. *American Educational Research Journal, 42,* 537–570.

Neuman, S. (1999). Books make a difference: A study of access to literacy. *Reading Research Quarterly, 34,* 286–311.

Organization for Economic Cooperation and Development. (2010). *The high cost of low educational performance: The long-run economic impact of improving educational outcomes.* Paris: Author.

Paracchini, S., Steer, C. D., Buckingham, L.-L., Morris, A. P., Ring, S., Scerri, T., et al. (2008). Association of the KIAA0319 dyslexia susceptibility gene with reading skills in the general population. *American Journal of Psychiatry, 165,* 1576–1584.

Pépin, M., & Loranger, M. (1999). Test d'Habiletés en Lecture [Reading Skills Test; Computer software]. Québec City, Canada: Réseau Psychotech.

Petrill, S. A., Deater-Deckard, K., Thompson, L., DeThorne, L. S., &

Schatschneider, C. (2006). Reading skills in early readers: Genetic and shared environmental influences. *Journal of Learning Disabilities, 39*, 48–55.

Puolakanaho, A., Ahonen, T., Aro, M., Eklund, K., Leppänen, P. H. T., Poikkeus, A.-M., et al. (2008). Developmental links of very early phonological and language skills to second grade reading outcomes: Strong to accuracy but only minor to fluency. *Journal of Learning Disabilities, 41*, 353–370.

Roth, F. P., Speece, D. L., & Cooper, D. H. (2002). A longitudinal analysis of the connection between oral language and early reading. *Journal of Educational Research, 95*, 259–272.

Scarborough, H. S. (1990). Very early language deficits in dyslexic children. *Child Development, 61*, 1728–1743.

Scarborough, H. S. (1998). Early identification of children at risk for reading disabilities: Phonological awareness and some other promising predictors. In B. K. Shapiro, P. J. Accardo, & A. J. Capute (Eds.), *Specific reading disability: A view of the spectrum* (pp. 75–119). Timonium, MD: York Press.

Scarborough, H. S. (2009). Connecting early language and literacy to later reading (dis)abilities: Evidence, theory, and practice. In F. Fletcher-Campbell, J. Soler, & G. Reid (Eds.), *Approaching difficulties in literacy development: Assessment, pedagogy and programmes* (pp. 23–38). London: Sage.

Sénéchal, M. (2006). Testing the home literacy model: Parent involvement in kindergarten is differentially related to Grade 4 reading comprehension, fluency, spelling, and reading for pleasure. *Scientific Studies of Reading, 10*, 59–87.

Sénéchal, M., & Cornell, E. (1993). Vocabulary acquisition through shared reading experiences. *Reading Research Quarterly, 28*, 360–374.

Shaywitz, S. E., Escobar, M. D., Shaywitz, B. A., Fletcher, J. M., & Makuch, R. (1992). Evidence that dyslexia may represent the lower tail of a normal distribution of reading ability. *New England Journal of Medicine, 326*, 145–150.

Silvén, M., Poskiparta, E., Niemi, P., & Voeten, M. (2007). Precursors of reading skill from infancy to first grade in Finnish: Continuity and change in a highly inflected language. *Journal of Educational Psychology, 99*, 516–531.

Snowling, M. J. (2000). Language and literacy skills: Who is at risk and why? In D. M. Bishop & L. B. Leonard (Eds.), *Speech and language impairments in children* (pp. 245–259). Philadelphia, PA: Psychology Press.

Snowling, M. J., Gallagher, A., & Frith, U. (2003). Family risk of dyslexia is continuous: Individual differences in the precursors of reading skill. *Child Development, 74*, 358–373.

St-Pierre, M.-C., Dalpé, V., Lefebvre, P., & Giroux, C. (2010). *Difficultés de lecture et d'écriture: Prévention et évaluation orthophonique auprès des jeunes* [Difficulties in reading and writing: Prevention and speech therapy evaluation among youth]. Québec City, Canada: Presses de l'Université du Québec.

Storch, S. A., & Whitehurst, G. J. (2002). Oral language and code-related precursors to reading: Evidence from a longitudinal structural model. *Developmental Psychology, 38*, 934–947.

Taipale, M., Kaminen, N., Nopola-Hemmi, J., Haltia, T., Myllyluoma, B., Lyytinen, H., et al. (2003). A candidate gene for developmental dyslexia encodes a nuclear tetratricopeptide repeat domain protein dynamically regulated in brain. *Proceedings of the National Academy of Sciences, 100,* 11553–11558.

Tallal, P. (2004). Improving language and literacy is a matter of time. *Nature Reviews Neuroscience, 5,* 721–728.

Tallal, P., Miller, S., Jenkins, B., & Merzenich, M. (1997). The role of temporal processing in developmental language-based learning disorders: Research and clinical implications. In B. Blackman (Ed.), *Foundations of reading acquisition* (pp. 49–66). Mahwah, NJ: Erlbaum.

Torppa, M., Lyytinen, P., Erskine, J., Eklund, K., & Lyytinen, H. (2010). Language development, literacy skills, and predictive connections to reading in Finnish children with and without familial risk for dyslexia. *Journal of Learning Disabilities, 43,* 308–321.

Tsao, F.-M., Liu, H.-M., & Kuhl, P. K. (2004). Speech perception in infancy predicts language development in the second year of life: A longitudinal study. *Child Development, 75,* 1067–1084.

Walker, D., Greenwood, C., Hart, B., & Carta, J. (1994). Prediction of school outcomes based on early language production and socioeconomic factors. *Child Development, 65,* 606–621.

Walker, K. M. M., Hall, S. E., Klein, R. M., & Phillips, D. P. (2006). Development of perceptual correlates of reading performance. *Brain Research, 1124,* 126–141.

Wechsler, D. (1989). *Wechsler Preschool and Primary Scale of Intelligence* (Rev. ed.). San Antonio, TX: Psychological Corporation.

Whitehurst, G., Arnold, D., Epstein, J., Angell, A., Smith, M., & Fischel, J. (1994). A picture book reading intervention in day care and home for children from low-income families. *Developmental Psychology, 30,* 679–689.

Zelazo, P. D., Jacques, S., Burack, J. A., & Frye, D. (2002). The relation between theory of mind and rule use: Evidence from persons with autism-spectrum disorders. *Infant and Child Development, 11,* 171–195.

Zhang, J., & McBride-Chang, C. (2010). Auditory sensitivity, speech perception, and reading development and impairment. *Educational Psychology Review, 22,* 323–338.

CHAPTER 6

Early Child Care Experiences and School Readiness

SYLVANA M. CÔTÉ, MARIE-CLAUDE GEOFFROY, and JEAN-BAPTISTE PINGAULT

Cognitive abilities and school success in early childhood predict subsequent health status and psychological well-being (Hertzman & Boyce, 2010; Koenen et al., 2009). Many countries have increased public investments in early child care services with the intention of providing all children with equal opportunities for school success. Such initiatives are based on the assumption that early educational child care services can promote cognitive growth and subsequent academic success for all children (High & the Committee on Early Childhood, 2008). It has also been argued that the provision of educational child care is particularly beneficial for disadvantaged children, because they may not receive adequate educational experiences in their home (Caughy, DiPietro, & Strobino, 1994; Côté, Doyle, Petitclerc, & Timmins, 2013).

There is experimental evidence that high-quality educational interventions in child care (or preschool settings) promote school readiness. Programs such as the Abecedarian or the Chicago Child–Parent Centers were shown to be effective in preparing children for better academic achievement and subsequent educational attainment (Anderson et al., 2003; Reynolds & Temple, 2008). It is not clear, however, whether child care services widely disseminated to the community with variable degrees of quality have effects that compare to those of educational interventions in child care or preschool settings designed to be of the highest quality. Furthermore, longitudinal studies also suggest that, under some conditions (e.g., type of care, intensity of care; type of sample), child care may have a negative impact on children's cognitive development. Thus, child care has tremendous potential for reducing social inequalities, but the conditions under which it may have positive and negative impacts need to be well understood in order to attain positive outcomes and avoid iatrogenic effects.

In this chapter, we review the empirical evidence regarding the associations between child care available to the community and children's cognitive development. We distinguish between two bodies of literature. The first is population-based studies investigating the associations between different features of child care use and children's cognitive development. Such studies typically rely on large population samples and compare children and families who used different type of child care settings (e.g., center care vs. family care), at various intensities (e.g., number of hours per week, number of years over the preschool years), initiated at different ages (e.g., infancy/toddlerhood). The second body of literature groups studies that are typically smaller and investigate the associations between the quality of child care and cognitive development. Such studies typically rely on smaller samples and compare children who receive care that varies in quality as assessed via extensive observations of the child care settings, including the quality of the physical environment, the material, and the interactions between children and caregivers/educators.

Defining Concepts: Child Care and School Readiness

We use *child care services* as a generic term for various forms of nonparental care arrangements experienced by preschool children, usually during the day when their parents are working or studying. A common distinction made between different forms of child care is that of formal versus informal child care. *Formal care* refers to child care services that are regulated by the public authority and include center care (also named day care, preschool, crèche, and nursery), which provides services to groups of children of similar ages in a nonresidential setting. Conversely, *informal care* describes unregulated child care services, including care by a relative (e.g., grandparent, sister or brother), a nanny, or a babysitter. Family child care, which serves a group of mixed-age children in a residential setting (other than the child's home) may be classified as either informal or formal child care depending on whether the services are registered by public authority and quality is controlled.

Many studies report on the associations between child care during the preschool years and cognitive skills during the preschool years, at school entry, or in middle childhood. These cognitive skills are not necessarily labeled "school readiness skills," although often they clearly are components of school readiness. For instance, many studies report on basic verbal skills (e.g., expressive and receptive vocabulary; Burchinal, Roberts, Nabors, & Bryant, 1996; Geoffroy et al., 2007, 2010; Waldfogel, Han, & Brooks-Gunn, 2002), knowledge of numbers and early mathematics abilities (Caughy, DiPietro, & Strobino, 1994; Côté, Doyle, et al., 2013; Magnuson, Meyers, Ruhm, & Waldfogel, 2004; Vandell & Ramanan, 1992), knowledge of letters and early reading abilities (Côté, Doyle, et al., 2013; Magnuson et al., 2004; Votruba-Drzal, Coley, & Chase-Lansdale, 2004), and general assessments of basic cognitive skills (e.g., colors, sizes, shapes, letters, numbers; Geoffroy et al., 2010). Those early cognitive skills predict later academic achievement (Boivin et al., Chapter 3, this volume; Duncan et al., 2007). In this chapter, we review studies of associations between child care and cognitive outcomes that represent cognitive school readiness.

Does Use of Child Care Services Contribute to Children's Cognitive School Readiness?

There is much controversy about the possible impact of child care on young children's cognitive development. Many are concerned that the use of child care, which has become a normative experience of early childhood (UNICEF, 2008), could compromise children's social and cognitive development. There is substantial heterogeneity in the research findings on this issue, and the direction and magnitude of the effects vary according to several important parameters, including the use of child care versus maternal work as predictor of child development, the age at which child care is initiated, the type of child care under consideration (e.g., formal vs. informal), and whether family characteristics moderate the associations between child care and cognitive outcomes. Although some studies found negative associations between early child care and language and cognitive outcomes (e.g., Brooks-Gunn, Han, & Waldfogel, 2002; Desai, Chase-Lansdale, & Michael, 1989), several others showed that child care is associated with meaningful benefits in terms of cognitive and school abilities (e.g., Caughy et al., 1994; Magnuson et al., 2004).

Variations in Findings on Child Care and Cognitive Development

Concerns about the impact of nonmaternal care early in life are rooted in the human and animal attachment literature, which suggests that maternal proximity and availability during infancy are essential to the offspring's healthy development (Belsky, 2001; Bowlby, 1951). Two bodies of literature have quantified the impact of maternal unavailability—or the fact that the mother is away from the child—on child development. Research in psychology tends to equate the amount of time that mothers are unavailable to the amount of *child care use,* while research in economics emphasizes *maternal employment* outside the home (cf. Burchinal & Clarke-Stewart, 2007). Child care use and maternal employment are only partially overlapping realities. That is, although most mothers who use child care are on the labor market, a substantial minority of them are not. The reverse is also true: Some working mothers find ways around not using child care services, for example, by working night shifts or working from home. Studies on child care use and maternal work have led to different conclusions about associations between maternal unavailability and children's cognitive development. Essentially, child care studies find that children who receive child care services have better cognitive outcomes, while maternal employment studies find that children of working mothers have poorer cognitive outcomes. In addition, there is evidence that the associations vary as a function of the socioeconomic status of the family. We review the results from child care and maternal employment studies in order to identify the sources of divergence in the findings.

Several studies have reported a negative association between early maternal work and the child's cognitive development (e.g., Baydar & Brooks-Gunn, 1991; Berger, Brooks-Gunn, Paxson, & Waldfogel, 2008; Brooks-Gunn et al., 2002; Han, Waldfogel, & Brooks-Gunn, 2001; Ruhm, 2004; Waldfogel et al., 2002). The negative associations are usually detected for maternal work in the first year postbirth, and are more pronounced for full-time employment than for part-time employment (Baydar & Brooks-Gunn, 1991; Brooks-Gunn et al., 2002; Hill, Waldfogel, Brooks-Gunn, & Han, 2005; Waldfogel et al., 2002). In at least one study, the mother's return to work in the second or third year was found to be negatively associated with the child's math and reading achievement at school entry (Ruhm, 2004).

The negative contribution of maternal employment appears limited to subgroups of participants, such as families in which mothers have high levels of education or in two-parent families (Brooks-Gunn et al., 2002; Gregg, Washbrook, Propper, & Burgess, 2005; Han et al., 2001; Harvey,

1999; Hill et al., 2005; Ruhm, 2004). For disadvantaged families (e.g., single mothers, mothers with low levels of education, or mothers with low levels of skills), maternal employment was not found to have these negative associations with child cognitive outcomes (Gregg et al., 2005; Han et al., 2001). There is also some evidence of positive effects of early child care for young children from socioeconomically disadvantaged families (Waldfogel et al., 2002). In summary, the research on maternal employment suggests that children from advantaged families may be affected negatively by maternal employment, while those from disadvantaged families may not, and may in some cases benefit from this experience.

Studies examining the role of child care use in cognitive development generally do not find negative associations, but rather find positive associations (Burchinal & Clarke-Stewart, 2007; Loeb, Bridges, Bassok, Fuller, & Rumberger, 2007; National Institute of Child Health and Human Services Early Child Care Research Network [NICHD ECCRN], 2000b, 2002a). However, in several studies, the positive associations with child care are limited to subgroups of the population. Studies have shown a beneficial contribution of child care for children of disadvantaged families (and not simply the absence of negative effects) (Caughy et al., 1994; Dearing, McCartney, & Taylor, 2009; Geoffroy et al., 2007, 2010; Magnuson et al., 2004; Peisner-Feinberg et al., 2001). For instance, in our work on a representative sample of Canadian children born between 1994 and 1996, we found that children from a socioeconomically disadvantaged background, but not children from well-off families, benefited from regular child care in their first year of life (Geoffroy et al., 2007). Positive putative impacts are also often reported among users of center-based care or formal child care services (Clarke-Stewart, Gruber, & Fitzgerald, 1994; Hansen & Hawkes, 2009; NICHD ECCRN, 2000a, 2000b, 2006), especially if this type of care is initiated in toddlerhood rather than infancy (Loeb et al., 2007; NICHD ECCRN, 2004).

In recent research using the Québec Longitudinal Study of Child Development (QLSCD), we provided evidence supporting the view that formal child care can be beneficial for children from disadvantaged backgrounds, but not (i.e., no association with outcomes) for children of well-off families. The QLSCD is a representative sample of children born in 1997–1998 in the Province of Québec, Canada, and includes detailed information on formal and informal child care attendance during the preschool years. In this study, formal child care included public and private centers and regulated family-based centers, whereas informal child care involved care by a relative or a babysitter. In Québec, family child care is generally provided by a registered caregiver, which means that the services are regulated and meet the same basic quality standards set by the government (e.g., child-to-caregiver ratio, trained caregiver, educational program) as other formal child care services. Specific to our discussion here, we compared the children of mothers with low levels of education (i.e., who did not complete a high school degree) to children of mothers with higher levels of education (i.e., who graduated from high school). Children from poorly educated and highly educated mothers exposed to formal care, informal care, or parental care were compared on two cognitive tests administered in kindergarten (e.g., receptive vocabulary: Peabody Picture Vocabulary Test [PPVT-R, Dunn & Dunn, 1981]; cognitive school readiness: Lollipop Test [Chew, 1989]), and on two achievement tests in first grade (e.g., mathematics: Number Knowledge Test [NKT]; reading: Kaufman Assessment Battery for Children [Kaufman & Kaufman, 1983]).

In general, the effect sizes for children of mothers with lower levels of education were much larger than those for children of more educated mothers. In addition, the effect sizes for children of mothers with low education were larger for formal care than for informal care.

Three specific results emerged from this study. First, children of mothers with low levels of education exhibited higher levels of receptive vocabulary and cognitive school readiness when they had been exposed to formal child care than did children from a similar background who experienced parental care. Second, informal child care was not associated with better outcomes for children of mothers with low levels of education, except for school readiness. Third, formal or informal child care was not associated with better or worse outcomes for children of mothers with higher levels of education.

Figure 6.1(a and b) illustrates the associations between formal and informal child care (vs. parental care) and cognitive scores among children of mothers with low and high levels of education, respectively. These associations are expressed in term of Cohen's *d* effect size, which represents standard deviations from the mean. It is generally agreed that a large effect size is equal to or greater than 0.80, a medium effect is equal to or greater than 0.50 but less than 0.80, and a small effect is equal to or greater than 0.20 but less than 0.50 (Cohen, 1988).

For children of mothers with low levels of education receiving formal or informal care, the effect sizes at 6 years were large for cognitive school readiness ($d > 0.80$). In addition, the long-term effect sizes associated with formal child care were maintained in first grade, as reflected by higher scores on mathematics ($d = 0.38$) and reading tests ($d = 0.48$) in second grade.

We performed the same type of comparison and found similar results in a large sample of families from the British Millennium Cohort Study (BMCS) in the United Kingdom. Figure 6.2(a and b) illustrates the size of the effects for children of mothers with low levels (who did not complete

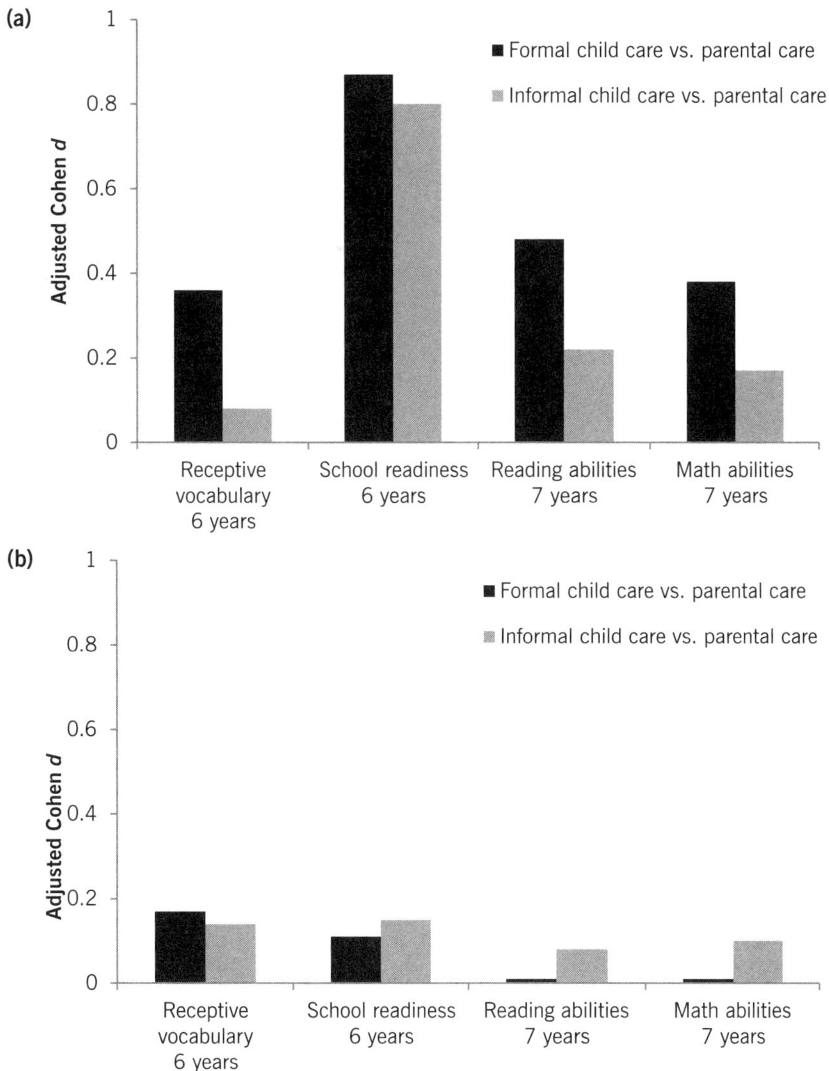

FIGURE 6.1. Associations (effect sizes, *d*) between child care services (CCS) and cognitive skills at 6–7 years in the Québec Longitudinal Study of Child Development (QLSCD). (a) Children of mothers with low levels of education. (b) Children of mothers with high levels of education. Cognitive tests were the Peabody Picture Vocabulary Test—Revised, Lollipop Test, Number Knowledge Test, and Kaufman Assessment Battery for Children, respectively. Effect sizes were adjusted for sex, birthweight, any breastfeeding, birth order, income, maternal age, maternal verbal skills, maternal depressive symptoms, home levels of stimulation, maternal overprotection, and perceived parental impact. Formal child care in the first 4 years of life includes center-based and family child care at home, whereas informal child care refers to unregulated care by relative/nanny/babysitter.

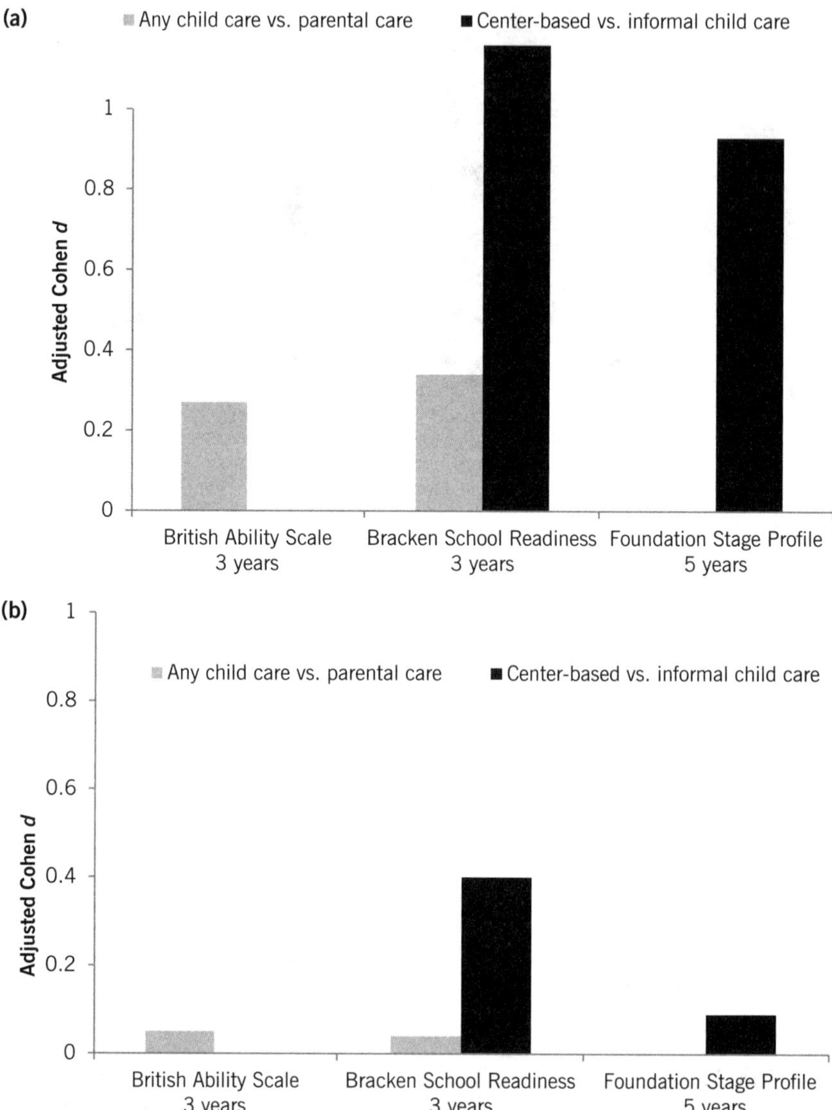

FIGURE 6.2. Associations (effect sizes, *d*) between child care and cognitive skills at ages 3 and 5 years in the British Millenium Cohort Study (n ~ 13,000). (a) Children of mothers with low levels of education. (b) Children of mothers with high levels of education. Informal child care at 9 months includes care by relative, nanny/child minder. The following control variables were included as covariates in all the models: any child care before age 3, center child care before age 3, any child care before age 5 (in BAS5, BAS7, FSP7 models only), center child care

mandatory schooling) and high levels of education, respectively, and who had received different types of child care at 9 months (Côté, Doyle, et al., 2013).

Specifically, we conducted two comparisons. In the first analysis, we contrasted children who received any type of formal and informal child care (34% of the sample) for a minimum of 9 hours per week to those who were in parental care (66% of the sample). In the second analysis, we compared children who experienced two types of child care: "center care versus informal care." This comparison was limited to the 34% of children who had received a minimum of 9 hours of child care per week, and compared children who had received center-based care (nurseries/crèches, 20%) to those who had received informal care (80%) by 9 months. Among children who had received informal care at 9 months, 61% received grandparental care; 21% were cared for by a nanny/child minder; and 18% were cared for by neighbors, relatives, or friends.

We found that child care at 9 months was associated with better cognitive development for certain outcomes, and that the association varied with the type of child care utilized and family risk as reflected by maternal education. The statistically significant contributions of any type of child care were small to moderate and limited to children of mothers with low levels of education. Compared with informal care (including family care, nanny/babysitter, relative), the significant contributions of center care were moderate overall but large for children of mothers with low education. The effects for center-based child care extended until school entry (5 years), but not beyond (age 7 years). While we found what could be seen as a short-term advantage of participating in any type of child care for children of mothers with low education, these results suggest that center-based child care increases further the likelihood of beneficial effects for these children.

---

before age 5 (in BAS5, BAS7, FSP7 only), child age (at time of assessment), child gender, maternal attachment at 9 months, maternal self-esteem at 9 months, HOME score at 3 years, the reading and teaching factors of parental time investment at 3 years, household income (at time of assessment), and maternal employment (at time of assessment). The FSP models also include a country dummy. The following variables, which were associated with (and potentially influenced) the infancy child care decision, were used to estimate the propensity scores matching models: child ethnicity, number of weeks of gestation, birthweight, birth by caesarean section, birth order, ever breastfed, planned pregnancy, attendance at antenatal classes, smoked during pregnancy, mother's age at the child's birth, mother was single at the birth of the child, mother's education level, mother's literacy difficulties, mother's social class, mother had a long-term chronic illness, and local authority housing at 9 months. *Note.* BAS, British Ability Scale; BSR, Bracken School Readiness; FSP, Foundation Stage Profile.

In summary, the findings from the QLSCD and the BMCS indicated positive and large contributions to school readiness of formal and center-care-based child care services for children of mothers with low levels of education. Quite interestingly, the effect sizes for children of mothers with low levels of education were similar to those obtained in randomized control trials of child care services programs for disadvantaged children, such as the Abecedarian and High/Scope Perry Preschool Study (Anderson et al., 2003; Reynolds & Temple, 2008). In both studies, we found smaller contributions for children of mothers with higher levels of education, but importantly, we did not find negative contributions of child care, even when initiated in infancy.

In the QLSCD (Geoffroy et al., 2010) and the BMCS (Côté, Doyle, et al., 2013), as in previous studies (Loeb et al., 2007; NICHD ECCRN, 2004), center-based or formal child care had larger impacts on cognitive outcomes than did informal child care. The characteristics of center-based settings may make them more likely to foster cognitive abilities than those of informal care settings. Informal care is usually family-based and aimed at providing a "home-like" setting that involves mostly free play. Infants receiving informal care are exposed to an environment less focused on structured activities compared to infants attending center-based child care. Center care is usually provided to groups of children of similar ages, and there is evidence that age segregation may promote higher quality care and education (NICHD ECCRN, 2004). Indeed, in groups of children of similar ages, the type of care and activities are more easily targeted to children's developmental needs. For instance, in mixed-age settings, younger children (toddlers) were found to receive less sensitive and supportive care than older children (preschoolers) (Kryzer, Kovan, Phillips, Domagall, & Gunnar, 2007). Children who experience center care have more exposure to an environment designed as an educational setting, and have access to a greater number and variety of toys and materials for children (Kisker & Maynard, 1991). Although we need to interpret these results cautiously given the correlational nature of the designs, this body of research suggests that child care helped disadvantaged children to compensate for what they lacked at home and to arrive at school better prepared.

Given the relevance of the type of child care for children's cognitive development, it may partly account for divergent findings between child care and maternal employment studies. Indeed, the type of child care that children receive while the mother is working is generally not considered in many maternal employment studies. In fact, the few studies that have examined the role of child care among children of working mothers tend to find results similar to those of child care studies. For instance, maternal employment was found to have negative effects on literacy when children were placed predominantly in the care of a friend or relative, but a positive effect when children were cared for in a center-based service (Gregg et al., 2005).

In summary, the evidence indicates that we need to be cautious about the type and intensity of child care services provided to young children. While there is evidence of positive contributions of formal child care for children from low socioeconomic status (SES) families, the evidence regarding informal child care is equivocal, especially among low-risk children. The reason why the type of child care is related to mixed outcomes is that it is only a rough proxy for child care quality. In order to understand more precisely the role of child care quality, we now turn to studies that have used detailed observations of child care settings to measure *process quality,* which refers to the proximal-level interactions and transactions among teachers, children, and materials (Bronfenbrenner & Morris, 1998), and encompasses the social, emotional, physical, and instructional quality of interactions with children aimed at promoting school readiness.

Does Quality of Child Care Matter?

While a relatively large number of studies have compared children on the basis of the intensity and type of child care they receive, few studies have compared children receiving child care of different quality. Examining quality in child care is important because the impact of child care may only be detected under high or low quality conditions. Examining the role of child care quality is also important as it may provide information on the aspects of care that could be targeted for further improvement of services.

Assessment of Child Care Quality

Child care quality studies have used tools to assess process quality at several levels of the classroom environment; from moment-to-moment displays of discrete behaviors to global characterizations of the overall setting (Pianta et al., 2005, p. 145). The Early Childhood Environmental Rating Scale—Revised (ECERS-R; Harms & Clifford, 1989), and its associated instruments, the Infant/Toddler Environmental Rating Scale (ITERS; Harms, Cryer, & Clifford, 2003) and the Family Day Care Rating Scale (FDCRS; Harms & Clifford, 1993), have been widely used to assess child care process quality (Perlman, Zellman, & Le, 2004). These observational instruments provide assessments of comparable dimensions in different settings (i.e., families vs. centers) and at different ages.

Using the ECERS-R, previous center-based studies identified two distinct quality factors—*Teaching and Interactions* and *Provisions for Learning*—that present the most appropriate psychometric properties (Burchinal, Cryer, Clifford, & Howes, 2002; Burchinal et al., 2000; Cassidy, Hestenes, Hegde, Hestenes, & Mims, 2005; Peisner-Feinberg et al., 1999, 2001; Perlman et al., 2004; Pianta et al., 2005). The *Teaching and Interactions* dimension reflects the warmth and adequacy of teacher–child interactions, as well as the richness and quality of language interactions in the classroom. The *Provisions for Learning* dimension reflects children's access to and use of appropriate learning materials.

Results from Child Care Quality Studies

Most studies of child care quality in diverse populations (i.e., not exclusively disadvantaged children) with a medium or long-term follow-up rely on small samples. There are, however, two notable exceptions—The Cost, Quality, and Child Outcomes in Child Care Centers Study (CQO, $N = 826$) and the NICHD Study of Early Child Care and Youth Development (SECCYD) (N = 1,364). The CQO study sampled child care centers, whereas the NICHD SECCYD sampled individual children, thus conducting child care quality assessments in a large variety of settings. Both studies were conducted in the United States and have shown modest, albeit significant, associations between higher child care quality and cognitive development (NICHD ECCRN, 2005; Peisner-Feinberg et al., 2001).

In the CQO, quality was assessed once, at the initiation of the study (child mean age of 4 years). Cognitive and academic outcomes were assessed yearly until children were 8 years of age (Peisner-Feinberg et al., 2001). Three main conclusions can be drawn from this study. First, the results indicate that the quality of children's experiences in typical child care centers predicts their development while they are in child care, and then their readiness for school in kindergarten. Children who attended higher quality child care centers performed better on measures of both cognitive skills (e.g., math and language abilities) and social skills (e.g., interactions with peers, problem behaviors) in child care and through the early transition into school. Furthermore, this association with child care quality was significant for children from a wide range of family backgrounds, and not just for disadvantaged children. Second, longitudinal analysis of children's performances indicated that child care quality before school entry continued to predict developmental outcomes at least through kindergarten, and in many cases, through the end of second grade. Child care quality predicted basic cognitive skills (language and math) and children's behavioral skills in the classroom (thinking/attention skills, sociability, problem behaviors, and peer relations), both of which reflect children's ability to take advantage of the opportunities available in school. Third, disadvantaged children were affected to a greater extent by the quality of child care experiences than other children. For some outcomes (math skills and problem behaviors), children whose mothers had lower levels of education were more sensitive to the negative effects of poor child care quality and received more benefits from high quality child care (Peisner-Feinberg et al., 1999).

In the NICHD SECCYD, child care quality was assessed yearly over the preschool years, and participants were followed from birth to adolescence. The NICHD study found significant positive associations between higher child care quality and language, math, and literacy skills during the preschool years and at school entry (Belsky, 2006). The significant predictions were shown to last into middle childhood (Dearing et al., 2009; Downer & Pianta, 2006; NICHD ECCRN, 2005) and adolescence (Vandell, Belsky, Burchinal, Steinberg, & Vandergrift, 2010). The more responsive and stimulating the care provided to the child, the better the child's cognitive–linguistic performance from 15 months onward (Belsky, 2006). The adolescent follow-up assessment (Vandell et al., 2010) confirmed that higher quality led to higher cognitive achievement in the long term. In childhood, as well as adolescent studies, however, most effect sizes were small.

Two additional findings from the NICHD study are worth reporting. First, there was evidence that the role of structural aspects of quality (e.g., caregiver–child ratio and caregiver training) was mediated by proximal processes of caregiver–child interaction (NICHD ECCRN, 2002a). That is, better structural characteristics of the child care environment led to better caregiver–child interactions, which in turn led to better outcomes in the children. In order to improve quality, further evidence of this type is needed to understand the mechanisms underlying its potential impact. Second, significant interactions were reported between poverty and child care quality (Dearing et al., 2009). Children from families with lower income appeared to benefit more from high-quality care (at 6–54 months of age), as seen in their math and reading achievement in middle school (4.5–11 years of age) than children from well-off families. Interestingly, for children receiving more episodes of high-quality child care, the negative association between low income and several achievement outcomes in middle school was no longer significant, thus highlighting the compensatory effect of high-quality child care (of significance to our discussion here is that this impact of high-quality care on low-income children's achievement was mediated by school readiness). However, this interaction effect was not consistently found in SECCYD reports, nor was it detected in the adolescent follow-up (Vandell et al., 2010). Finally, in the SECCYD as in the CQO, at-risk children benefited more from high-quality child care; however, contrary to the CQO, at-risk children from SECCYD were not more sensitive to the negative effects of poor-quality child care.

Some smaller international studies have also provided support for the association between process child care quality and cognitive development. In a Chilean study of private and public child care centers (approximately 400 children), higher scores on the ITERS/ECERS predicted better vocabulary and reading scores at school entry (Herrera, Mathiesen, Merino, & Recart, 2005). In a Swedish study (*N*= 123), child care quality prior to school entry predicted higher math abilities at 8 years (Broberg, Wessels, Lamb, & Hwang, 1997). In a Bermudian study, child care quality was related to children's concurrent development while in child care, but not in the long-term (Chin-Quee & Scarr, 1994).

Quality over Time: Is There Evidence for a Timing Effect?

In a longitudinal approach, repeated measures are important for methodological and conceptual reasons. At the methodological level, multiple measures reduce measurement error, and this is particularly relevant for a phenomenon with potentially important time variations such as child care quality. At the conceptual level, there may be true variations in child care quality over time, which may be meaningfully related to variations in child outcomes. Thus, repeated assessments can both reduce measurement error and provide important information on true variation in child care quality. However, few studies have measured child care quality at multiple times over the preschool years and accounted for change in child care quality.

Although many reports from the NICHD SECCYD treated the repeated measures of child care quality as an average across time (e.g. from 6 months through 54 months), some addressed the question of whether the timing of quality was important. For instance, the NICHD and Duncan (2003) compared the contribution of early (6, 15, and 24 months) and late (36 and 54 months) quality in child care, and showed that both periods were significantly and independently associated with PreK cognitive and preacademic achievement scores. In addition, two studies using hierarchical linear modeling (HLM) showed that both initial levels of quality and increase in quality over time were related to higher preacademic skills (Hirsh-Pasek & Burchinal, 2006; NICHD ECCRN, 2002b). In one report, Hirsh-Pasek and Burchinal (2006) used a trajectory group-based approach and found no significant associations between the four patterns of global quality they identified and child outcomes. However, it is possible that the limited amount of variability in the patterns of quality over time could explain the null findings (Hirsh-Pasek & Burchinal, 2006).

In a study using a group-based methodological approach (Jones, Nagin, & Roeder, 2001; Nagin, 1999), we examined the patterns of variation in quality in various child care settings (some family-based, others center-based) over the preschool years. The sample (N = 257) comprised children receiving child care in the Montréal (Canada) region (Côté, Mongeau, et al., 2013). This method allows for identifying distinct patterns of quality over time, thereby providing a dynamic measure of quality (i.e., one that may vary with age). A notable advantage is that this approach can identify groups of children exposed to distinct levels of quality grounded on their distribution over time, rather than based on an arbitrary cutoff. Hence, this approach provides information on the proportion of children similarly exposed to various levels of quality without the imposition of a predefined criterion for defining the size of the group or the level of quality.

Using this approach, we found that a substantial proportion of children were exposed to high and progressively ascending levels of quality of *Teaching and Interactions* (59%), whereas a smaller group (41%) was exposed to low and stable quality. Conversely, on the *Provision for Learning* dimension, only a minority of children (24.3%) was exposed to high and stable quality, while the majority was exposed to lower quality (75.7%). Figure 6.3(a and b) illustrates the quality trajectories on the *Teaching and Interaction* and *Provision for Learning* dimensions, respectively (Côté, Mongeau, et al., 2013).

How does the level of quality experienced by children in the distinct trajectory groups correspond to the ITERS/ECERS/FDCRS guidelines for quality? These guidelines suggest that a quality score below 2.9 reflects poor quality; whereas a score between 3 and 4.9 signals minimal quality; and a score above 5, good to excellent quality. Thus, according to the ITERS/ECERS/FDCRS guidelines, children in the low groups were exposed to poor or barely minimal levels of quality. Such low levels reflect none to very little age-appropriate stimulation of child development, and a relatively unpleasant emotional climate in the care environment. Children in the high trajectories were exposed to minimal to good quality according to the ITERS/ECERS/FDCRS guidelines for quality. Despite the relatively low levels of quality, the high and ascending quality trajectory of *Teaching and Interactions* was associated with higher cognitive scores on numeracy (NKT), receptive vocabulary (PPVT-R), and school readiness (Lollipop) at age 4 years compared to the lower trajectory, with effect sizes in the small to medium range. In bivariate analyses, both the higher *Teaching and Interactions* and *Provision for Learning* trajectories were associated with higher cognitive scores, but in multivariable analyses, only the *Teaching and Interactions* had an independent contribution. Figure 6.4 illustrates the Cohen d effect sizes for cognitive outcomes by

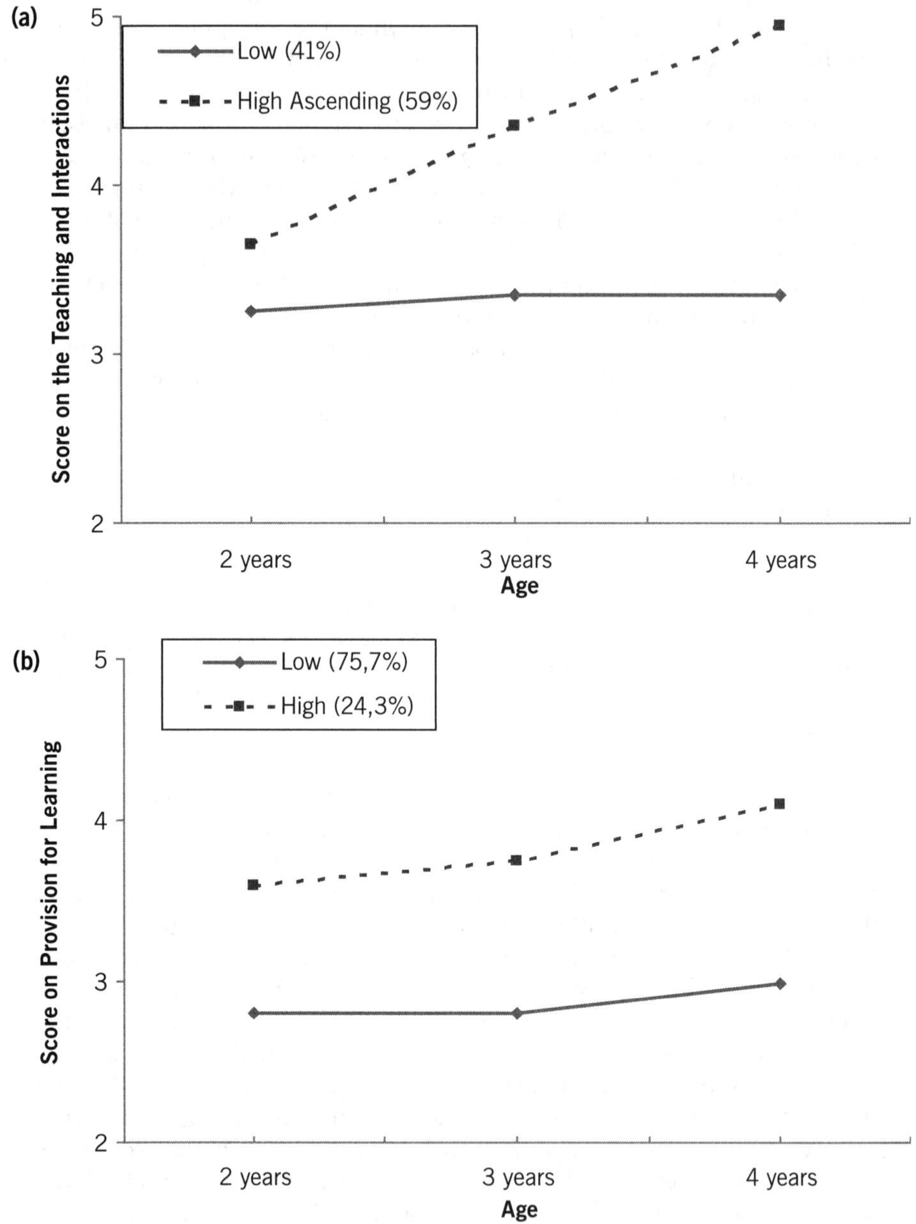

FIGURE 6.3. Quality trajectories on the (a) *Teaching and Interactions,* and (b) *Provision for Learning* dimensions.

quality trajectory for the *Teaching and Interactions* and *Provision for Learning* (high ascending vs. low) dimensions, respectively.

The *Teaching and Interactions* dimension reflects quality of the interplay between the educator and the children, that is, the extent to which the educator uses the material or his or her skills to promote children's participation and learning (Harms, Clifford, & Cryer, 1998). High quality indicates an emphasis on using verbal interactions in stimulation of language development, conflict resolution, and in the general interactions and greetings exchanged with children. The results point to the role that child care educators play in supporting communication via personal conversations with children, encouraging reasoning throughout daily activities, providing a balance between listening and talking, and supporting positive interactions during peer interactions, as well as during child–adult interactions.

The *Provision for Learning* dimension reflects the availability, accessibility, and diversity of activities that children can initiate in an autonomous way (e.g., fine motor skills activities, artistic expression, body movement, symbolic play, science). The fact that this dimension did not contribute to cognitive scores when the quality of *Teaching and Interactions*

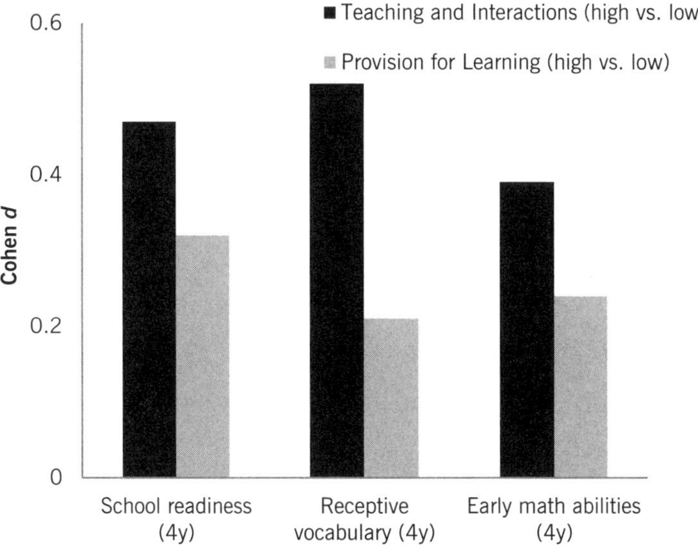

FIGURE 6.4. Cognitive outcomes at 4 years by quality of Trajectory of *Teaching and Interactions* and *Provision for Learning* (Cohen's *d*). Cognitive tests were the Lollipop Test, Peabody Picture Vocabulary Test–Revised, and Number Knowledge Test, respectively.

was accounted for may be due to a number of reasons. First, there was a relatively high correlation between the two quality factors (r = .77). Second, there were few children in the high level *Provision for Learning* quality group (i.e., 24.3%), thus reducing the power to detect an association. Third, the overall quality—even of the high trajectory—was minimal. Although a recent study suggested that achievement of minimal quality standards is necessary to contribute to preacademic gains (Burchinal, Vandergrift, Pianta, & Mashburn, 2010), these results suggest that minimal quality on the *Provision for Learning* dimension may not be sufficient. The significant association between *Teaching and Interaction* and cognitive outcomes rather suggests that a moderate level of quality is necessary to obtain a positive impact. Improvements in quality could potentially lead to higher impact on the development of cognitive abilities.

In summary, several studies have shown that higher-quality child care is associated with better cognitive outcomes in the children, but that the associations are of small magnitude. Specific aspects of quality appear to be more relevant than others—dimensions reflecting the quality of the interactions between children and educators are particularly correlated with cognitive outcomes. However, the conclusions we can draw from existing child care quality studies are limited by the facts that studies relied on samples of small or medium sizes and did not include long-term follow-up. In addition, quality child care studies are affected by the same methodological problems as population-based studies. These methodological problems include the selection of families into child care services, the nonrandomness of missing data, and the relative lack of studies using samples from outside North America. We discuss these methodological problems in the next section and propose ways to address them.

Methodological Problems in Child Care Research and Ways to Address Them

The Social Selection Problem

A major conceptual and methodological issue in child care research is the possibility that the self-selection of families into child care or of mothers in maternal work explains part of the observed relationship with children's outcomes. By *self-selection*, we mean that only families or individuals with certain characteristics succeed in having access to child care services or to employment. Studies that examine child outcomes associated with maternal employment typically control for a wide range of characteristics that distinguish families with an employed mother from those with a nonemployed mother. Quite similarly, child care studies control for characteristics that distinguish families that use child care from those that do not. These characteristics typically include factors such as parenting and cognitive skills, levels of stimulation in the home, and income (Geoffroy et al., 2012; Gregg et al., 2005). In addition, family characteristics such as ethnicity (Early & Burchinal, 2001; NICHD ECCRN, 1997), whether the child has other siblings (Singer, Fuller, Keiley, & Wolf, 1998), and maternal beliefs about the effects of maternal employment (NICHD ECCRN, 1997), have been suggested as potential selection factors. Apart from family characteristics, the decision to work or to use child care may also depend on the child's characteristics. For instance, mothers of children with a difficult temperament may be less likely to work than mothers of children with an easy temperament (Lerner & Galambos, 1986). Despite efforts to include all potential confounding selection factors as statistical controls, unmeasured confounders may bias the results.

Recent studies have attempted to reduce the social selection bias by using methods that go beyond controlling for confounding factors. For instance, Jaffee, Van Hulle, and Rodgers (2011) recently used a sibling design to compare children within the same family who have had different child care experiences. Consistent with previous studies, between-family comparisons indicated that early child care was associated with higher achievement scores in childhood and adolescence. However, within-family comparisons failed to detect differences between siblings whose early child care experiences differed. The study concluded that the timing of entry to child care in the first 3 years was not associated with children's outcomes.

A few studies have applied propensity score matching to investigate the association between maternal employment and children's development (e.g., Berger et al., 2008; Hill et al., 2005). *Propensity score matching* is a method designed to identify effects in the presence of selection bias (Dehejia & Wahba, 2002; Rosenbaum & Rubin, 1983) by matching subjects who receive a treatment (in this case, child care) with subjects who have similar characteristics but do not receive the treatment (in this case, they receive maternal care). The first step is to estimate a propensity score defined as the predicted probability of treatment (i.e., child care) based on regression using a set of pretreatment variables (e.g., maternal education, maternal employment and family income prior to the birth of the child). The score is then used to create a comparison group that is as similar as possible to the treatment group, but that is not exposed to the treatment. The usefulness of the propensity score matching approach in developmental psychology has recently been highlighted as a step further toward causal inference (Foster, 2010).

In studies examining the impact of maternal work on cognitive development, both propensity score matching and regression analyses were used. Berger et al. (2008) found that maternal employment in the first year of children's lives was associated with detrimental effects on vocabulary size for white children, but no association was found for black or Hispanic 3-year-olds. Hill and colleagues (2005) found small but significant negative effects on children's cognitive outcomes for full-time maternal employment in the first year postbirth, as compared with employment postponed until after the first year.

We recently examined selection into child care among children of the BMCS (Côté, Doyle, et al., 2013), and found strong selection effects in the use of child care, especially center-based child care. Children exposed to higher levels of family and maternal risk characteristics were much more likely to receive parental care or informal child care. The magnitude of the effects obtained with regression analyses was largely in line with that obtained with propensity score matching analyses. However, in two instances, we detected significant interactions between maternal education and center-based child care using the propensity score matching strategy that we did not detect using regression. This suggests that the assumptions of regression may not be tenable in the presence of strong selection effects, and may thus conceal group differences, pointing to the importance of controlling for social selection. However, even with propensity score matching, the possibility that unmeasured factors affect the results remains.

Thus, the most robust evidence for the view that child care can promote school readiness will come from randomized control trials in which the impact on school readiness is verified under strict conditions of control. Because the selection problem is mainly reflected in low participation rates in disadvantaged families, large-scale trials with random assignment of disadvantaged families to child care services are needed. These would be ethically acceptable if the services being offered meet the conditions that are known to foster positive child development. These include services of high quality that can be used with moderate intensity (e.g., part-time to full-time) and offer flexible schedules. High-quality services are usually found in center-based settings that meet safety requirements and are equipped with age-appropriate material. The services should be offered by qualified educators, who provide a warm, stimulating, and age-appropriate educational environment. In addition, the services should be easily accessible by the parents. Such services should have a double function: fostering child development and freeing time for the parent for work or respite.

The Missing Value Problem

Attrition is inherent to any longitudinal study, and this creates a missing value problem as participants lost to follow-up usually differ in important ways from those who remain in the study. One strategy to reduce the bias created by attrition is to use multiple imputations (i.e., to fill in missing values with predictions based on observed data). A multiple imputations approach, as compared with a complete case approach, was found to make important differences in the conclusion drawn from the results of a maternal employment study (Hill et al., 2005) as well as a child care study (Côté, Doyle, et al., 2013). In the maternal employment study, maternal employment was found to have no negative effects in the subgroup most affected by attrition and therefore by imputation, whereas it did using the complete case approach. Hence, imputation reduced the negative impact of maternal employment by supplementing the subgroup in which there was no negative effect—the subgroup of disadvantaged families (Hill et al., 2005). In the child care study, none of the maternal education × child care interactions reached significance using the complete case approach, while four interactions suggesting a beneficial effect of child care for children of mothers with low levels of education reached significance with multiple imputation. In this case, multiple imputations made it possible to keep more disadvantaged children (who are typically disproportionately affected by attrition) in the analyses, and therefore provided adequate power for testing interactions between maternal education and child care. Both studies underlie the importance, in future longitudinal child care studies, to account for attrition by using multiple imputations. They also suggest that the positive impact of child care in a segment of the population disproportionately affected by attrition or missing values—disadvantaged families—may have been underestimated.

Emphasis on North American Studies

The bulk of the studies on child care or maternal employment were conducted in North America, mostly in the United States. As results may differ in settings where the provision, users, and quality of child care differ, it is crucial to examine the extent to which the findings are similar in other cultures/countries. For example, differences between the United States and the United Kingdom may be particularly important, as return-to-work patterns differ markedly in these two countries (Crosby & Hawkes, 2007). For instance, in the United States, approximately 40% of new mothers are back at work within 3 months, while this number is 8% in the United Kingdom (Berger & Waldfogel, 2004). Furthermore, 70% of the U.K. mothers who return to work by 6 months work part-time compared with only 40% in the United States. These differential patterns of the return to work and the associated differential patterns of child care use not only illustrate the need for studies from various countries but also highlight the importance of international comparisons in child care.

Studies comparing the patterns of use and user profiles across countries or regions differing in social policy and financing of early child care can shed light on the strategies facilitating access to those most in need. If, in addition, such studies include information about child care quality, then the comparison could provide information on patterns of use and user profiles for various child care quality and provide information about the strategies most likely to lead to poor or good quality.

Experimental Studies

The most robust evidence for the view that child care promotes school readiness comes from randomized control trials in which the quality of child care is systematically manipulated and the impact on school readiness can be verified under strict conditions of control. Such studies are detailed elsewhere in this book and are not reviewed here. However, it is worth noting that most of these experimental studies focus on formal child care and, in particular, the provision of educational interventions in center-based settings. Interestingly, this type of intervention seems indeed the most likely to make a positive contribution to cognitive school readiness, as reported in this chapter.

Summary and Conclusion

Accumulating evidence from epidemiological and experimental studies tends to demonstrate that child care services can be effective in promoting school readiness. However, several questions of significance require additional attention. First, the long-term impact of child care is still underdocumented. While a few long-term evaluations of well-controlled randomized trials of early childhood educational interventions have shown enduring impacts, the long-term effects of widely disseminated child care services provided at community, regional, and state levels are largely unknown. The bulk of the evidence on the long-term impact comes from a single study—the NICHD SECCYD. The study has a relatively small sample size (N = 1,364 at adolescent follow-up; Vandell et al., 2010) with the usual rate of attrition. Over time, short-term effects can fade away or latent effects can emerge. Hence, conclusions regarding the long-term impact of any particular child care services require such long-term studies.

Second, child care quality has been shown to be particularly important. However, the mechanisms of influence of different aspects of quality are still poorly understood. There is evidence that the impact of structural aspects of quality is mediated by the quality of child–caregiver interactions. The specific aspects of both structural and interactional dimensions of quality that have a greater impact, and the way they operate, should be better understood in order to tailor adequate programs. Furthermore, monitoring of quality over time and assessments of the impact of quality at different periods are crucial. Indeed, quality of care may or may not be more important at specific developmental levels (e.g., infancy) than others. Patterns of evolution of quality during preschool (e.g., rising or declining) may also be important determinants of child outcomes. Therefore, quality should be assessed repeatedly over time. Finally, additional research is needed to highlight the conditions under which the promises of child care will be fulfilled; that is, which children at what age benefit most from child care, and the dose and quality necessary to achieve long-term, sizable effects. Ideally, as mentioned earlier, these questions should be examined within large randomized control trials in order to avoid the problem of social selection.

Services and Policy Implications

In this chapter, we have presented evidence that child care services seem to favor children's cognitive school readiness under certain conditions. First, the evidence indicates that formal (but not informal) child care and the inclusion of educational interventions are needed to achieve this goal. Second, high-quality services, particular in regard to teaching and interactions (e.g., warmth of teacher–child interaction or richness of language interactions) are associated with greater gains. Third, disadvantaged children seem to benefit more from a high-quality child care experience than do children who are not socioeconomically disadvantaged. Taken together, these findings indicate that investment in high-quality, center-based settings, particularly for more disadvantaged children, should lead to better school readiness. From a skills formation perspective, such a policy would represent a sound economic investment (Heckman, 2006) and might also contribute to reduction of the intergenerational reproduction of social inequalities (Deming, 2009). For service providers, the evidence suggests both the need to insist on a continuous investment in quality and an effort to enroll and retain disadvantaged children. However, a word of caution is necessary, because the causal nature and the magnitude of the positive contribution of child care to children's cognitive outcomes is still open to debate (Jaffee et al., 2011; U.S. Department of Health and Human Services, 2010).

Furthermore, in order to fulfill the promises of child care, two important obstacles must be taken into account. First, social selection is a major threat to the efficiency of child care interventions at a population level. Indeed, disadvantaged children are less likely to be enrolled.

In order to be efficient, child care policies should be designed to maximize the enrollment of disadvantaged children. Social selection issues are largely dependent on actual national policies. For instance, social selection issues in Norway and the United States differ largely (Bekkhus, Rutter, Maughan, & Borge, 2011). Recent changes in Sweden demonstrated how a shift in family policy may exacerbate social selection: Home child care was rendered economically more interesting for disadvantaged families, which created an incentive, in particular for immigrant women, to stay at home and take care of their children instead of using public child care (Tunberger & Sigle-Rushton, 2011). Consequently, such policies can reinforce class disparities in the long-term.

The second threat to the usefulness of child care interventions is the possibility that their contributions might fade out with time. Indeed, several studies have reported that the positive contributions of child care to cognitive school readiness fade out in the school years (Deming, 2009; Schweinhart et al., 2005; Schweinhart & Weikart, 1997; Weikart & Schweinhart, 1992). One explanation may be that the maintenance of a positive effect of child care interventions in elementary school seems to depend on school quality. For instance, in a randomized controlled trial in Head Start settings, only children who later went to high-quality schools showed enduring effects of the early intervention; the positive effect was not maintained for children in low-quality schools (Zhai, Raver, & Jones, 2012). To mitigate this concern, long-term positive contributions of child care were still reported, even in studies in which the fading effect was observed (Deming, 2009; Schweinhart et al., 2005; Schweinhart & Weikart, 1997; Weikart & Schweinhart, 1992). However, to sustain and/or enhance the positive impact of early child care interventions in not only cognitive school readiness but also elementary school and later on, a continuous investment in disadvantaged children's education may be required.

To conclude, investment in high-quality, center-based child care appears to be a wise policy to promote short-term cognitive readiness and long-term social inclusion, and thus may be beneficial for the economy and social cohesion (Deming, 2009; Heckman, 2006). However, investment in high-quality education may have to be maintained during children's schooling to favor their development and address the consequences of social inequalities.

REFERENCES

Anderson, C. A., Berkowitz, L., Donnerstein, E., Huesmann, L. R., Johnson, J. D., Linz, D., et al. (2003). The influence of media violence on youth. *Psychological Science in the Public Interest, 4*(3), 81–110.

Baydar, N., & Brooks-Gunn, J. (1991). Effects of maternal employment and child-care arrangements on preschoolers' cognitive and behavioral outcomes: Evidence from the Children of the National Longitudinal Survey of Youth. *Developmental Psychology, 27*(6), 932–945.

Bekkhus, M., Rutter, M., Maughan, B., & Borge, A. I. H. (2011). The effects of group daycare in the context of paid maternal leave and high-quality provision. *European Journal of Developmental Psychology, 8*(6), 681–696.

Belsky, J. (2001). Emanuel Miller Lecture: Developmental risks (still) associated with early child care. *Journal of Child Psychology and Psychiatry, 42*(7), 845–859.

Belsky, J. (2006). Early child care and early child development: Major findings of the NICHD Study of Early Child Care. *European Journal of Developmental Psychology, 3*(1), 95–110.

Berger, L., Brooks-Gunn, J., Paxson, C., & Waldfogel, J. (2008). First-year maternal employment and child outcomes: Differences across racial and ethnic groups. *Children and Youth Services Review, 30*(4), 365–387.

Berger, L. M., & Waldfogel, J. (2004). Maternity leave and the employment of new mothers in the United States. *Journal of Population Economics, 17*(2), 331–349.

Bowlby, J. (1951). *Maternal care and mental health.* Geneva: World Health Organization.

Broberg, A. G., Wessels, H., Lamb, M. E., & Hwang, C. (1997). Effects of day care on the development of cognitive abilities in 8-year-olds: A longitudinal study. *Developmental Psychology, 33*(1), 62–69.

Bronfenbrenner, U., & Morris, P. A. (1998). The ecology of developmental process. In R. M. Lerner & W. Damon (Eds.), *Handbook of child psychology* (5th ed., Vol. 1, pp. 993–1028). Cambridge, MA: Harvard University Press.

Brooks-Gunn, J., Han, W. J., & Waldfogel, J. (2002). Maternal employment and child cognitive outcomes in the first three years of life: The NICHD Study of Early Child Care. *Child Development, 73*(4), 1052–1072.

Burchinal, M. R., & Clarke-Stewart, K. A. (2007). Maternal employment and child cognitive outcomes: The importance of analytic approach. *Developmental Psychology, 43*(5), 1140–1155.

Burchinal, M. R., Cryer, D., Clifford, R. M., & Howes, C. (2002). Caregiver training and classroom quality in child care centers. *Applied Developmental Sciences, 6*(1), 2–11.

Burchinal, M. R., Roberts, J. E., Nabors, L. A., & Bryant, D. M. (1996). Quality of center child care and infant cognitive and language development. *Child Development, 67*(2), 606–620.

Burchinal, M. R., Roberts, J. E., Riggins, R., Jr., Zeisel, S. A., Neebe, E., & Bryant, D. (2000). Relating quality of center-based child care to early cognitive and language development longitudinally. *Child Development, 71*(2), 338–357.

Burchinal, M., Vandergrift, N., Pianta, R., & Mashburn, A. (2010). Threshold analysis of association between child care quality and child outcomes for low-income children in pre-kindergarten programs. *Early Childhood Research Quarterly, 25*(2), 166–176.

Cassidy, D. J., Hestenes, L. L., Hegde, A., Hestenes, S., & Mims, S. (2005). Measurement of quality in preschool child care classrooms: An exploratory and confirmatory factor analysis of the Early Childhood Environment Rating Scale—Revised. *Early Childhood Research Quarterly, 20*(3), 345–360.

Caughy, M. O., DiPietro, J. A., & Strobino, D. M. (1994). Day-care participation as a protective factor in the cognitive development of low-income children. *Child Development, 65*(2), 457–471.

Chew, A. L. (1989). *The Lollipop Test: A diagnostic training test of school readiness.* Atlanta, GA: Humanics Psychological Test Corporation.

Chin-Quee, D. S., & Scarr, S. (1994). Lack of early child care effects on school-age children's social competence and academic achievement. *Early Development & Parenting, 3*(2), 103–112.

Clarke-Stewart, K. A., Gruber, C. P., & Fitzgerald, L. M. (1994). *Children at home and in day care.* Hillsdale, NJ: Erlbaum.

Cohen, J. (1988). *Statistical power analysis for the behavioral sciences* (2nd ed.). Hillsdale, NJ: Erlbaum.

Côté, S. M., Doyle, O., Petitclerc, A., & Timmins, L. (2013). Child care in infancy and cognitive performance until middle childhood in the Millennium Cohort Study. *Child Development, 84*(4), 1191–1208.

Côté, S. M., Mongeau, C., Japel, C., Xu, Q., Séguin, J. R., & Tremblay, R. E. (2013). Child care quality and cognitive development: Trajectories leading to better pre-academic skills. *Child Development,* 84(2), 752–766

Crosby, D. A., & Hawkes, D. D. (2007). Cross-national research using contemporary birth cohort studies: A look at early maternal employment in the UK and USA. *International Journal of Social Research Methodology, 10*(5), 379–404.

Dearing, E., McCartney, K., & Taylor, B. A. (2009). Does higher quality early child care promote low-income children's math and reading achievement in middle childhood? *Child Development, 80*(5), 1329–1349.

Dehejia, R. H., & Wahba, S. (2002). Propensity score-matching methods for nonexperimental causal studies. *Review of Economics and Statistics, 84*(1), 151–161.

Deming, D. (2009). Early childhood intervention and life-cycle skill development: Evidence from Head Start. *American Economic Journal: Applied Economics, 1*(3), 111–134.

Desai, S., Chase-Lansdale, P. L., & Michael, R. T. (1989). Mother or market?: Effects of maternal employment on the intellectual ability of 4-year-old children. *Demography, 26*(4), 545–561.

Downer, J. T., & Pianta, R. C. (2006). Academic and cognitive functioning in first grade: Associations with earlier home and child care predictors and with concurrent home and classroom experiences. *School Psychology Review, 35*(1), 11–30.

Duncan, G. J., Dowsett, C. J., Claessens, A., Magnuson, K., Huston, A. C., Klebanov, P., et al. (2007). School readiness and later achievement. *Developmental Psychology, 43*(6), 1428–1446.

Dunn, L. M., & Dunn, L. M. (1981). *Peabody Picture Vocabulary Test–Revised (PPVT-R).* Circles Pines, MN: American Guidance Services.

Early, D. M., & Burchinal, M. R. (2001). Early childhood care: Relations with family characteristics and preferred care characteristics. *Early Childhood Research Quarterly, 16*(4), 475–497.

Foster, E. M. (2010). Causal inference and developmental psychology. *Developmental Psychology, 46*(6), 1454–1480.

Geoffroy, M.-C., Côté, S. M., Borge, A., Larouche, F., Séguin, J. R., & Rutter, M. (2007). Association between nonmaternal care in the first year of life and children's receptive language skills prior to school entry: The moderating role of the socioeconomic status. *Journal of Child Psychology and Psychiatry, 48*(5), 490–497.

Geoffroy, M.-C., Côté, S. M., Giguere, C.-E., Dionne, G., Zelazo, P. D., Tremblay, R. E., et al. (2010). Closing the gap in academic readiness and achievement: The role of early child care. *Journal of Child Psychology and Psychiatry, 51*(12), 1359–1367.

Geoffroy, M.-C., Séguin, J. R., Lacourse, É., Boivin, M., Tremblay, R. E., & Côté, S. M. (2012). Parental characteristics associated with child care use during the first 4 years of life: Results from a representative cohort of Québec families. *Canadian Journal of Public Health, 103*(1), 76–80.

Gregg, P., Washbrook, E., Propper, C., & Burgess, S. (2005). The effects of a mother's return to work decision on child development in the UK. *Economic Journal, 115*(501), F48–F80.

Han, W.-J., Waldfogel, J., & Brooks-Gunn, J. (2001). The effects of early maternal employment on later cognitive and behavioral outcomes. *Journal of Marriage and Family, 63*(2), 336–354.

Hansen, K., & Hawkes, D. (2009). Early child care and child development. *Journal of Social Policy, 38*(2), 211–239.

Harms, T., & Clifford, R. M. (1989). *Family Day Care Rating Scale*. New York: Teachers College Press.

Harms, T., & Clifford, R. M. (1993). Studying educational settings. In B. Spodek (Ed.), *Handbook of research on the education of young children* (pp. 477–492). New York: Macmillan.

Harms, T., Clifford, R. M., & Cryer, D. (1998). *Early Childhood Environment Rating Scale* (Revised ed.). New York: Teachers College Press.

Harms, T., Cryer, D., & Clifford, R. M. (2003). *Infant/Toddler Environment Rating Scale: Book revised edition*. New York: Teachers College Press.

Harvey, E. (1999). Short-term and long-term effects of early parental employment on children of the National Longitudinal Survey of Youth. *Developmental Psychology, 35*(2), 445–459.

Heckman, J. J. (2006). Skill formation and the economics of investing in disadvantaged children. *Science, 312*(5782), 1900–1902.

Herrera, M. A., Mathiesen, M. E., Merino, J. M., & Recart, I. (2005). Learning contexts for young children in Chile: Process quality assessment in preschool centres. *International Journal of Early Years Education, 13*(1), 13–27.

Hertzman, C., & Boyce, T. (2010). How experience gets under the skin to create gradients in developmental health. *Annual Review of Public Health, 3* (1), 329–347.

High, P. C., & the Committee on Early Childhood. (2008). School readiness. *Pediatrics, 121*(4), E1008–E1015.

Hill, J. L., Waldfogel, J., Brooks-Gunn, J., & Han, W. J. (2005). Maternal employment and child development: A fresh look using newer methods. *Developmental Psychology, 41*(6), 833–850.

Hirsh-Pasek, K., & Burchinal, M. (2006). Mother and caregiver sensitivity over time: Predicting language and academic outcomes with variable- and person-centered approaches. *Merrill–Palmer Quarterly-Journal of Developmental Psychology, 52*(3), 449–485.

Jaffee, S. R., Van Hulle, C., & Rodgers, J. L. (2011). Effects of nonmaternal care in the first 3 years on children's academic skills and behavioral functioning in childhood and early adolescence: A sibling comparison study. *Child Development, 82*(4), 1076–1091.

Jones, B. L., Nagin, D. S., & Roeder, K. (2001). A SAS procedure based on mixture models for estimating developmental trajectories. *Sociological Methods and Research, 29,* 374–393.

Kaufman, N., & Kaufman, A. S. (1983). *Kaufman Assessment Battery for Children.* Circle Pines, MN: American Guidance Service.

Kisker, E. E., & Maynard, R. (1991). Quality, cost, and parental choice of child care. In D. M. Blau (Ed.), *The economics of child care* (pp. 127–143). New York: Russell Sage Foundation.

Koenen, K. C., Moffitt, T. E., Roberts, A. L., Martin, L. T., Kubzansky, L., Harrington, H., et al. (2009). Childhood IQ and adult mental disorders: A test of the cognitive reserve hypothesis. *American Journal of Psychiatry, 166*(1), 50–57.

Kryzer, E. M., Kovan, N., Phillips, D. A., Domagall, L. A., & Gunnar, M. R. (2007). Toddlers' and preschoolers' experience in family day care: Age differences and behavioral correlates. *Early Childhood Research Quarterly, 22*(4), 451–466.

Lerner, J. V., & Galambos, N. L. (1986). Temperament and maternal employment. *New Directions for Child Development, 31,* 75–88.

Loeb, S., Bridges, M., Bassok, D., Fuller, B., & Rumberger, R. W. (2007). How much is too much?: The influence of preschool centers on children's social and cognitive development. *Economics of Education Review, 26*(1), 52–66.

Magnuson, K. A., Meyers, M. K., Ruhm, C. J., & Waldfogel, J. (2004). Inequality in preschool education and school readiness. *American Educational Research Journal, 41*(1), 115–157.

Nagin, D. S. (1999). Analyzing developmental trajectories: A semiparametric, group-based approach. *Psychological Methods, 4*(2), 139–157.

National Institute of Child Health and Human Development (NICHD), & Duncan, G. J. (2003). Modeling the impact of child care quality on children's preschool cognitive developement. *Child Development, 74*(5), 1454–1475.

NICHD Early Child Care Research Network (ECCRN). (1997). Familial factors associated with the characteristics of nonmaternal care for infants. *Journal of Marriage and the Family, 59*(2), 389–408.

NICHD ECCRN. (2000a). Characteristics and quality of child care for toddlers and preschoolers. *Applied Developmental Science, 4*(3), 116–135.

NICHD ECCRN. (2000b). The relation of child care to cognitive and language development. *Child Development, 71*(4), 960–980.

NICHD ECCRN. (2002a). Early child care and children's development prior to school entry: Results from the NICHD study of early child care. *American Educational Research Journal, 39*(1), 133–164.

NICHD ECCRN. (2002b). The interaction of child care and family risk in relation to child development at 24 and 36 months. *Applied Developmental Science, 6*(3), 144–156.

NICHD ECCRN. (2004). *Trajectories of physical aggression from toddlerhood to middle school* (Serial No.278 69-4). Malden, MA: Blackwell.

NICHD ECCRN. (2005). Early child care and children's development in the primary grades: Follow-up results from the NICHD study of early child care. *American Educational Research Journal, 42*(3), 537–570.

NICHD ECCRN. (2006). Child-care effect sizes for the NICHD study of early child care and youth development. *American Psychologist, 61*(2), 99–116.

Peisner-Feinberg, E. S., Burchinal, M. R., Clifford, R. M., Culkin, M. L., Howes, C., Kagan, S. L., et al. (1999). *The children of the Cost, Quality, and Outcomes Study go to school: Public report.* Chapel Hill: FPG Child Development Center, University North Carolina at Chapel Hill.

Peisner-Feinberg, E. S., Burchinal, M. R., Clifford, R. M., Culkin, M. L., Howes, C., Kagan, S. L., et al. (2001). The relation of preschool child-care quality to children's cognitive and social developmental trajectories through second grade. *Child Development, 72*(5), 1534–1553.

Perlman, M., Zellman, G. L., & Le, V.-N. (2004). Examining the psychometric properties of the Early Childhood Environment Rating Scale—Revised (ECERS-R). *Early Childhood Research Quarterly, 19*(3), 398–412.

Pianta, R., Howes, C., Burchinal, M., Bryant, D., Clifford, R., Early, D., et al. (2005). Features of pre-kindergarten programs, classrooms, and teachers: Do they predict observed classroom quality and child–teacher interactions? *Applied Developmental Science, 9*(3), 144–159.

Reynolds, A. J., & Temple, J. A. (2008). Cost-effective early childhood development programs from preschool to third grade. *Annual Review of Clinical Psychology, 4*, 109–139.

Rosenbaum, P. R., & Rubin, D. B. (1983). The central role of the propensity score in observational studies for causal effects. *Biometrika, 70*(1), 41–55.

Ruhm, C. J. (2004). Parental employment and child cognitive development. *Journal of Human Resources, 39*(1), 155–192.

Schweinhart, L. J., Montie, J., Xiang, Z., Barnett, W. S., Belfield, C. R., & Nores, M. (2005). *Lifetime effects: The High/Scope Perry Preschool study through age 40.* Ypsilanti, MI: High/Scope Press.

Schweinhart, L. J., & Weikart, D. P. (1997). The High/Scope Preschool Curriculum Comparison study through age 23. *Early Childhood Research Quarterly, 12*(2), 117–143.

Singer, J. D., Fuller, B., Keiley, M. K., & Wolf, A. (1998). Early child-care selection: Variation by geographic location, maternal characteristics, and family structure. *Developmental Psychology, 34*(5), 1129–1144.

Tunberger, P., & Sigle-Rushton, W. (2011). Continuity and change in Swedish family policy reforms. *Journal of European Social Policy, 21*(3), 225–237.

UNICEF. (2008). *The child care transition* (Innocenti Report Card 8). Florence, Italy: UNICEF Office of Research.

U.S. Department of Health and Human Services. (2010). *Head Start impact study: Final report.* Washington, DC: Author.

Vandell, D. L., Belsky, J., Burchinal, M., Steinberg, L., & Vandergrift, N. (2010). Do effects of early child care extend to age 15 years?: Results from the NICHD Study of Early Child Care and Youth Development. *Child Development, 81*(3), 737–756.

Vandell, D. L., & Ramanan, J. (1992). Effects of early and recent maternal employment on children from low-income families. *Child Development, 63*(4), 938–949.

Votruba-Drzal, E., Coley, R. L., & Chase-Lansdale, P. (2004). Child care and low-income children's development: Direct and moderated effects. *Child Development, 75*(1), 296–312.

Waldfogel, J., Han, W. J., & Brooks-Gunn, J. (2002). The effects of early maternal employment on child cognitive development. *Demography, 39*(2), 369–392.

Weikart, D. P., & Schweinhart, L. J. (1992). High/Scope preschool program outcomes. In J. McCord & R. E. Tremblay (Eds.), *Preventing antisocial behavior: Interventions from birth to adolescence* (pp. 67–86). New York/London: Guilford Press.

Zhai, F., Raver, C. C., & Jones, S. M. (2012). Academic performance of subsequent schools and impacts of early interventions: Evidence from a randomized controlled trial in Head Start settings. *Children and Youth Services Review, 34*(5), 946–954.

PART III

SUPPORTING SCHOOL READINESS WITH EVIDENCE-BASED PROGRAMS AND PRACTICES

CHAPTER 7

The Role of Language and Literacy Interventions in School Readiness

BARBARA A. WASIK and ANNEMARIE H. HINDMAN

One of the most critical tasks facing children in the early school years is learning to read. In order to become fluent readers by grade 4, children need to establish foundational skills long before formal reading instruction begins. Of particular importance are strong language skills, which are necessary for understanding instruction and, ultimately, for making sense of what they read. Unfortunately, many children, including a disproportionate number of those living in poverty, enter school lacking the necessary reading readiness skills and begin school on a trajectory of failure (Hart & Risley, 1995; Lee & Burkam, 2002). To address this problem, considerable attention and resources have been devoted to developing and evaluating effective preschool language and preliteracy interventions (Jackson et al., 2007; Preschool Curriculum Evaluation Research Consortium [PCERC], 2008). These programs represent the United States' frontline efforts to provide children who are at risk for reading difficulty and school failure with the skills they need to be ready for and successful in school.

In this chapter we first briefly describe the collection of foundational skills that support reading development, with a focus on the unique role of language and vocabulary. We then discuss the extent to which early schooling experiences promote these skills and review prominent early, vocabulary-focused interventions, the majority of which are professional development models for teachers. Finally, we focus on one successful intervention: Exceptional Coaching for Early Language and Literacy (**ExCELL**), reviewing empirical research on this model and highlighting remaining questions and directions for future research.

THEORETICAL AND EMPIRICAL FOUNDATIONS FOR EARLY LITERACY INTERVENTIONS

Learning to read is arguably the most important undertaking that children face in the first years of school. Reading—including decoding words and making sense of their meaning—is a multifaceted task that requires children to simultaneously integrate many skills; as a result, in order to learn to read, children must acquire a collection of foundational competencies. These foundational skills include print awareness, letter and letter-sound knowledge, phonological sensitivity, and oral language skills such as syntax and semantics (National Early Literacy Panel [NELP], 2009; Storch & Whitehurst, 2002; Whitehurst & Lonigan, 1998).

Before children can decode or make sense of their first printed word, they must develop the awareness that print is a special form of communication that carries meaning and is governed by particular language rules and conventions. Through repeated exposures to print, children learn that words, unlike pictures, are read; that letters make up words; and that reading follows a specific pattern of directionality and use of punctuation (although those logistics depend on each culture's particular rules). In addition, children must develop phonological sensitivity. In particular, it is essential that children become increasingly aware of the sounds in language, beginning with recognizing and producing similarities of sounds in words, to identifying chunks (syllables) of sounds in words, to finally being able to recognize the phonemes (the smallest unit of sounds) in words. Children also need to recognize the names and shapes of letters, as well as the specific sound(s) or phoneme(s) with which letters are associated.

Although all of these preliteracy skills are important and lay the critical foundation for reading, the development of oral language skills is particularly central to learning to read. Comprehension is the main goal of reading. Decoding is of little benefit unless children can understand the meaning of individual words and then synthesize sentences into whole ideas. Children must have well-developed vocabularies and experience with language in order to process the syntax and semantics that they have read. In addition, without strong language skills, children struggle at home and school to understand instruction on letters, sounds, and other early reading competencies (Hammer, Farkas, & Maczuga, 2010; Heinrichs et al., 2011; Hindman, Skibbe, Miller, & Zimmerman, 2010). Moreover, when children begin to read words, those with well-developed language and vocabularies can focus their cognitive energy on the considerable challenge of figuring out the word through decoding and/or recognition strategies, while using their word knowledge more readily to make sense of the text (and, quite possibly, leverage their understanding to make strategic guesses about words that are difficult to decode) (Byrnes, 2008). Conversely, children with weaker language and vocabulary knowledge will face greater difficulty. For example, when reading a story about animals of the desert, a child who knows what a *camel* is can immediately understand that word after decoding it and quickly proceed to the next word in the sentence, whereas a peer with limited vocabulary skills may be able to decode or recognize the word but not be able rapidly to make meaning of the sentence. Children must use all of these skills simultaneously while synthesizing the meaning of text in order to comprehend what is read. Limited language and especially vocabulary skills interfere in multiple ways with the primary goal of reading: comprehension (Snow, Burns, & Griffin, 1998).

The Early Achievement Gap in Vocabulary Development

Unfortunately, year after year, national datasets in the United States indicate that many children, including a high proportion of children from low-income backgrounds, demonstrate limited vocabulary and oral language skills in early childhood. For example, in nationally representative studies of the Family and Child Experiences Survey (FACES; Administration for Children and Families [ACF], 2011) and the Early Childhood Longitudinal Study–Kindergarten Cohort (ECLS-K; National Center for Education Statistics [NCES], 2011), data show that children in poverty enter preschool and kindergarten with language and vocabulary skills nearly a full standard deviation below the national average (ACF, 2011; Lee & Burkam, 2002). This gap widens over time (e.g., Lee, 2011; Stanovich, 1986), and by fourth grade, half of the children in poverty cannot read with even basic fluency, compared to just 25% of those from middle-income backgrounds (National Assessment of Educational Progress [NAEP], 2010).

Theoretical and Empirical Foundations of Language Development Interventions

Given the import of language and vocabulary development—and particularly the need to address the persistent and pernicious vocabulary gap that separates children from low- and middle-income backgrounds—many research efforts in recent decades have examined how children learn and can be taught words. The predominant theory regarding word learning in early education draws on Vygotsky's (1978) work, which suggests that children learn language, including vocabulary, in the context of social interactions with more skilled interlocutors, including parents, teachers, and peers. These expert conversational partners scaffold, or strategically support, children's knowledge of word meanings, guiding them toward complete understanding of the definitions and pronunciations of words.

The empirical literature on the precise scaffolds and situations that support vocabulary development is vast and increasingly unambiguous. With the exception of relatively rare fast mapping, children need multiple (i.e., between four and 14), meaningful exposures to learn about new words and the patterns of grammar and syntax that govern the use of these words (Elley, 1989; Hoff, 2000). Moreover, not all exposures are equally effective; instead, several supports increase the probability that children will understand and remember a new word. First, children learn best when new words are presented to them in a meaningful context, such as rich conversation, a story, or an in-depth study of a theme, rather than in isolation through tools such as flashcards (Ruston & Schwanenflugel, 2010). Connections to children's background knowledge may be particularly important. Second, although children are remarkably skilled at deriving the meanings of words through implicit instruction, their knowledge is best scaffolded with clear definitions and explanations in child-friendly language, including images, props, or other unambiguous stimuli (Lugo-Neris, Jackson, & Goldstein, 2010). When appropriate, information focusing on the function of a novel object might be particularly memorable (Booth, 2006). Third, distributed exposure to new words over time, spiraling toward increasingly sophisticated content, supports word learning (Zipoli, Coyne, & McCoach, 2011). Finally, having the opportunity to use and receive feedback on the meaning and pronunciation of new words is critical (Beck & McKeown, 2007; Coyne, McCoach, & Kapp, 2007; Coyne, Simmons, Kame'enui, & Stoolmiller, 2004).

Exposure to Vocabulary in Early Childhood Settings

There is considerable evidence that families vary in the degree to which they expose children to new words, with low-income families (who often face multiple risks and stressors) using fewer words at home, providing a smaller variety of different words, and offering children less frequent opportunities to use language and receive feedback on that language (Dickinson & Tabors, 2001; Hart & Risley, 1995). This inequity of experiences places particular pressure on schooling experiences to provide highly effective vocabulary instruction for all children, but particularly those in poverty, during the school transition period. Unfortunately, accumulating evidence indicates that early childhood school settings offer little focus on vocabulary, especially compared to time spent on letters, sounds, and conventions of print. In a review of preschool curricula, Neuman and Dwyer (2009) concluded that vocabulary instruction was virtually nonexistent and that "strategies that introduce young children to new words and entice them to engage in meaningful contexts through semantically related activities are much needed" (p. 384). In the absence of this guidance, descriptive classroom studies show that early childhood teachers spend an average of only 5 minutes per day explicitly developing oral language and vocabulary skills (Beck & McKeown, 2007; Biemiller, 2001; Cunningham, Zibulsky, Stanovich, & Stanovich, 2009; Juel, Biancarosa, Coker, & Deffes, 2003). Much of the language exchanged is of a managerial nature, even during potentially vocabulary-intensive activities such as book reading (Dickinson, 2001; Hindman, Connor, Jewkes, & Morrison, 2008; Hindman, Wasik, & Erhart, 2012). Not surprisingly, data suggest that the effects of most early childhood classrooms on vocabulary are minimal (Pianta, Belsky, Houts, Morrison, & the National Institute of Child Health and Human Development Early Child Care Research Network [NICHD-ECCRN], 2007; Skibbe, Connor, Morrison, & Jewkes, 2011).

Language- and Vocabulary-Building Interventions

In response to the need to provide effective word-learning opportunities, especially for children from underresourced households and communities, a number of interventions aimed at early childhood language and literacy settings (i.e., preschool and kindergarten) have been carefully studied. In virtually all of the available research on preschool and kindergarten vocabulary instruction, investigators used storybooks as the meaningful context from which vocabulary was drawn. Storybooks represent uniquely powerful tools in the effort to build vocabulary, as they provide rich information about words children are not likely to encounter in their daily lives (e.g., *camels, elephants*), accompanied by pictures that help to explain these words (Hoff, 2010; Ganea, Pickard, & DeLoache, 2008; Mol, Bus, de Jong, & Smeets, 2008). Not only can books bring novel words into children's lives, but when words are central to the narrative of a book, they are often used multiple times in the book and can figure heavily into conversations about the book between and among adults and children. Moreover, books can be revisited many times, so that children can engage in distributed practice with these new words (Beck & McKeown, 2007). Notably, individual word meanings may become especially salient for children as the story becomes highly familiar and, thus, demands less attention from children as they hear the book being read. Finally, books can serve as springboards for the integration of vocabulary words in conversations before, during, and after the reading, as well as for follow-up activities featuring these words. This approach is consistent with the work of Wasik and colleagues (Wasik & Bond, 2001; Wasik, Bond, & Hindman, 2006), demonstrating that if teachers engineer interactive storybook readings and coordinated extension activities around the same core set of words, preschoolers' vocabularies increase.

In the well-researched Text Talk intervention, Beck and McKeown (2007) conducted a series of important studies that evaluated the impact of what they termed "rich instruction" in kindergarten and first grade. During read-aloud time, teachers contextualized, defined, and provided examples of target words from the read-aloud books; furthermore, they used words in sentences and invited children to judge whether they were used correctly, and encouraged children to repeat and talk about the words. Results showed that children who received this rich instruction learned significantly more of the words than those without such instruction, and that children who received a greater amount of rich instruction doubled the gains of those with less exposure. The resulting Text Talk intervention functions as a supplemental vocabulary program for students in grades K–3.

In much the same vein, Coyne and colleagues' work tested the effectiveness of extended vocabulary instruction in kindergarten (Coyne et al., 2007; Coyne, McCoach, Loftus, Zipoli, & Kapp, 2009). In this model, researchers worked with young children, explicitly defining and providing contextual information about new words on multiple occasions across varied contexts. Researchers also provided game-like tasks that encouraged children to use the words in meaningful ways. For example, researchers said, "I'll tell you about some things. If you think it is strong, say 'That's sturdy!' If you think it's not very strong, say, 'That's not sturdy.'" Children were then asked open-ended questions that encouraged extension of and elaboration on initial responses. Children in this explicit vocabulary instruction condition learned more words than peers exposed to the same words but without explicit guidance. Critically, learning was maintained after delayed posttesting, suggesting that children had successfully encoded these new words and made them a part of their vocabularies. Finally, using a similar routine of activities, Biemiller and Boote (2006) also found that kindergartners and first graders learned more novel words when teachers provided two or more read-alouds of books that featured new words and explained the meanings of these words. Consistent findings were also discovered in a study by Silverman and Crandell (2010).

Thus, a consensus is emerging that explicit, relevant instruction accompanied by opportunities to practice new words in meaningful ways can support word learning in early childhood settings, including among children in poverty who face the highest risks for vocabulary challenges and, thus, reading difficulties. However, this work has focused on children's acquisition of words, with little regard for how best to train teachers to implement these language-building instructional strategies. For example, Coyne et al. (2009) had researchers deliver the book readings, while Beck and McKeown (2007) and Biemiller and Boote (2006) had teachers deliver highly structured experiences for children over a short span of time with fairly limited and focused professional development. These studies focused on the value of the intervention for children's learning rather than on how to ensure that teachers could deliver this high-quality instruction independently, with fidelity, over time.

This gap is important, because there is ample evidence in the literature that even well-designed programs do not necessarily support vocabulary learning when placed in the field with minimal support from researchers. For example, the Preschool Curriculum Evaluation Research (PCER) program (PCERC, 2008) evaluated more than a dozen well-crafted preschool curricula and assessed children on a variety of preliteracy skills, including alphabet knowledge, phonological sensitivity, and vocabulary. Of all of the programs evaluated, only one program had effects on vocabulary, and the same program had effects on alphabet knowledge and phonological sensitivity. In addition, one other program raised alphabet knowledge. Together these data suggest that even with the substantial pool of resources available to PCER participants, it was difficult to advance teachers' skills in helping children get ready to read, and particularly challenging to help teachers build the unconstrained skill of vocabulary. In order to engender lasting, significant improvements in vocabulary and language instruction in preschool and kindergarten, especially for children in poverty, it is necessary to build on this research base to identify what teachers need to learn and do so as to deliver instruction with these effective features consistently and independently. In doing so, teachers can prepare children with the readiness skills needed for the task of learning to read.

Effective Professional Development for Teachers around Vocabulary

At present, the strongest literature on professional development around teachers' language and vocabulary instruction features preschool teachers but illuminates components that are likely to be effective among kindergarten and first-grade teachers. Effective professional development provides accurate *conceptual information* about how children's skills develop, as well as *procedural information* about what practices (e.g., identifying and defining target words in a meaningful context and providing repeated exposure to and use of new words) should be implemented in the classroom (Dickinson & Brady, 2006; Jackson et al., 2007). Research on professional development for preschool teachers as a tool for changing educators' conceptual and procedural knowledge and, by extension, children's skills has focused on coaching (e.g., Joyce & Showers, 1981, 1982; Showers & Joyce, 1996), and the popularity of this method has recently escalated (Landry, Anthony, Swank, & Monseque-Bailey, 2009; Neuman & Cunningham, 2009).

The International Reading Association (IRA; 2004) defines a *literacy coach* as "a reading specialist who focuses on providing professional development for teachers by giving them the additional support needed to implement various instructional programs and practices." However, this definition is broad, and institutions and interventions differ on key topics, such as how coaches are trained and monitored, how much time they spend with teachers, what strategies they train teachers to use, and how they monitor teachers. While research suggests that either face-to-face meetings between coaches and teachers or Web-mediated interactions support change in teachers' practices (Adger, Hoyle, & Dickinson, 2004; Dickinson & Caswell, 2007; Neuman & Cunningham, 2009; Pianta, Mashburn, Downer, Hamre, & Justice, 2008), most studies have *not* examined the impact of teacher professional development on child outcomes.

In the few studies that have drawn this important connection, significant effects on children's language outcomes are rare. For example, a recent evaluation of a random selection of Early Reading First projects (Jackson et al., 2007) showed that much of the training had positive impacts on teachers' classroom practices, including their language and literacy environments, instructional practices, and use of assessment, and that children who participated in Early Reading First programs had stronger print and letter knowledge than those whose teachers did not receive this training. On average, however, children were no different from nonintervention peers on language skills, including vocabulary and phonological awareness. In other Early Reading First programs children have shown improvements in phonemic awareness and emergent writing but, again, not in expressive language skills (DeBaryshe & Gorecki, 2007). For example, Powell, Diamond, Burchinal, and Koehler (2010) designed and implemented a well-developed language and literacy coaching intervention. According to Powell et al., the professional development emphasized classroom strategies to improve children's oral language skills and code-focused skills, particularly phonological awareness and letter knowledge.

Oral language outcomes included vocabulary knowledge, listening comprehension skills, and syntactic knowledge, and key techniques featured teaching practices (e.g., asking questions) that elicited and expanded children's use of language. In addition, teachers were given printed copies and demonstrations of phonological awareness activities developed by Adams, Foorman, Lundberg, and Beeler (1998) and were encouraged to emphasize letter sounds when teaching letter names and to use writing to promote letter knowledge (Diamond, Gerde, & Powell, 2008). After teachers received intensive training and coaching, and viewed videos of exemplary teacher practices, significant increases in children's alphabet knowledge and phonological awareness were found, yet with no effects on their vocabulary skills.

In contrast, several interventions, including that of the Center for Improving the Readiness of Children for Learning and Education (CIRCLE; Landry, Swank, Smith, Assel, & Gunnewig, 2006; Landry et al., 2009) and the ExCELL program (Wasik et al., 2006; Wasik & Hindman, 2011b) have been linked to children's vocabulary development. Both CIRCLE and ExCELL have professional development interventions that include training on development of children's oral language, phonological sensitivity, alphabet knowledge, and writing skills. Like other programs, these interventions provided intensive training, including group workshops and several hours of individualized coaching per month (4 hours per month in CIRCLE and 12 hours per month in ExCELL), to help teachers refine their understanding of new ideas and implement related practices in their classrooms. However, one factor that CIRCLE and ExCELL did include that may not have been part of the other effective programs was progress-monitoring tools to follow children's learning over time. Finally, ExCELL teachers also received supplemental materials modeling explicit strategies to enhance language and vocabulary in their instruction. In both CIRCLE and ExCELL, teachers who participated showed moderate-to-large growth in the quality of their classroom language practices, such as asking open-ended questions, modeling complex language for children, and providing meaningful feedback on children's language. In turn, children experienced moderate-to-large gains on alphabet and phonological awareness, as well as small-to-moderate gains in language growth, including vocabulary.

Given the need to make such learning opportunities available to the wider community of preschool and kindergarten teachers and students, we describe the ExCELL program in greater detail below, including the precise conditions under which ExCELL engenders the greatest gains for participants. Furthermore, we highlight remaining questions about the specific mechanisms through which ExCELL operates on teachers and children.

Exceptional Coaching for Early Language and Literacy

ExCELL is a comprehensive professional development model designed to increase teachers' use of research-based strategies to promote language and preliteracy development in preschoolers. Using research-based strategies, ExCELL focuses on developing oral language and vocabulary, as well as phonological sensitivity, alphabet knowledge, and emergent writing skills in preschool children. ExCELL includes (1) intensive training, including monthly, 3-hour group training and weekly coaching sessions; (2) materials such as lesson plans and books for thematic units of study, including activities that support language and literacy development; and (3) ongoing assessment of both teachers and children to monitor learning and, when necessary, target areas of difficulty. ExCELL has been implemented in over 75 Baltimore City, Maryland, Head Start classrooms.

In the group training, a coach provides teachers with a rationale for focusing on a particular aspect of early language and literacy (e.g., asking open-ended questions during book reading) and explains how this practice supports children's learning. Then, the coach describes and models a series of techniques for teachers to use when implementing this practice in the classroom. Finally, teachers plan how they will use these techniques in their own classrooms. During the 3 weeks after the training, a coach visits each teacher's classroom each week. During this time, the coach works individually with the lead teacher and follows a specified sequence of activities: (1) modeling specific strategies from the training; (2) videotaping the teacher using these strategies; (3) assessing the teacher's efforts, using a fidelity of implementation measure; and (4) providing explicit feedback to the teacher on his or her classroom practices and particularly his or her use of instructional language in the classroom. Thus, teachers receive individualized guidance based on ongoing assessments of their classroom performance.

There are five training modules in ExCELL (see Wasik & Hindman, 2011a). These include oral language development, viewed as the foundation for the subsequent models, as well as book reading, alphabet knowledge, phonological sensitivity, and writing. The training for each module is divided further into specific issues related to the broader topic. For example, the oral language development module includes three trainings: (1) an introduction to research explaining why oral language establishes a solid foundation for young children's reading skills and how creating opportunities for conversations promotes oral language development; (2) questioning strategies that include asking open-ended questions and questions that allow children to "fill-in" missing information; and (3) specific strategies for modeling rich language, providing meaningful feedback to children during a conversation, and expanding children's language by recasting what they say in a more rich, elaborate way. Each training is conducted in a 3-hour session with a group of 10–20 teachers after the end of the school day. Teachers are also given lesson plans that include recommended activities for oral language, alphabet knowledge, phonological sensitivity, and writing. However, teachers are encouraged but not obligated to follow the lesson plans with fidelity.

Findings from ExCELL

In order to understand the impact of ExCELL on both teachers and children, we conducted a series of randomized controlled evaluations (Wasik et al., 2006; Wasik & Hindman, 2011a, 2011b). Teachers and children in the ExCELL program were compared to teachers and children who received the "business as usual" Head Start professional development and curriculum. These studies addressed efficacy questions (e.g., the degree to which ExCELL training had a positive impact on teacher and child outcomes), mechanisms of change (e.g., how changes in teachers' practices affected changes in child outcomes), and moderators of change (e.g., how children's characteristics affected their learning during ExCELL).

ExCELL's Impact on Teachers

ExCELL professional development trains teachers to implement research-based strategies in order to increase children's language and preliteracy skills. Observers rated teachers on the Instructional Support domain of the Classroom Assessment Scoring System–PreK (CLASS-PreK; Pianta, LaParo, & Hamre, 2007), which measures the overall quality of classroom instruction, including concept development, language modeling, and feedback that teachers provide to children. In addition, all intervention classrooms were observed using a program-specific fidelity measure gauging the degree to which teachers implemented ExCELL as intended. In addition, teachers' classrooms were observed using the Literacy Environment Checklist of the ELLCO toolkit (Smith, Dickinson, Sangeorge, & Anastasopoulos, 2002), which assessed the availability and use of language- and literacy-building resources such as books and writing materials. Finally, to assess these effects, in the fall and again in the spring, teachers were administered a teacher belief and knowledge survey, designed to assess their ideas about language and literacy.

The findings from randomized controlled trials suggest that teachers in ExCELL significantly outperformed their peers in the "usual practice" control group on teacher quality and language interactions (Wasik & Hindman, 2011b). Specifically, ExCELL teachers provided better scaffolding for concept development and more quality feedback to support children's language development compared to teachers in the control group. The most significant effects on the CLASS Instructional Support domain were found in language modeling, as ExCELL teachers engaged in more frequent conversations, asked more open-ended questions, and used more advanced vocabulary words. For all subscales of the CLASS, intervention participation was linked to a gain of approximately one standard deviation, a large effect. In summary, ExCELL professional development was effective in improving the quality of teachers' instruction and language interactions, an important finding in light of research showing that these language modeling opportunities create a context for children to develop language and vocabulary skills (Bowers & Vasilyeva, 2011).

Teachers in ExCELL classrooms also provided children with more access to literacy experiences, as measured by the ELLCO. While ExCELL and control classrooms showed no differences in availability and use of books—likely because the ExCELL project provided the same materials to all classrooms, whether teachers received training or not—ExCELL classrooms provided children with more writing materials and made more frequent use of these tools. This difference in writing presents an interesting finding. In ExCELL, teachers were trained to conceptualize writing as a technique that allows children to call on their language skills to construct messages and then employ alphabet knowledge and phonemic awareness to write this message down. The control teachers did not receive any writing training as part of their professional development. This disparity in access to information about writing could have resulted in differences in the classroom practices in ExCELL and control classrooms.

In an attempt to understand at an even more specific level how ExCELL affected important teacher practices, we examined how teachers' book-reading practices changed after the intervention. In our own work (Wasik & Bond, 2001; Wasik et al., 2006) and in early childhood research (Marulis & Neuman, 2010; Mol et al., 2008), book reading is often identified as a central activity in the development of young children's language and literacy skills. Analysis of a book-reading activity—using the same book in both the ExCELL and control classrooms in the spring after training had occurred—revealed interesting differences in teachers' use of language-building techniques. Given that ExCELL teachers were found to use higher-quality language in the classroom (including concrete and abstract comments and questions) as measured by the CLASS tool, similar findings were expected during book reading. This, however, did not occur; instead, analyses revealed no statistical differences between ExCELL and control teachers in the number of questions and comments teachers made about either concrete or abstract information during the book reading, using the same book. It is important to note that the number was high in both conditions (with teachers making an average of 40 concrete remarks and 25 abstract remarks), suggesting that both groups of teachers were engaging children in discussion of texts. There were, however, significant differences in how teachers allowed children to talk, with teachers in the intervention offering children more opportunities to use one-word and multiword utterances during the book reading. Currently, we are conducting a follow-up study to explore the quality of the questions that teachers asked during reading to determine whether there were differences across conditions, and particularly whether teachers with ExCELL training asked more questions specifically focused on vocabulary in the book. We are also examining whether children in the intervention used target vocabulary words more frequently in their responses.

ExCELL's Impact on Children

Beyond understanding the impact of ExCELL on teacher skills, it is also essential to explore how professional development is linked to child outcomes. A series of measures was administered to children in ExCELL and control classrooms at the start and at the end of the year in order to determine the program's impact on child outcomes. All children were assessed on the Peabody Picture Vocabulary Test–III (PPVT-III; Dunn & Dunn, 1997), a "gold standard" measure of receptive language skills. In addition, a progress-monitoring measure designed to tap into the specific vocabulary highlighted in ExCELL classrooms was administered three times per year to all children in these classrooms. From all of the words related to themes that the classroom had studied since the last progress-monitoring assessment, 10 words were selected randomly to be used on the assessment (e.g., *cow, leaves, farm*). Teachers did not know which words were selected. Picture cards were created to depict these 10 randomly selected vocabulary words. Children were shown each of the 10 picture vocabulary cards and asked to name what they saw in the picture (tapping expressive vocabulary). For any items that they could not correctly identify, children were next shown a card with that image, as well as three others, and asked to point to that item (i.e., receptive vocabulary). Finally, while vocabulary was a particular focus of ExCELL, other language and literacy skills were assessed. Among 4-year-olds, alphabet knowledge and phonological skills were assessed using subtests of the Phonological Awareness Literacy Screening–PreK (PALS-PreK; Invernizzi, Sullivan, Meier, & Swank, 2004). Specifically, children were asked to identify each upper- and lowercase letter of the alphabet, as well as the rimes and onsets of words.

The findings from the randomized controlled studies indicate that children in ExCELL classrooms significantly outperformed children in the control classrooms on standardized vocabulary measures (PPVT-III).

Specifically, the final hierarchical linear model (HLM) revealed that children in the intervention outperformed their peers in the spring (beta = 3.57, p = .04), controlling for children's fall vocabulary skills, as well as their age, gender, and disability status, and their teacher's education and classroom exposure to public preschool (Wasik & Hindman, 2011a, 2011b). Beyond everything else in the model, participation in the intervention explained 17% of the variance between classrooms in children's vocabulary skills, an effect of moderate size.

This finding is significant for several reasons. First, changes in children's vocabulary performance on standardized assessments have been difficult for even well-designed interventions to demonstrate, as evidenced by the many null associations in the PCER evaluation (PCERC, 2008). It is also important to note that these effects emerged on a measure that is age-normed, meaning that a typically developing child would not be expected to increase his or her standardized score over the 9-month school year (i.e., a child who began the year with a score of 100, the national average, and learned as much as his or her peers over the year, would conclude the year with a score of 100). Thus, children in ExCELL not only kept pace with expected growth but also actually exceeded the predicted or typical rate of word learning. Given the importance of early vocabulary in later reading (Dickinson & Porche, 2011), these findings are critical in helping to inform teacher training.

Similar positive results were found for the curriculum-specific progress-monitoring data. Children in the ExCELL program learned more than 75% of the target words presented on the curriculum-based progress-monitoring measure (Wasik, Hindman, & Jusczyk, 2009). These findings suggest that children were, in fact, learning the words that were presented in class, as well as acquiring more general vocabulary as measured by the PPVT-III. It appears that the strategies that teachers were implementing in the classroom promoted the increased pace of vocabulary knowledge acquisition observed in the children.

One question of importance that needs to be addressed is whether ExCELL has differential impacts on children with different abilities. In many interventions, a Matthew effect emerges, such that children who begin the intervention with more skills are better able to take advantage of instruction and acquire even more knowledge as the intervention goes on (Lee, 2011; Stanovich, 1986). At the same time, children who have the fewest skills make the smallest gains and exit the intervention with the lowest skills—often with the gap between the groups widening as a result of exposure to the program. To address this question, we examined the differential effects of ExCELL on children with varied skill levels. The results (see Hindman, Erhart, & Wasik, 2012) suggest that children who entered ExCELL with the lowest language skills grew more than children with higher language skills. We suggest several reasons for this finding. First, the use of progress monitoring informs teachers about what vocabulary specific children are learning. Along with coaches, teachers review the findings of the progress monitoring and make adaptations in their instruction. One adaptation in ExCELL was to place children with similar skills in the same small groups and focus explicit instruction on the vocabulary and language skills with which they were struggling. This attention to children who were struggling in class may provide one explanation for this finding. In addition, ExCELL professional development guides teachers in developing a wide range of vocabulary, focusing on both complex vocabulary words (labeled as Tier Two and Tier Three vocabulary words by Beck & McKeown, 2007) as well as simple vocabulary (labeled as Tier One words). Tier One vocabulary comprises relatively common words that, in fact, many young children (especially those from underresourced homes or communities) may not know. These words are often overlooked in instruction, even though they are critical for children's oral language comprehension. Finally, another plausible explanation is that young children with limited language skills are not frequently given opportunities to talk and use language. In ExCELL, teachers are trained to provide all children with opportunities to use language and communicate their ideas and needs in a meaningful context. Although this is a more difficult part of the intervention to measure, the findings from the CLASS data do indicate that ExCELL classrooms provide enhanced opportunities for children to hear and use language. Thus, positive effects for children with limited language skills could grow from the relatively greater opportunities that these children enjoy in ExCELL to participate in and practice with discourse.

Beyond vocabulary to other important, early, reading-related skills, findings also indicate that children in ExCELL classrooms performed significantly better on phonological sensitivity measures. Our analyses indicate that, over and above the collection of covariates, the intervention made a significant contribution to children's skills (beta = 2.04, $p < .01$), explaining 26% of the variance between classrooms, a large association. This finding is consistent with the fact that children who acquire more vocabulary words and learn more about language also become increasingly sensitive to the different sounds that comprise words (Metsala & Walley, 1998).

Interestingly, children in ExCELL and control classrooms made significant gains in letter knowledge over the course of the year, although there were no differences between these conditions in the number of letters learned. This finding may reflect the fact that the unique and powerful role of letter knowledge as a predictor of subsequent child literacy learning has been widely publicized in the last decade, and that teachers in Head Start and other programs have received extensive training on letter instruction. Thus, even without intensive ExCELL professional development, Head Start centers may provide effective instruction in this area. Another possible point of consideration behind this finding is that relative to the abstract language-related skills of vocabulary and sound awareness, letter learning is essentially a paired-associates task and can often be accomplished through repetition. Thus, less professional development may be necessary for this content area.

FUTURE QUESTIONS TO EXPLORE

The findings from ExCELL are promising and suggest that professional development can impact teachers' instructional practices and, in turn, children's language and preliteracy outcomes. However, as we consider providing ExCELL to teachers on a wider scale, several important questions remain.

Perhaps the most critical question concerning ExCELL is which components of the professional development are most important for improving the quality of teacher–child language interactions. In its current form, ExCELL provides very intensive support to teachers, including weekly observations and coaching, and monthly training. Although the costs of this professional development, considering its positive results, are far lower than the costs of children entering school not ready to read and embarking on a trajectory of school failure (Camili, Vargas, Ryan, & Barnett, 2010), school district budgets are shrinking, and few have the resources to provide professional development of this intensity. Therefore, in our current work, we are trying to identify what components are both necessary and sufficient to change teachers' practices and increase children's language skills.

Based on our previous work (Wasik & Bond, 2001; Wasik et al., 2006), we are exploring the role that book reading can play in enhancing teachers' skills. We acknowledge that considerable research has questioned the impact of book reading on children's language development (Marulis & Neuman, 2010; Scarborough & Dobrich, 1995). However, we consider language-rich book readings and follow-up activities with salient target vocabulary as the nexus for classroom language and literacy development efforts (Hoff, 2010; Wasik & Bond, 2001). It may be possible to focus ExCELL professional development on book-reading and follow-up activities, and achieve the same teacher and child results with more streamlined content. In addition, recent work on professional development has shown the positive impact of using videos and remote coaching to improve teachers' skills and practice (Pianta et al., 2008; Powell et al., 2010). Although face-to-face, *in situ,* individualized coaching is very powerful, ExCELL coaches report that one of their most effective tools is having teachers view videos of themselves while they (coaches) provide feedback on the video. Training could be further streamlined if coaches provided feedback on videos through a secure website rather than traveling to sites.

In ExCELL, all teachers were provided with the same amount, or dose, of training. One issue that needs to be explored is whether all teachers, despite the varying levels of knowledge and skills with which they enter the intervention, need the same amount and type of training. Perhaps training could be individualized for teachers. For example, teachers might take an initial assessment and videotape themselves conducting a variety of activities in their classroom (e.g., book reading, morning message, center activities) before training begins. Experienced coaches could review these videos to identify specific strengths and weaknesses for each teacher. An individualized training program could then be designed to meet that teacher's particular needs. This strategy would optimize the use of coaches' resources, providing intensive basic coaching to teachers with the lowest skills, while affording more advanced training for more skilled teachers.

Finally, the issue of sustainability is critical to any effective intervention. One of the reasons that ExCELL focuses on teachers' conceptual understanding of topics—the *why* of implementing specific strategies and practices rather than simply providing scripts or routines—is to ensure that teachers understand the rationale behind these techniques and permanently incorporate them into their teaching. To determine whether teachers continued to use the strategies in which they were trained, teachers in ExCELL were assessed on the CLASS and ELLCO 1 year after the training was completed. Preliminary findings indicate that ExCELL teachers continued to maintain high scores on these measures of classroom quality. In addition, ExCELL teachers continued to score high on program-specific fidelity measures, suggesting that they also continued to implement ExCELL even after training ended.

Summary and Conclusions

In summary, there is widespread recognition that developing vocabulary in the preschool years is critical for the rapid acquisition of formal reading skills. Theoretical frameworks and empirical data suggest that vocabulary is best fostered through multiple, meaningful exchanges with others in the course of conversations and other formal and informal instructional exchanges. The ExCELL professional development model is one program that has demonstrated positive effects on teachers' practices and children's outcomes. Research on this and other models is ongoing, providing new information that promises to help close the vocabulary achievement gap between low-income children and their more advantaged peers at its narrowest point, before the start of formal schooling.

References

Adams, M. J., Foorman, B. R., Lundberg, I., & Beeler, T. (1998). *Phonemic awareness in young children: A classroom curriculum.* Baltimore: Brookes.

Adger, C. T., Hoyle, S. M., & Dickinson, D. K. (2004). Located learning in inservice eduation for preschool teachers. *American Educational Research Journal, 41,* 867–900.

Administration for Children and Families (ACF). (2011). *Family and Child Experiences Dataset.* Retrieved October 1, 2011, from *www.researchconnections.org/childcare/resources/14345.*

Beck, I. L., & McKeown, M. G. (2007). Increasing young low-income children's oral vocabulary repertoires through rich and focused instruction. *Elementary School Journal, 107,* 251–271.

Biemiller, A. (2001). Teaching vocabulary: Early, direct, and sequential. *The American Educator, 25*(1), 24–28.

Biemiller, A., & Boote, C. (2006). An effective method for building meaning vocabulary in primary grades. *Journal of Educational Psychology, 98,* 44–62.

Booth, A. E. (2006). Object function and categorization in infancy: Two mechanisms of facilitation. *Infancy, 10*(2), 145–169.

Bowers, E., & Vasilyeva, M. (2011). The relation between teacher input and lexical growth of preschoolers. *Applied Psycholinguistics, 32,* 221–241.

Byrnes, J. P. (2008). *Cognitive development and learning in instructional contexts* (3rd ed.). New York: Allyn & Bacon.

Camilli, G., Vargas, S., Ryan, S., & Barnett, W. S. (2010). Meta-analysis of the effects of early education interventions on cognitive and social development. *Teachers College Record, 112,* 579–620.

Coyne, M. D., McCoach, D. B., & Kapp, S. (2007). Vocabulary intervention for kindergarten students: Comparing extended instruction to embedded instruction and incidental exposure. *Learning Disability Quarterly, 30,* 74–88.

Coyne, M. D., McCoach, D. B., Loftus, S., Zipoli, R., Jr., & Kapp, S. (2009). Direct vocabulary instruction in kindergarten: Teaching for breadth versus depth. *Elementary School Journal, 110,* 1–18.

Coyne, M. D., Simmons, D. C., Kame'enui, E. J., & Stoolmiller, M. (2004). Teaching vocabulary during shared storybook readings: An examination of differential effects. *Exceptionality, 12,* 145–162.

Cunningham, A. E., Zibulsky, J., Stanovich, K. E., & Stanovich, P. J. (2009). How teachers would spend their time teaching language arts: The mismatch between self-reported and best practices. *Journal of Learning Disabilities, 42,* 418–430.

DeBaryshe, B. D., & Gorecki, D. M. (2007). An experimental validation of a preschool emergent literacy curriculum. *Early Education and Development, 18,* 93–110.

Diamond, K. E., Gerde, H. K., & Powell, D. R. (2008). Development in early literacy skills during the pre-kindergarten year in Head Start: Relations between growth in children's writing and understanding of letters. *Early Childhood Research Quarterly, 23,* 467–478.

Dickinson, D. K. (2001). Book reading in preschool classrooms: Is recommended practice common? In D. K. Dickinson & P. O. Tabors (Eds.), *Beginning literacy with language: Young children learning at home and school* (pp. 175–203). Baltimore: Brookes.

Dickinson, D. K., & Brady, J. P. (2006). Toward effective support for language and literacy through professional development. In M. J. Zaslow & I. Martinez-Beck (Eds.), *Critical issues in early childhood professional development* (pp. 141–170). Baltimore: Brookes.

Dickinson, D., & Caswell, L. (2007). Building support for language and early literacy in preschool classrooms through in-service professional development: Effects of the Literacy Environment Enrichment Program (LEEP). *Early Childhood Research Quarterly, 22,* 243–260.

Dickinson, D. K., & Porche, M. V. (2011). Relation between language experiences in preschool classrooms and children's kindergarten and fourth-grade language and reading abilities. *Child Development, 82,* 870–886.

Dickinson, D. K., & Tabors, P. O. (Eds.). (2001). *Beginning literacy with language: Young children learning at home and school.* Baltimore: Brookes.

Dunn, L. M., & Dunn, L. M. (1997). *Peabody Picture Vocabulary Test–III* (3rd ed.). Circle Pines, MN: American Guidance Services.

Elley, W. B. (1989). Vocabulary acquisition from stories. *Reading Research Quarterly, 24,* 174–187.

Ganea, P. A., Pickard, M. B., & DeLoache, J. S. (2008). Transfer between picture books and the real world by very young children. *Journal of Cognition and Development, 9,* 46–66.

Hammer, C. S., Farkas, G., & Maczuga, S. (2010). The language and literacy development of Head Start children: A study using the Family and Child Experiences Survey database. *Language, Speech, and Hearing Services in Schools, 41,* 70–83.

Hart, B., & Risley, T. R. (1995). *Meaningful differences in the everyday experience of young American children.* Baltimore: Brookes.

Hayes, B. K., & Hennessy, R. (1996). The nature and development of nonverbal implicit memory. *Journal of Experimental Child Psychology, 63,* 22–43.

Henrichs, J., Rescorla, L., Schenk, J. J., Schmidt, H. G., Jaddoe, V. W. V., Hofman, A., et al. (2011). Examining continuity of early expressive vocabulary development: The Generation R Study. *Journal of Speech, Language, and Hearing Research, 54,* 854–869.

Hindman, A. H., Connor, C. M., Jewkes, A. M., & Morrison, F. J. (2008). Untangling the effects of shared book reading: Multiple factors and their associations with preschool literacy outcomes. *Early Childhood Research Quarterly, 23,* 330–350.

Hindman, A. H., Erhart, A. M., & Wasik, B. A. (2012). Reducing the Matthew effect: Lessons from the ExCELL Head Start intervention. *Early Education and Development, 23*(5), 781–806.

Hindman, A. H., Skibbe, L. E., Miller, A., & Zimmerman, M. (2010). Ecological contexts and early learning: Contributions of child, family, and classroom factors during Head Start to literacy and mathematics growth through first grade. *Early Childhood Research Quarterly, 25*, 235–250.

Hindman, A. H., Wasik, B. A., & Erhart, A. M. (2012). Shared book reading and Head Start preschoolers' vocabulary learning: The role of book-related discussion and curricularconnections. *Early Education and Development, 23*(4), 451–474.

Hoff, E. (2000). *Language development* (2nd ed.). New York: Wadsworth.

Hoff, E. (2010). Context effects on young children's language use: The influence of conversational setting and partner. *First Language, 30*, 461–472.

International Reading Association (IRA). (2004). *The role and qualifications of the reading coach in the United States.* Newark, DE: Author. Retrieved April 13, 2013, from *www.reading.org/downloads/resources/545standards2003.*

Invernizzi, M., Sullivan, A., Meier, J., & Swank, L. (2004). *PALS Pre-K Phonological Awareness Screening.* Charlottesville: University of Virginia.

Jackson, R., McCoy, A., Pistorino, C., Wilkinson, A., Burghardt, J., Clark, M., et al. (2007). *National evaluation of Early Reading First: Final report.* Washington, DC: U.S. Government Printing Office.

Joyce, B. R., & Showers, B. (1981). Transfer of training: The contribution of "coaching." *Journal of Education, 163*, 163–172.

Joyce, B., & Showers, B. (1982). The coaching of teaching. *Educational Leadership, 40*, 4–8.

Juel, C., Biancarosa, G., Coker, D., & Deffes, R. (2003). Walking with Rosie: A cautionary tale of early reading instruction. *Educational Leadership, 60*, 12–18.

Landry, S. H., Anthony, J. L., Swank, P. R., & Monseque-Bailey, P. (2009). Effectiveness of comprehensive professional development for teachers of at-risk preschoolers. *Journal of Educational Psychology, 101*, 448–465.

Landry, S. H., Swank, P. R., Smith, K. E., Assel, M. A., & Gunnewig, S. B. (2006). Enhancing early literacy skills for preschool children: Bringing a professional development model to scale. *Journal of Learning Disabilities, 39*, 306–325.

Lee, J. (2011). Size matters: Early vocabulary as a predictor of language and literacy competence. *Applied Psycholinguistics, 32*, 69–92.

Lee, V. E., & Burkam, D. (2002). *Inequality at the starting gate: Social background differences in achievement as children begin school.* Washington, DC: Economic Policy Institute.

Lugo-Neris, M. J., Jackson, C. W., & Goldstein, H. (2010). Facilitating vocabulary acquisition of young English language learners. *Language, Speech, and Hearing Services in Schools, 41*, 314–327.

Marulis, L. M., & Neuman, S. B. (2010). The effects of vocabulary intervention on young children's word learning: A meta-analysis. *Review of Educational Research, 80*, 300–335.

Metsala, J. L., & Walley, A. C. (1998). Spoken vocabulary growth and the segmental restructuring of lexical representations: Precursors to phonemic awareness and early reading ability. In J. L. Metsala & L. C. Ehri (Eds.), *Word recognition in beginning literacy* (pp. 89–120). Mahwah, NJ: Erlbaum.

Mol, S. E., Bus, A. G., de Jong, M. T., & Smeets, D. J. H. (2008). Added value of dialogic parent-child book readings: A meta-analysis. *Early Education and Development, 19*, 7–26.

National Assessment of Educational Progress (NAEP). (2010). *The nation's report card: Reading.* Retrived October 1, 2011, from *www.ed.gov/nces.*

National Center for Education Statistics (NCES). (2011). Early Childhood Longitudinal Study—Kindergarten Cohort. Retrieved October 1, 2011, from *www.ed.gov/ecls.*

National Early Literacy Panel (NELP). (2009). *Developing early literacy: Report of the National Early Literacy Panel.* Washington, DC: National Institute for Literacy.

Neuman, S. B., & Cunningham, A. E. (2009). The impact of professional development and coaching on early language and literacy instructional practices. *American Educational Research Journal, 46*, 532–566.

Neuman, S. B., & Dwyer, J. (2009). Missing in action: Vocabulary instruction in pre-k. *The Reading Teacher, 62*, 384–392.

Pianta, R. C., Belsky, J., Houts, R., Morrison, F. J., & NICHD-ECCRN. (2007). Opportunities to learn in America's elementary classrooms. *Science, 315*, 1795–1796.

Pianta, R. C., LaParo, K. M., & Hamre, B. K. (2006). *Classroom Assessment Scoring System (CLASS).* Baltimore: Brookes.

Pianta, R., Mashburn, A. J., Downer, J. T., Hamre, B. K., & Justice, L. M. (2008). Effects of web-mediated professional development resources on teacher–child interactions in pre-kindergarten classrooms. *Early Childhood Research Quarterly, 23*, 431–451.

Powell, D. R., Diamond, K. E., Burchinal, M. R., & Koehler, M. J. (2010). Effects of an early literacy professional development intervention on Head Start teachers and children. *Journal of Educational Psychology, 102*, 299–312.

Preschool Curriculum Evaluation Research Consortium (PCERC). (2008). *Effects of preschool curriculum programs on school readiness (NCER 2008–2009).* Washington, DC: National Center for Education Research, Institute of Education Sciences, U.S. Department of Education. Washington, DC: U.S. Government Printing Office.

Ruston, H. P., & Schwanenflugel, P. J. (2010). Effects of a conversation intervention on the expressive vocabulary development of prekindergarten children. *Language, Speech, and Hearing Services in Schools, 41*, 303–313.

Scarborough, H. S., & Dobrich, W. (1994). On the efficacy of reading to preschoolers. *Developmental Review, 14*, 245–302.

Showers, B., & Joyce, B. (1996). The evolution of peer coaching. *Educational Leadership, 53*, 12–16.

Silverman, R., & Crandell, J. D. (2010). Vocabulary practices in prekindergarten and kindergarten classrooms. *Reading Research Quarterly, 45*, 318–340.

Skibbe, L. E., Connor, C. M., Morrison, F. J., & Jewkes, A. M. (2011). Schooling effects on preschoolers' self-regulation, early literacy, and language growth. *Early Childhood Research Quarterly*, 26, 42–49.

Smith, M. W., Dickinson, D. K., Sangeorge, A., & Anastasopoulos, L. (2002). *Early Language and Literacy Classroom Observation (ELLCO) toolkit, research edition*. Baltimore: Brookes.

Snow, C. E., Burns, M. S., & Griffin, P. (1998). *Preventing reading difficulties in young children*. Washington, DC: National Academy Press.

Stanovich, K. E. (1986). Matthew effects in reading: Some consequences of individual differences in the acquisition of literacy. *Reading Research Quarterly, 21*, 360–406.

Storch, S. A., & Whitehurst, G. J. (2002). Oral language and code-related precursors to reading: Evidence from a longitudinal structural model. *Developmental Psychology, 38*, 934–947.

Vygotsky, L. (1978). *Mind in society: The development of higher mental processes*. Cambridge, MA: Harvard University Press.

Wasik, B. A., & Bond, M. A. (2001). Beyond the pages of a book: Interactive book reading and language development in preschool classrooms. *Journal of Educational Psychology, 93*, 243–250.

Wasik, B. A., Bond, M. A., & Hindman, A. H. (2006). The effects of a language and literacy intervention on Head Start children and teachers. *Journal of Educational Psychology, 98*, 63–74.

Wasik, B. A., & Hindman, A. H. (2011a). Identifying critical components of effective language and literacy coaching of preschool teachers. In D. K. Dickinson & S. B. Neuman (Eds.), *Handbook of early literacy: Volume 3* (pp. 322–336). New York: Guilford Press.

Wasik, B. A., & Hindman, A. H. (2011b). Low-income children learning language and early literacy skills: The effects of a teacher professional development model on teacher and child outcomes. *Journal of Educational Psychology, 103*, 455–469.

Wasik, B. A., Hindman, A. H., & Jusczyk, A. M. (2009). Using curriculum specific progress monitoring to determine Head Start children's vocabulary development. *National Head Start Association: Dialog Journal, 12*, 257–275.

Whitehurst, G. J., & Lonigan, C. J. (1998). Child development and emergent literacy. *Child Development, 69*, 848–872.

Zipoli, R. P., Coyne, M. D., & McCoach, D. B. (2011). Enhancing vocabulary intervention for kindergarten students: Strategic integration of semantically related and embedded word review. *Remedial and Special Education, 32*, 131–143.

CHAPTER 8

Promoting Math Readiness through a Sustainable Prekindergarten Mathematics Intervention

PRENTICE STARKEY, ALICE KLEIN, and LYDIA DEFLORIO

Educators are increasingly concerned about the low level of mathematics performance of American students on national as well as international assessments of mathematics (Kilpatrick, Swafford, & Findell, 2001; National Center for Education Statistics, 2011; National Mathematics Advisory Panel, 2008). Disparities in mathematics achievement are especially pronounced for students from low-income and linguistic-minority backgrounds (Rampey, Dion, & Donahue, 2009), and there is compelling evidence that this socioeconomic status (SES)-related achievement gap in mathematics emerges prior to school entry (Starkey & Klein, 2008). Research has revealed that low-income preschool and kindergarten children possess less extensive mathematical knowledge than their middle-income peers (Griffin, Case, & Siegler, 1994; Jordan, Huttenlocher, & Levine, 1992; Starkey & Klein, 1992; Starkey, Klein, & Wakeley, 2004). Furthermore, unless these SES-related math differences are addressed early through effective educational interventions, this achievement gap will persist and increase over time, especially for at-risk children (Anunola, Leskinen, Lerkkanen, & Nurmi, 2004; Entwisle & Alexander,

1989; Morgan, Farkas, & Wu, 2009; Rathbun & West, 2004). Thus, there is a need to enhance the early mathematics learning of economically disadvantaged children.

The Need for Early Mathematics Intervention

A substantial body of research has shown that children from different socioeconomic backgrounds enter elementary school at different levels of readiness to learn mathematics (Clements, Sarama, & DiBiase, 2004; Ginsburg, Klein, & Starkey, 1998; National Research Council, 2009; West, Denton, & Germino-Hausken, 2000). Moreover, cross-cultural research on young children's mathematical development in China and the United States found that an SES-related gap in math knowledge was evident by 3 years of age in both countries (Starkey & Klein, 2008). What happens to this gap, however, differs between the countries. This gap widens during the preschool years in the United States, but it narrows in China. One factor that may contribute to the narrowing of the gap in China is that public preschools implement a national curriculum, which includes math, beginning at age 3. In contrast, most public preschool programs in the United States do not utilize effective mathematics curricula (Preschool Curriculum Evaluation Research Consortium, 2008; U.S. Department of Health and Human Services, 2010). The existence of this math gap at age 3 raises the possibility that, like some SES-related language gaps (Hart & Risley, 1995), it begins forming at an even earlier age, before most children enter preschool. This suggests that SES differences in children's home learning environments contribute to these early gaps, and in fact, such differences have been found both for language (Hart & Risley, 1995) and for mathematics (Starkey & Klein, 2008).

Research has also shown that early mathematical knowledge is of more general importance than was previously thought. A meta-analysis of several large, longitudinal studies found that children's mathematical knowledge in kindergarten is the strongest predictor of later school achievement–stronger than early literacy knowledge, attention skills, or social-emotional development (Duncan et al., 2007; Duncan & Magnuson, 2011). Thus, it is clear that the acquisition of early mathematical knowledge by all children must be a major educational priority.

Additional evidence of the need for an early intervention comes from the literature on mathematical learning difficulties. Not only are mathematical difficulties as persistent as reading difficulties, but also the long-term consequences are just as severe. Long-term trajectories in mathematics achievement measured on children prior to formal school entry, and through the first few years of elementary school, clearly show that children who start school doing poorly in mathematics continue to struggle in third and fourth grade (Bodovski & Farkas, 2007; Duncan et al., 2007; Hanich, Jordan, Kaplan, & Dick, 2001; Morgan et al., 2009). For children with severe math difficulties, the consequences are particularly dire. For example, children entering and exiting kindergarten below the 10th percentile at both time points, a large majority of whom are low-SES children, have a 70% chance of scoring below the 10th percentile 5 years later. Their mathematics achievement is 1 standard deviation below that of their peers who scored above the 10th percentile in kindergarten. This difference grows to 2 standard deviations by grade 5 (Morgan et al., 2009).

The persistence of the math achievement gap not only prevents students from developing deep proficiency and understanding of critical mathematical concepts taught in kindergarten, but it also may prevent them from acquiring the more advanced mathematical concepts and content they will encounter in later grades. For example, a student's limited understanding of whole number places his or her understanding of advanced topics, such as rational number and algebra, in serious jeopardy as he or she progresses through the grades (Milgram, 2005; Wu, 1999), potentially prohibiting access to future educational and employment opportunities (National Science Board, 2008).

In light of these considerations, the summary by the National Research Council (2009) is apt: "All young Americans must learn to think mathematically, and they must think mathematically to learn" (p. 16). Thus, a focused early mathematics intervention is needed during the critical preschool years in order to ensure that children from low-income backgrounds develop a solid foundation of informal mathematical knowledge prior to receiving formal mathematics instruction in school.

Early Math Standards and Guidelines

The existence of a sizable SES-related gap is a significant problem when schools attempt to implement mathematics standards. All math standards have a starting point. In the United States, the new Common Core State Standards for Mathematics begin in kindergarten (e.g., Common Core Standards Initiative, 2010) and the older National Council of Teachers of Mathematics standards begin with a grade band from prekindergarten through grade 2 (e.g., National Council of Teachers of Mathematics, 2000, 2006). Writers of math standards assume, at least implicitly, that a wide range of children possess a sufficient foundation of mathematical knowledge at school entry to participate fully in instruction based on these initial math standards. The validity of this assumption, however, is questionable given the evidence for a significant SES-related gap prior to school entry. Schools and teachers are left with the problem of how to teach standards-based mathematics curricula to children who are not ready to learn them. This provides further support for the argument that an early math intervention is needed to help schools bridge this math readiness gap.

Early Mathematics Instruction

It is widely accepted that intervention is easier and more effective when conducted earlier in life than later (e.g., Lazar & Darlington, 1982; Ramey & Campbell, 1984). At present, however, most public preschool programs in the United States spend little time on mathematics. In a recent study of 730 prekindergarten and kindergarten classrooms, prekindergarten children spent only 6% of their school day engaged in math learning (LaParo et al., 2009). Likewise, many preschool programs do not use effective mathematics curricula. Several recent rigorous evaluations of preschool curricula frequently used in Head Start and state preschool programs found that these curricula did not have a significant effect on the math knowledge of low-SES 4-year-olds over the prekindergarten year (Preschool Curriculum Evaluation Research Consortium, 2008; U.S. Department of Health and Human Services, 2010). Therefore, due to the existence of a SES-related math gap in young children and the dearth of effective early mathematics curricula, we undertook the development and evaluation of an early math intervention.

The Pre-K Mathematics Intervention

The first step was to develop and evaluate a set of home math activities for low-income families with prekindergarten children (Starkey & Klein, 2000). Head Start families were randomly assigned to treatment or control conditions. Parent–child dyads attended a series of biweekly classes in which parents were shown how to engage in math activities with their children and they were provided with math materials to use at home. Significantly more growth in mathematical knowledge was found in treatment children than in control children. The second step was to develop and evaluate a set of small-group math activities for use in prekindergarten classrooms (Starkey et al., 2004). A quasi-experimental design included low- and middle-SES 4-year-olds who engaged in the classroom math activities (treatment condition) and a similar sample of children who did not (business-as-usual comparison condition). Again, significantly more growth in mathematical knowledge was demonstrated by treatment children than by comparison children at each level of SES.

The third step was to integrate the home and classroom components and publish the integrated curriculum as *Pre-K Mathematics* (Klein & Starkey, 2002, 2004). This curricular intervention consists of small-group math activities, with objects for children to manipulate, for teachers to use in classrooms and a related set of math activities for parent–child dyads to use at home. Activities with closely related mathematical content are organized into units and sequenced to help children construct and connect mathematical knowledge. The mathematical content focuses on number and operations, space and geometry, patterns/functions, and informal measurement. Examples of content include counting, one-to-one correspondence, and one- and two-set addition and subtraction (number and operation units), iteration of ordered sets (pattern/function unit), analysis of two- and three-dimensional forms (space and geometry unit), and nonstandard length measurement (measurement unit). Several key features of the intervention are designed to be developmentally sensitive to children's learning needs. Downward extensions of math activities (e.g., problems involving very small sets) are provided for children who are not ready for a given activity, and upward extensions (e.g., concrete arithmetic problems with larger addends or subtrahends) are provided for children who complete an activity without needing help. Furthermore, suggestions for scaffolding of learning and development by teachers and parents are provided to support children who experience difficulty with a part of an activity. Teachers record children's learning of each math activity and monitor their progress over the course of the school year.

Model of Causation

The relation between the mathematics intervention and children's mathematical knowledge can be explained with a causal model (Figure 8.1). The main elements of the model are (1) the curricular intervention, which includes mathematics content—the active ingredients in activities needed to promote change in children's mathematical knowledge; (2) professional development support in mathematics for teachers; (3) proximal (teacher) outcomes resulting from this support; (4) mediation of mathematical content, modeled as child engagement in curricular activities, as influenced by teachers' math practices; and (5) child outcomes, which are changes in children's knowledge that result from the intervention.

The active ingredients in the intervention are modeled as the mathematics content from the curriculum, Pre-K Mathematics. Intensive and frequent professional development is the primary means through which teachers become able to deliver the curriculum activities with both

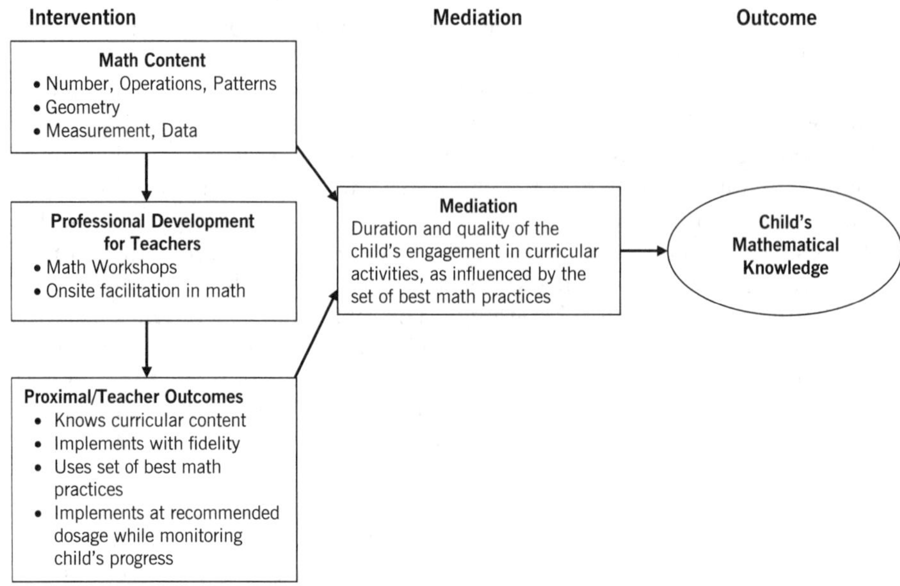

FIGURE 8.1. Causal model.

fidelity and understanding (cf. Shulman, 2000) and at the recommended "dosage" (frequency) children need. Math-focused workshops and on-site training aligned with the mathematics curriculum are designed to enable teachers: (1) to learn the essential mathematics content comprising the scope and sequence of the math curriculum; (2) to implement the curriculum with fidelity; (3) to use a set of best math practices to present mathematically focused, small-group activities; and (4) to use a curriculum plan to ensure that children are provided with the recommended sequence of math activities, while monitoring their progress and conducting periodic reviews of the activities. It is expected that this professional training for teachers will change their mathematics practices and enhance children's learning opportunities. In particular, teachers will utilize the set of best math practices to ensure children's engagement with mathematics content from the curriculum. Children's mental mathematical activities are necessary to produce cognitive change, but teachers' practices can influence the duration and type of activities in which children engage. Thus, best practices by teachers, and analogous practices by parents, enable children receiving this curricular intervention to spend more time engaged in critical mathematical learning, relative to children in "usual practice" classrooms that are not using this intervention.

Evaluations of Effectiveness

The integrated curricular intervention was evaluated in two efficacy studies as part of the Preschool Curriculum Evaluation Research Consortium (2008). A randomized controlled study was conducted in public preschool programs in California and New York. It was found that Pre-K Mathematics was highly effective at enhancing low-SES children's mathematical knowledge, when compared with a business-as-usual control group (Klein, Starkey, Clements, Sarama, & Iyer, 2008). Based on this study and a subsequent study, Pre-K Mathematics was reviewed by the U. S. Department of Education's What Works Clearinghouse. It has been assigned the highest rating of effectiveness (++), with the greatest extent of evidence (medium to large).

Evaluation of effectiveness at scale is among the most rigorous tests of effectiveness for educational interventions. Some promising early childhood programs have produced attenuated or no effects when implemented on a larger scale (Farran, 1990, p. 508; Gilliam, Ripple, Zigler, & Leiter, 2000). Loss of effectiveness can result from a loss of implementation fidelity (e.g., Elias, Zins, Graczyk, & Weissberg, 2003) or content dosage (Borman, Hewes, Overman, & Brown, 2002; Klinger, Ahwee, Pilonieta, & Menendez, 2003). In view of this possibility, our next step was to determine whether Pre-K Mathematics continues to be effective when implemented on a larger scale than is customary for public preschool curriculum adoption (e.g., an entire Head Start program) and at a distance from the developer (Starkey, Klein, DeFlorio, & Swank, in press). In the previous efficacy study, teacher volunteers had been assigned to treatment and control conditions, and project trainers were used to provide on-site support to teachers. Our more rigorous scale-up study used the curriculum adoption procedures actually used in programs, specifically, that all teachers are required by program administrators to implement the new curriculum programwide. Also, in contrast to the efficacy study's use of university-affiliated project trainers to provide on-site support, the scale-up study used a trainer-of-trainers approach, whereby project trainers provided training to local trainers who were employees or contractors with the participating programs. Another objective was to determine whether the intervention would be effective when implemented in varied contexts. Classrooms were randomly assigned to treatment (math intervention) or business-as-usual control conditions. Contextual variation included type of preschool program (state-funded prekindergarten vs. Head Start), length of program day (half-day vs. full day), state (California and Kentucky/Indiana), and demographics of parent population (ethnically diverse, low-income, urban families in California and predominantly rural, low-income, white families in Kentucky and Indiana).

This scale-up project comprised two studies, a Main Study and a Sustainability Study. The research design of the Main Study was a cluster randomization in which 94 classrooms at 63 preschool sites were randomly assigned to the treatment and control conditions. The total sample for the study included 744 prekindergarten children. Two measures were used to assess growth in children's mathematical knowledge. The Child Math Assessment (CMA) measures preschool children's informal mathematical knowledge in the content areas of number, arithmetic operations, space and geometry, measurement, and patterns (Starkey et al., 2004). It comprises nine tasks, with multiple problems per task, and is administered individually in one 20-minute session. The Test of Early Mathematics Ability–Third Edition (TEMA-3) is a standardized measure of informal and formal number and operations knowledge (Ginsburg & Baroody, 2003). It is administered to children individually in one 20- to 30-minute session. The intervention was again found to be effective. Children's mathematical knowledge was assessed at pretest and posttest of the prekindergarten year. Nested analyses found that significantly greater gains in mathematical knowledge were experienced by treatment children, relative to control children, on both the CMA (effect size [ES] = 0.83) and the TEMA (ES = 0.45). Moreover, the intervention effect was consistent across states and program types. There was no significant effect of state or program type, and no significant interaction of time with state or program type. This indicates that the Pre-K Mathematics intervention was robust across the varied preschool contexts included in this study. Moreover, treatment effects were found to persist into kindergarten.

The Main Study demonstrated that the Pre-K Mathematics intervention was effective when implemented at a customary level of scale for curriculum adoptions by public preschool programs. This study focused on programs' first year of implementation. An important subsequent question was whether programs sustain their implementation on a long-term basis with sufficient fidelity and treatment dosage to provide educational benefits to the children. This issue of sustainability was addressed in a subsequent study of the second year of implementation (designated as the Sustainability Study). Programs were asked to hold the Main Study teachers in their experimental conditions for an additional year of implementation. Although project staff monitored teachers' implementation, program staff members (teachers, internal facilitators, and program administrators) were responsible for ensuring continued use of the curriculum. Except where otherwise noted, the measures and data collection procedures mirrored those used in the first year of implementation, thus allowing for comparisons of the quality of implementation by teachers and child outcomes in the first versus second year of implementation.

The hypothesis and research questions that were addressed included the following:

- *Hypothesis 1.* The math intervention will lead to increased mathematical knowledge in treatment children, relative to control children, by the end of the prekindergarten year.
- *Research Question 1.* Will math outcomes for treatment children at the end of the prekindergarten year be similar during the first and second years of implementation?
- *Research Question 2.* Children are given verbal directions during all math intervention activities. Will the math intervention influence children's ability to follow verbal directions?
- *Research Question 3.* Will teachers sustain their implementation of the intervention with a comparable degree of fidelity and similar dosage levels as observed in the Main Study?
- *Research Question 4.* Will treatment teachers' sustain their use of best mathematics practices?
- *Research Question 5.* Will the hypothesized effects of the intervention on children's mathematical knowledge persist in elementary school?

METHOD

Participants

Teacher Participants

A total of 85 teachers participated in this study. Thirty-nine of the initial 48 treatment teachers who participated in the Main Study continued implementation of Pre-K Mathematics for a second year. The remaining nine teachers were no longer teaching in prekindergarten classrooms, thus were not able to continue participation. The control group was comprised of the same 46 teachers as the Main Study. Teachers in the treatment group reported a mean of 16 years teaching experience, and teachers in the control group reported a mean of 13 years teaching experience. In regard to teacher education, 59% of treatment teachers and 54% of control teachers reported having BA degrees or higher.

Child Participants

Children were randomly selected from the participating classrooms (approximately eight per classroom), balanced for age and gender, yielding a sample of 683 children. The California sample comprised 357 low-income, ethnically diverse, urban children. The Kentucky/Indiana sample comprised 326 low-income, predominantly European American, rural children. All were age-eligible to enter kindergarten the following year. Mean age at pretest in prekindergarten was 4.37 years (range, 3.82–5.04 years) for treatment children and 4.44 years (range, 3.86–4.99 years) for control children. The ethnic composition of the sample was 53% European American, 19% Hispanic/Latino, 15% African American, 4% Asian American, and 9% multiethnic/other. Most children (86%) spoke English fluently, and the remainder spoke Spanish. Attrition during the prekindergarten year was similar for treatment and control children, 11 and 9%, respectively, and occurred primarily due to family mobility.

Research Design

Classrooms remained in the same conditions as in the first year of implementation, when randomization had resulted in the assignment of 94 classrooms (48 treatment and 46 control) at 63 preschool sites. Teacher attrition resulted in the loss of one site and nine treatment classrooms from the first year of implementation to the second year. Consequently, the Sustainability Study design included 85 classrooms (39 treatment and 46 control) at 62 preschool sites. Children's mathematical knowledge was assessed using a pretest/posttest design.

Intervention

The Pre-K Mathematics intervention included 26 small-group classroom activities and 16 home activities. Teachers followed a curriculum plan and usually conducted activities with groups of four children in the language of the classroom. Teachers implemented curriculum activities twice per week for approximately 20 minutes, with time during a third day reserved for review or making up absences. Assessment record sheets that accompanied each math activity enabled teachers to record individual children's learning of specific math content. Teachers also used a curriculum-based progress-monitoring form to monitor individual children's progress toward mastery over the course of the school year. Cumulative review was conducted periodically during weeks reserved for review. Teachers followed the curriculum plan during implementation of the home component of the intervention. They sent home math activities to parents at the same time that small-group classroom activities with related content were conducted. Parents received a letter about the activity, materials, and a picture strip depicting a parent–child dyad conducting the activity in English or Spanish.

Professional Development

Program trainers provided refresher workshops in the fall and spring with their respective teachers to review the procedures for documenting dosage and mastery, as well as to practice some of the activities identified the previous year as being more difficult to implement. All 39 treatment teachers participated in the fall workshop, and 38 treatment teachers participated in the spring workshop. Treatment teachers continued to receive on-site training and facilitation and technical assistance from their program trainers throughout the school year.

Curriculum Implementation Measures

Implementation Fidelity. To determine whether treatment teachers sustained their implementation of the intervention at a level comparable to their implementation in the first year of the study, bi-weekly observations of implementation were conducted. Program trainers conducted an average of 9.95 fidelity visits (range, 5–21) per classroom over the school year. At each observation, fidelity of implementation was evaluated on five dimensions: (1) adherence to the schedule of activities set in the curriculum plan; (2) use of all materials, including manipulative objects for children, needed to conduct the activity; (3) presentation of the principal problems or parts of the activity; (4) provision of developmental adjustments (scaffolding, downward extensions, and upward extensions) needed by individual children in the group; and (5) use of assessment record sheets to record the performance of individual children on the activity. Each observation resulted in an overall fidelity score, ranging from 0 to 1.00. A fidelity score between .90 and 1.00 was considered to be high.

Classroom Curriculum Dosage. As in the first year of implementation, the goal was for each child to be exposed twice per week to each of 26 curriculum activities for a total of 52 planned doses per year. The number of doses children actually received was calculated from teachers' assessment record sheets (Klein & Starkey, 2002; 2004).

Home Curriculum Dosage. Information on use of Pre-K Mathematics home activities was obtained through a home math activity checklist completed by parents. Parents were asked to report whether they had received these activities from their child's teacher and, if so, how often they used the activities with their child.

Progress Monitoring. Children's mastery of the mathematical concepts embedded into each small-group activity was documented using the

Pre-K Mathematics Math Mastery form (Klein & Starkey, 2000, 2004), which treatment teachers updated after each small-group lesson.

Assessment Procedures

The same child and classroom measures were used in the Sustainability Study as in the Main Study in order to compare math outcomes resulting from teachers' first versus second year of implementation of Pre-K Mathematics.

Child Assessments in Prekindergarten

Children's mathematical knowledge was assessed using the CMA and TEMA-3 in the fall and spring of the prekindergarten year. In addition, the Woodcock–Johnson Tests of Achievement–III (WJ-III) Understanding Directions subtest was administered at both time points. This subtest assessed children's ability to follow oral directions to point to different parts of pictures. To obtain a true baseline of children's math knowledge, the curriculum plan was set for the first small-group math activity to be conducted immediately after all children had been pretested in the fall, and for the final activity to be completed just prior to posttesting at the end of the program year.

Classroom and Home Learning Environment Measures

The Early Mathematics Classroom Observation (EMCO) a classroom observation instrument, was administered in fall and again in spring to measure differences in math practices of treatment and control teachers. This made it possible to detect effects of the training on teachers' math practices. The EMCO assessed the nature and amount of mathematics support teachers provided in their classrooms. The observation began during the arrival of children and lasted 3–4 hours. An observation was made of all teacher-participant activities in which there was mathematical content. The observer recorded the mathematical content, number of children present, and duration of the activity. Activities were categorized as (1) *focal* math activities in which the primary goal of the activity was children's mathematics learning (e.g., an activity focused on the names of numerals) or (2) embedded math activities in which the primary goal was nonmathematical (e.g., a cooking project in which children measured ingredients at one point). By recording the duration and number of children present during each teacher-participant math activity, the EMCO made it possible to calculate the average amount of time children received math support during a school day.

Classroom math materials were catalogued using the Numeracy Environment Checklist (NEC) during the same observation sessions as the EMCO. Observers recorded whether classrooms had a math learning center and the number and types of child-accessible math materials found anywhere in the indoor or outdoor areas used by the class. Finally, information about the home learning environment was obtained by administering a home math environment questionnaire to parents in the winter of the prekindergarten year.

Kindergarten Follow-Up

To determine whether the effects of the intervention were sustained over time, the TEMA-3 was administered in the spring of the kindergarten year. Also, kindergarten teachers, blind to the children's experimental condition during the prekindergarten year, evaluated each child's mathematical skills by completing a Uniform Report Card for each child in the spring of the kindergarten year. Teacher ratings on the Uniform Report Card yielded two types of scores: (1) teacher's rating of children's overall mathematical ability, and (2) the mean rating of children's ability on 14 skills across the domains of number, arithmetic, space and geometry, measurement, and pattern knowledge. In addition, these teachers were asked to complete a Math Instructional Survey to provide information on the mathematical practices utilized in their classrooms.

RESULTS

Child Math Outcomes in the Prekindergarten Year

As in the Main Study, both CMA composite scores and TEMA-3 raw scores were used in analyses to determine the impact of intervention on growth of mathematical knowledge. A set of analyses tested the main hypothesis (see Hypothesis 1) that the Pre-K Mathematics intervention would lead to increased mathematical knowledge in treatment children, as compared to control children, by the end of the prekindergarten year. These analyses required the use of multilevel models, because observations (pretest, posttest) were nested within students, students were nested within classrooms, and classrooms were nested within schools.

By centering the time variable at the posttest, level difference between the intervention groups could be determined at the posttest. In addition, a model centering at the pretest was computed in order to determine that there were no differences between groups at the pretest. Effects sizes were estimated by determining the difference between the two intervention groups divided by the pretest standard deviation.

Effects of potential covariates and moderators (child gender and age at pretest, state, and type of preschool program) were tested to see whether they accounted for significant variation in the model and were included in tests of the condition effect if they were significant. Then, the condition effect, its interaction with time, and any other significant interactions were added to determine the effect of the intervention and whether its effect was moderated by these covariates.

CMA Scores

A three-level ANOVA of children's CMA scores, with observations nested within children, and children nested within classrooms, revealed no differences at pretest but a significant condition × time interaction, $F(1, 527) = 68.82$, $p < .0001$ (ES = 0.70), indicating a greater increase in mathematical knowledge for treatment children than for control children during teachers' second year of implementation (Figure 8.2). Treatment children's mean composite scores increased from .30 ($SD = 0.16$) at pretest to .58 ($SD = 0.20$) at posttest, an increase of 93%. Control children's mean composite scores increased less—from .32 ($SD = 0.17$) at pretest to .45 ($SD = 0.19$) at posttest, an increase of only 40%. Differences between the mean scores of treatment and control children were greater for children in state preschool than for children in Head Start, $F(1, 527) = 5.32$, $p < .05$, with an effect size of 0.89 in state preschool compared to 0.50 in Head Start. There were no differences by program type in Kentucky/Indiana, but in California, state preschool children outperformed children in Head Start, $F(1,522) = 3,4.57$, $p < .05$. One possible explanation for this interaction stems from enrollment policy differences between California state

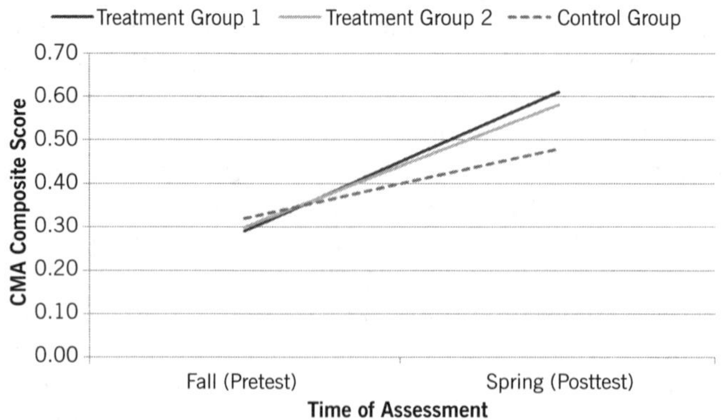

FIGURE 8.2. Effects of the intervention on children's CMA scores.

preschools and Head Start programs. Family income limits, and hence family SES, is slightly higher in the state preschools than in Head Start programs.

TEMA-3 Scores

A three-level ANOVA of children's TEMA-3 scores, with observations nested within children, and children nested within classrooms, also revealed a significant condition × time interaction favoring treatment children, $F(1, 527) = 34.57$, $p < .0001$ (ES = 0.45) (Figure 8.3). Treatment children's mean raw scores increased from 7.26 (SD = 5.42) at pretest to 14.78 (SD = 6.92) at posttest, an increase of 104%. Control children's raw scores increased less–from 7.05 (SD = 5.07) at pretest to 12.49 (SD = 6.64) at posttest, an increase of only 77%. There were no significant interactions including program type, but there was a condition × state interaction. Differences between the raw scores of treatment and control children at posttest were greater for children in Kentucky/Indiana than in California, $F(1, 527) = 3.93$, $p < .05$ (ES = 0.60 in Kentucky/Indiana and 0.30 in California). There were no differences by condition at pretest.

Comparison of Math Outcomes during Teachers' First and Second Year of Implementation

The next set of analyses compared children's math outcomes during the first versus second year of implementation by treatment teachers (Research Question 1). Again, mixed multilevel models, with observations nested

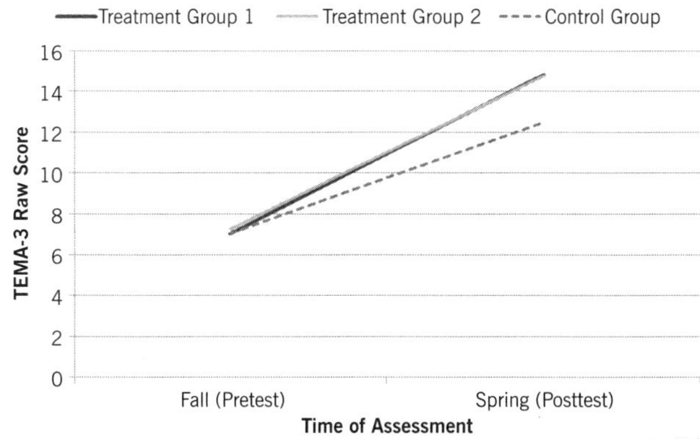

FIGURE 8.3. Effects of the intervention on children's TEMA-3 scores.

within students, and students nested within classrooms, were used to compare growth in treatment children's CMA and TEMA-3 scores during the first and second years of implementation. There were no significant differences between the two treatment groups on the CMA or TEMA-3 at pretest or posttest. During the first year of implementation, treatment children's mean composite scores on the CMA increased from .29 (SD = 0.17) at pretest to .61 (SD = 0.19) at posttest, an increase of 110%. Their raw scores on the TEMA-3 increased from 7.02 (SD = 4.94) at pretest to 14.82 (SD = 6.95) at posttest, an increase of 111%.

WJ-III Understanding Directions Subtest Scores

This language subtest assessed children's ability to follow oral directions (Research Question 2). A three-level repeated measures analysis of variance (ANOVA) using children's WJ-III scores revealed a strong condition × time interaction, $F(1, 606) = 20.27$, $p < .0001$ (ES = 0.51). Scores of treatment children did not differ by condition at pretest, but gains by treatment children were greater than those by control children. Treatment children's mean scores increased from 447.23 (SD = 13.12) at pretest to 456.55 (SD = 12.74) at posttest. Control children's raw scores increased from 450.37 (SD = 12.67) at pretest to 455.28 (SD = 11.43) at posttest. Main effects were found for age, $F(1, 606) = 200.69$, $p < .0001$, with older children scoring higher than younger children, and state, $F(1, 606) = 10.31$, $p < .005$, with children in Kentucky/Indiana scoring higher than children in California. Thus, as was found with the TEMA-3 math assessment, greater gains were found for rural children from Kentucky/Indiana than for urban children in California. Further research is needed to determine whether these differential gains are due to state differences in the samples or implementation.

Teachers' Implementation of the Curriculum

To determine whether teachers were able to sustain their implementation of the intervention with a comparable degree of fidelity and similar dosage levels as observed in the Main Study (Research Question 3), descriptive data on fidelity, classroom dosage, home dosage, and progress monitoring were compared.

Fidelity. Fidelity did not significantly differ in the first and second years of implementation, .91 versus .93, respectively. Thus, teachers sustained an implementation that was high quality and conformed to what was intended by the developers.

Classroom Curriculum Dosage. Teachers in one program were unable to complete the final curriculum activity prior to posttest assessments due to school days lost due to inclement weather. Consequently, the 26th activity was not included in analyses of implementation data. The average percentage of doses of small-group math activities that children actually received was 88% (43.8 of the 50 included in the analysis), excluding additional doses above two for the same activity during their second year of implementation. In comparison, children received 85% of the recommended dose in the first year. Thus, teachers sustained their delivery of curriculum activities.

Home Curriculum Dosage. On average, parents reported using 54% (8.7 of 16) Pre-K Mathematics home activities, with a range of 0–16 activities used by families. During the first year of implementation, parents reported using a similar percentage of home math activities, 61%.

Progress Monitoring. According to teachers' curriculum-based progress-monitoring records, children mastered approximately 65% (16.2 of 25) of the small-group math activities during the second year of implementation. Children mastered a similar percentage, 71%, during the first year.

Teachers' Mathematics Practices

In the first year of implementation, it was found that treatment teachers, relative to control teachers, spent more time on math instruction overall and more time engaged in instruction that utilized a set of best math practices. These math practices were emphasized in the written Pre-K Mathematics curriculum, as well as in the training experiences provided to teachers and local trainers. This set of best practices included greater use of small-group math activities, focal (mathematically explicit) activities, and scaffolding. In the second year of implementation, treatment teachers, relative to control teachers, continued to spend more time engaged in math instruction compared to control teachers, $F(1,77) = 19.394$, $p < .0001$. Treatment teachers also continued to use the set of best math practices (Research Question 4). Specifically, they devoted more instructional time to small-group math activities, $F(1,77) = 74.176$, $p < .0001$, focal math activities, $F(1,77) = 24.305$, $p < .0001$, and provided children with scaffolding for math learning more, $F(1,77) = 26.040$, $p < .0001$ compared to control teachers (Figure 8.4). As in the first year of implementation, there were no significant differences by condition in the amount of instructional time devoted to whole-group math activities, embedded math activities (i.e., nonmathematical activities with some math embedded in them, such as measurement embedded within a cooking project), or math activities in which children were not provided with scaffolding, all *p*s > .05 (Figure 8.4).

Classroom observations using the NEC found that 80% of treatment classrooms had dedicated centers for math learning, compared to 74% of these same treatment classrooms in the Main Study. Computers were present in all classrooms, and math software was available for the children to use in 77% of these.

Kindergarten Follow-Up

The next set of analyses examined whether the effects of the intervention on children's mathematical knowledge persisted into elementary school (Research Question 5). Children's mathematical knowledge in kindergarten was measured by the TEMA-3. In spring of the kindergarten year, mean raw scores were 30.01 ($SD = 8.33$) for treatment children and 25.67 ($SD = 8.42$) for control children. TEMA-3 raw scores at prekindergarten pretest (Time 1), prekindergarten posttest (Time 2), and kindergarten (Time 3) were analyzed using a repeated measures mixed model. Main effects were found for condition, $F(1, 1{,}398) = 21.93$, $p < .0001$, indicating

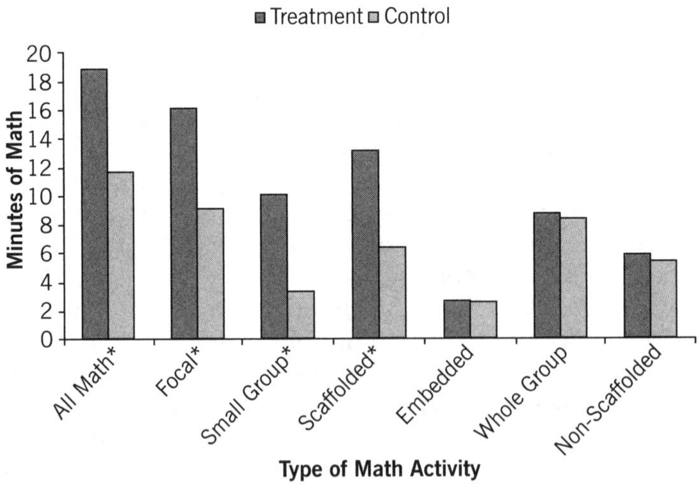

FIGURE 8.4. Amount of time per child that treatment and control teachers engaged in specific types of math practices. Significant intervention–control group differences are indicated by * ($p < .05$).

that treatment children scored higher than control children across the three time points, and time, $F(1, 1{,}398) = 27.86$, $p < .0001$, indicating that children's scores increased over time. There was also a significant condition by time interaction, $F(1, 1{,}398) = 34.65$, $p < .0001$. Tests between condition at each time point revealed no differences by condition at Time 1, but treatment children demonstrated significantly greater mathematical knowledge at Time 2, $F(1, 1{,}398) = 20.37$, $p < .0001$, and Time 3, $F(1, 1{,}398) = 38.44$, $p < .0001$.

Uniform Report Card Ratings

Teacher ratings of children's mathematical ability on the Uniform Report Card provide further evidence that the effects of the intervention persisted into kindergarten. Ratings of treatment and control children's overall mathematical ability were compared using a three-level ANOVA. Kindergarten teachers gave higher ratings of children's overall math ability to treatment children ($M = 2.18$; $SD = 0.55$) than to control children ($M = 2.07$; $SD = 0.64$), $F(1, 545) = 5.77$, $p < .05$. Teachers also rated children's ability on 14 mathematical skills, spanning the domains of number, arithmetic, space/geometry, measurement, and pattern knowledge. The mean rating across these skills was also higher for treatment children ($M = 2.00$; $SD = 0.46$) compared to control children ($M = 1.82$; $SD = 0.50$), $F(1, 547) = 21.245$, $p < .0001$.

Math Instruction in Kindergarten

The Math Instruction Survey was used to obtain data on mathematics instruction provided to project children. Kindergarten teachers reported teaching mathematics, on average, 32 minutes per day (range, 0–90 minutes) in whole groups, 16 minutes per day (range, 0–48 minutes) in small groups, and 7 minutes per day (range, 0–40 minutes) to individuals. The amount of math instruction provided by teachers in whole groups, small groups, or to individuals was not significantly correlated with children's TEMA-3 scores.

Summary and Conclusions

This study was conducted to determine whether a curricular math intervention, Pre-K Mathematics, for economically disadvantaged children is effective and sustainable when implemented at a level of scale that is customary for public preschool programs.

Can Public Preschool Programs Sustain High-Quality Instructional Practices?

In the sustainability year, treatment teachers were able to continue to implement Pre-K Mathematics with a high degree of fidelity, to deliver a good dose of small-group math activities in their classrooms, and to get parents to provide a fair-to-good dose of home math activities. Comparison of teachers' fidelity and dosage levels during their first and second years of implementation revealed similar–and acceptable–levels both years. Teachers sustained their use of a set of best mathematics practices that had been emphasized in their professional training, and with support from program trainers, teachers monitored and recorded children's progress in math across the prekindergarten year.

Can Public Preschool Programs Sustain an Effective Implementation?

The principal hypothesis–that the math intervention would lead to increased mathematical knowledge in participating children by the end of the prekindergarten year– was clearly supported. Furthermore, treatment effects, as measured both by standardized assessment and by children's teachers, persisted in the kindergarten year. Thus, programs were able to sustain an effective implementation when implementing at a customary, program-wide level of scale.

It is also noteworthy that children benefited in another way from participation in the math intervention. In an important communication skill, understanding and following verbal directions from adults, treatment children showed more improvement than did control children. To speculate, this could explain, at least in part, the finding that children's math knowledge in kindergarten is a strong predictor of achievement in general in elementary school (Duncan et al., 2007; Duncan & Magnuson, 2011). Given that the experience of learning math enhances children's ability to understand and follow verbal directions, this enhanced ability could, in turn, help children achieve in other content areas.

Recommendations for Policymakers

Public preschool programs could be required to implement mathematics curricula that are of proven effectiveness. It should be recognized, however, that programs need resources to implement mathematics curricula effectively over a sustained period of time. To build capacity in early math, program trainers as well as preschool teachers will require additional professional development in early math (Starkey, 2007). For programs to experience a high level of sustained program quality and child outcomes, they may need to have administrative or training staff monitor implementation fidelity and dosage, and be prepared to help teachers meet implementation challenges as needed. It is also recommended that program personnel forge a closer working relationship with parents, such as by having teachers send math readiness materials home to parents and discuss in parent–teacher conferences or home visits the importance of supporting children's early math learning. We believe that these changes are necessary to prepare economically disadvantaged children for elementary school mathematics.

Acknowledgments

The research reported in this chapter was supported by the Institute of Education Sciences, U.S. Department of Education, through Grant No. R305K050004 to WestEd. The opinions expressed are those of the authors and do not represent views of the U.S. Department of Education. We thank Victoria Molfese, Dennis Molfese, and Elizabeth T. Brown for their work on the project in Kentucky; Kiyome Inouye, Alison Paskal, Stacey Koo, Amber Busby, Christina Mulcahy, Annie Paladino, Simone Shane, and Sophie Vogel for their assistance with the project in California; and Paul Swank for data analyses.

References

Anunola, K., Leskinen, E., Lerkkanen, M. K., & Nurmi, J. E. (2004). Developmental dynamics of math performance from preschool to grade 2. *Journal of Educational Psychology, 96*, 699–713.

Bodovski, K., & Farkas, G. (2007). Mathematics growth in early elementary school: The roles of beginning knowledge, student engagement and instruction. *Elementary School Journal, 108*, 115–130.

Borman, G., Hewes, G., Overman, L., & Brown, S. (2002). *Comprehensive school reform and student achievement: A meta-analysis* (Report No. 59). Baltimore: Center for Research on the Education of Students Placed At Risk.

Clements, D. H., Sarama, J., & DiBiase, A. M. (Eds.). (2004). *Engaging young children in mathematics: Standards early childhood mathematics education.* Mahwah, NJ: Erlbaum.

Common Core Standards Initiative. (2010). *Common core state standards for mathematics* [On-line]. Available from *www.corestandards.org/files/k12mathstandards.pdf.*

Duncan, G. J., Dowsett, C. J., Claessens, A., Magnuson, K., Huston, A. C., Klebanov, P., et al. (2007). School readiness and later achievement. *Developmental Psychology, 43*, 1428–1446.

Duncan, G. J., & Magnuson, I. K. (2011). *The long reach of early childhood poverty.* Washington, DC: Brookings.

Elias, M. J., Zins, J. E., Graczyk, P. A., & Weissberg, R. P. (2003). Implementation, sustainability, and scaling up of social-emotional and academic innovations in public schools. *School Psychology Review, 32*(3), 303–319.

Entwisle, D. R., & Alexander, K. L. (1989). Early schooling as a "critical period" phenomenon. *Research in the Sociology of Education and Socialization, 8*, 27–55.

Farran, D. C. (1990). Effects of intervention with disadvantaged and disabled children: A decade review. In S. J. Meisels & J. P. Shonkoff (Eds.), *Handbook of early childhood intervention* (pp. 501–539). New York: Cambridge University Press.

Gilliam, W. S., Ripple, C. H., Zigler, E. F., & Leiter, V. (2000). Evaluating child and family demonstration initiatives: Lessons from the comprehensive child development program. *Early Childhood Research Quarterly, 15*(1), 41–59.

Ginsburg, H. P., & Baroody, A. (2003). *Test of Early Mathematics Ability (TEMA-3)* (3rd. ed.). Austin, TX: Pro-Ed.

Ginsburg, H. P., Klein, A., & Starkey, P. (1998). The development of children's mathematical thinking: Connecting research with practice. In W. Damon (Series Ed.) & I. E. Sigel & K. A. Renninger (Vol. Eds.), *Handbook of child psychology: Vol. 4. Child psychology in practice* (5th ed., pp. 401–476). New York: Wiley.

Griffin, S., Case, R., & Siegler, R. S. (1994). Rightstart: Providing the central conceptual prerequisites for first formal learning of arithmetic to students at-risk for school failure. In K. McGilly (Ed.), *Classroom lessons: Integrating cognitive theory and classroom practice* (pp. 24–49). Cambridge, MA: Bradford Books/MIT Press.

Hanich, L., Jordan, N. C., Kaplan, D., & Dick, J. (2001). Performance across different areas of mathematical cognition in children with learning disabilities. *Journal of Educational Psychology, 93*, 615–626.

Hart, B., & Risley, T. R. (1995). *Meaningful differences in the everyday experience of young American children*. Baltimore: Brookes.

Jordan, N. C., Huttenlocher, J., & Levine, S. C. (1992). Differential calculation abilities in young children from middle- and low-income families. *Developmental Psychology, 28*, 644–653.

Kilpatrick, J., Swafford, J., & Findell, B. (2001). *Adding it up: Helping children learn mathematics*. Washington, DC: National Academy Press.

Klein, A., & Starkey, P. (2002). *Pre-K Mathematics Curriculum*. Glenview, IL: Scott Foresman.

Klein, A., & Starkey, P. (2004). *Scott Foresman–Addison Wesley Mathematics: Pre-K* (2nd ed.). Glenview, IL: Pearson/Scott, Foresman.

Klein, A., Starkey, P., Clements, D., Sarama, J., & Iyer, R. (2008). Effects of a prekindergarten mathematics intervention: a randomized experiment. *Journal of Research on Educational Effectiveness, 1*, 155–178.

Klinger, J., Ahwee, S., Pilonieta, P., & Menendez, R. (2003). Barriers and facilitators on scaling up research-based practices. *Exceptional Children, 69*, 411–429.

LaParo, K. M., Hamre, B. K, Locasale-Crouch, J., Pianta, R. C., Bryant, D., Early, D., et al. (2009). Quality in kindergarten classrooms: Observational evidence for the need to increase children's learning opportunities in early childhood classrooms. *Early Childhood Research Quarterly, 20*, 657–692.

Lazar, I., & Darlington, R. (1982). Lasting effects of early education: A report from the Consortium for Longitudinal Studies. *Monographs of the Society for Research in Child Development, 47* (2–3, Serial No. 195).

Milgram, J. (2005). *The mathematics pre-service teachers need to know.* Stanford, CA: Department of Mathematics, Stanford University.

Morgan, P. L., Farkas, G., & Wu, Q. (2009). Five-year growth trajectories of kindergarten children with learning difficulties in mathematics. *Journal of Learning Disabilities, 42*(4), 306–321.

National Center for Education Statistics. (2011). The condition of education 2011. [Available online at *http://nces.ed.gov/pubsearch/pubinfo.asp?pubid=2011033*].

National Council of Teachers of Mathematics. (2000). *Principles and standards for school mathematics.* Reston, VA: Author.

National Council of Teachers of Mathematics. (2006). *Curriculum focal points for prekindergarten through grade 8 mathematics.* Reston, VA: Author.

National Mathematics Advisory Panel. (2008). *Final report of the National Mathematics Advisory Panel.* Washington, DC: U.S. Department of Education.

National Research Council. (2009). *Mathematics learning in early childhood: Paths toward excellence and equity* (Committee on Early Childhood Mathematics, Christopher T. Cross, Taniesha A. Woods, & Heidi Schweingruber, Eds., Center for Education, Division of Behavioral and Social Sciences and Education). Washington, DC: National Academies Press.

National Science Board. (2008). *Science and Engineering Indicators 2008* (Vols. I & II). Arlington, VA: National Science Foundation.

Preschool Curriculum Evaluation Research Consortium. (2008). *Effects of preschool curriculum programs on school readiness* (NCER 2008–2009). Washington, DC: National Center for Education Research, Institute of Education Sciences, U.S. Department of Education.

Ramey, C., & Campbell, F. (1984). Preventive education for high-risk children: Cognitive consequences of the Carolina Abecedarian Project. *American Journal of Mental Deficiency, 88,* 512–523.

Rampey, B. D., Dion, G. S., & Donahue, P. L. (2009). *NAEP 2008 Trends in Academic Progress* (NCES 2009-479). Washington, DC: National Center for Education Statistics, Institute of Education Sciences, U.S. Department of Education.

Rathbun, A., & West, J. (2004). *From kindergarten through third grade: Children's beginning school experience.* Available from *http://nces.ed.gov/pubsearch/pubsinfo.asp?pubid=2-4-7#.*

Shulman, L. S. (2000). Teacher development: Roles of domain expertise and pedagogical knowledge. *Journal of Applied Developmental Psychology, 21,* 129–135.

Starkey, P. (2007). Mathematical development in economically disadvantaged children. *National Head Start Association Dialogue Briefs, 10*(2), 1–7.

Starkey, P., & Klein, A. (1992). Economic and cultural influences on early mathematical development. In F. L. Parker, R. Robinson, S. Sombrano, C. Piotrowski, J. Hagen, S. Randolph, & A. Baker (Eds.), *New directions in child and family research: Shaping Head Start in the 90s* (pp. 440–443). New York: National Council of Jewish Women.

Starkey, P., & Klein, A. (2000). Fostering parental support for children's mathematical development: An intervention with Head Start families. *Early Education and Development, 11*, 659–680.

Starkey, P., & Klein, A. (2008). Sociocultural influences on young children's mathematical knowledge. In O. N. Saracho & B. Spodek (Eds.), *Contemporary perspectives on mathematics in early childhood education* (pp.253–276). Charlotte, NC: Information Age.

Starkey, P., Klein, A., DeFlorio, L., & Swank, P. (in press). Scaling up a Pre-K Mathematics intervention in public preschool programs. *Journal of Educational Psychology.*

Starkey, P., Klein, A., & Wakeley, A. (2004). Enhancing young children's mathematical knowledge through a prekindergarten mathematics intervention. *Early Childhood Research Quarterly, 19*(1), 99–120.

U.S. Department of Health and Human Services, Administration for Children and Families, Office of Planning, Research and Evaluation. (2010). Head Start Impact Study: Final Report. Retrieved from *www.acf.hhs.gov/sites/default/files/opre/hs_impact_study_final.pdf.*

West, J., Denton, K., & Germino-Hausken, E. (2000). *America's kindergarteners.* Washington, DC: National Center for Education Statistics, U.S. Department of Education.

Wu, H. (1999). Basic skills versus conceptual understanding. *American Educator, 23*(3), 14–19, 50–52.

CHAPTER 9

The Development of Self-Regulatory Skills and School Readiness

CHRISTINE PAJUNAR LI-GRINING, JACLYN LENNON, MARIA MARCUS, VALERIE FLORES, and KELLY HAAS

Families' economic status is associated with wide disparities in children's academic achievement; this linkage creates particular concern given that almost 25% of preschool-age children in the United States live below the poverty line (National Center for Children in Poverty, 2012). Longitudinal studies document that later scholastic achievement is linked closely with children's academic skills in kindergarten, fueling efforts to enrich preschool education for at-risk children in order to promote their future success (Duncan et al., 2007). One target area for early education efforts is the growth of language, literacy, and quantitative skills that will support academic learning (Lonigan, 2006). Also, future school success requires children to develop the social-emotional skills necessary for cooperation and positive interaction with teachers and classmates.

Children's school readiness in the dual domains of academic and social skills relies heavily on the development of self-regulation skills, or children's ability to manage their behavior, attention, and emotions in voluntary and adaptive ways (Blair & Razza, 2007). This chapter provides an overview of the development of young children's self-regulation skills, and efforts to promote self-regulation with preschool interventions. A central focus is on the design and impact of the Chicago School Readiness Project

(CSRP), an intervention program designed to improve low-income children's preparedness for school by fostering their self-regulation.

Defining Self-Regulation

Self-regulation reflects the extent to which children are able to control impulses (i.e., stop themselves from a reactive or habitual response) and shift focus (i.e., plan and engage in alternative thoughts or behaviors; Blair & Razza, 2007). As such, self-regulation skills underlie the capacity to delay gratification, inhibit inappropriate behaviors, focus attention, and engage in effective problem solving (Diamond & Lee, 2011). It has long been recognized that there are individual differences in children's capacity for self-regulation. Theorists speculate that the roots of self-regulation are biological and associated with individual temperament, which includes activity level, extraversion, and emotional reactivity (Rothbart, Sheese, & Posner, 2007). Temperamental variations in reactivity are often described as the "bottom-up" determinants of self-regulation, as they represent the strength of the dominant impulses that individuals must inhibit in order to exert volitional control; also, children develop "top-down" cognitive structures that allow them to exert increasing levels of control over those involuntary impulses (Bierman & Torres, in press; Raver, 2012).

Temperament theorists describe "effortful control" as the core self-regulatory capability to suppress a dominant response and to execute a subdominant one instead (Rothbart et al., 2007). Effortful control is a function of both "bottom-up" involuntary emotional reactions and "top-down" voluntary efforts to modulate such reactions. Reactivity includes individual differences in children's tendencies to experience negative emotions such as anger. Self-regulation involves differences in children's ability to manage anger. Reflecting biological underpinnings, effortful control is moderately stable over the course of early childhood, with longitudinal correlations ranging between .30 and .70 among children from a range of socioeconomic backgrounds (Cohen, 1992; Kochanska & Knaack, 2003; Li-Grining, 2007).

The development of self-regulation during early childhood has been studied extensively by cognitive-developmental neuroscientists, who focus on the measurement of developing higher-order cognitive processes termed *executive functions*, that are implicated in the self-regulation of learning, emotions, and behavior. Children's executive function skills comprise working memory, inhibitory control, and cognitive flexibility (Diamond & Lee, 2011). *Working memory* refers to the ability to hold instructions and information in short-term memory and draw on it for immediate use. *Inhibitory control* refers to the ability to resist temptation, overcome the tendency to respond in an automatic or habitual manner, and instead respond in an alternative, subdominant way. *Cognitive flexibility* refers to the ability to adjust to differences and changes in rules and expectations, within and across contexts, such as shifting attention in order to understand a problem from a new perspective.

There is overlap between the research literatures on children's executive function and temperament, as both focus centrally on understanding the development of self-regulation skills in early childhood (Rothbart et al., 2007). Many of the tasks used to assess executive function are designed to be neutral emotionally, and are sometimes referred to as "cool EF" tasks. On the other hand, some executive function skills, such as inhibitory control, may also be drawn upon when a child seeks to regulate him- or herself in an emotionally charged task (sometimes referred to as "hot EF" tasks). In this type of task, both inhibitory control (a higher-order executive function) and the strength of the child's behavioral impulses and emotional reactivity (aspects of temperament) influence children's capacity for self-regulation. For example, the process of demonstrating inhibitory control might involve modulating emotional reactions in order to adhere to rules and expectations at school (Ursache, Blair, & Raver, 2012).

Linkages between Preschoolers' Self-Regulation and Broader Development

Self-regulation (which includes effortful control and executive function skills) has been linked to higher academic skills among children of various socioeconomic backgrounds. For example, in a cross-sectional investigation, preschoolers' effortful control was moderately correlated with higher scores on measures of phonemic awareness, print knowledge, and vocabulary (Allan & Lonigan, 2011). Longitudinal, positive linkages have also been found between preschoolers' earlier effortful control and later quantitative skills, with small correlations ranging from r = .22–.27 (Cohen, 1992; Li-Grining, Votruba-Drzal, Bachman, & Chase-Lansdale, 2006). Additionally, modest, positive links between young children's executive function skills and their math, literacy, and vocabulary have been detected across the preschool year (McClelland et al., 2007). In general, small, positive links to kindergarteners' academic skills have been found as well (Blair & Razza, 2007). Specifically, preschoolers' executive function and effortful control predict kindergarteners' math skills, and preschoolers' effortful control accounts for a significant amount of variance in kindergarteners' letter knowledge. Moreover, longer-term studies have found that preschoolers' executive function skills modestly predict first graders' greater math achievement (Clark, Pritchard, & Woodward, 2010) and sixth graders' higher academic grades (Jacobson, Williford, & Pianta, 2011).

Prior research has examined associations between preschoolers' self-regulation and behavior problems as well. Cross-sectional, moderate associations between preschoolers' better executive function and lower hyperactive behavior have been detected (Espy, Sheffield, Wiebe, Clark, & Moehr, 2011). Preschoolers' executive function skills have also modestly predicted lower levels of problem behaviors in sixth grade (Jacobson et al., 2011). In addition, small, concurrent correlations between preschoolers' greater effortful control and lower externalizing and internalizing behavior have been found (Allan & Lonigan, 2011). Given the role of children's self-regulation in their broader development, we next turn to predictors of individual differences in children's self-regulatory competence.

The Development of Children's Self-Regulation

As children get older, children's effortful control and executive function skills tend to improve. Basic executive function skills first emerge during the latter part of the first year, and become more complex and efficient during early childhood (Wiebe et al., 2011). Growth in executive function then continues into adolescence (Marcovitch & Zelazo, 2009). When effortful control has been measured using delay of gratification tasks, effortful control scores increase across the early childhood years but in smaller increments over time (Kochanska, Murray, & Harlan, 2000; Li-Grining, 2007). Among children with lower initial scores on observations of attention and behavioral persistence, ratings continue to rise during middle childhood (Zhou et al., 2007). Besides individual characteristics such as age, environmental factors also predict children's self-regulatory competence.

The Role of Parenting in the Development of Self-Regulation

The parenting context particularly appears to be closely associated with the development of self-regulation. Experiences of disrupted parenting have been linked to lower levels of executive function in young children. For example, preschoolers who experience maltreatment and placement in foster homes display lower levels of inhibitory control than preschoolers without exposure to this trauma (Pears, Fisher, Bruce, Kim, & Yoerger, 2010).

Living in poverty is also associated with delayed development of preschoolers' executive function and effortful control (Li-Grining, 2007; Wiebe et al., 2011). Poverty-related stress may jeopardize children's self-regulation by compromising parents' psychological well-being and quality of caregiving (Blair & Raver, 2012). Additionally, exposure to poverty-related stressors may shape brain chemistry and neural connectivity in ways that directly pose risks to children's self-regulation. That is, elevated stress and heightened emotions may decrease the efficiency at which higher cognitive processes perform by placing greater demands on children's executive function skills, which are marshaled to dampen emotions and reactions to stress (Ursache et al., 2012). In turn, children's dysregulated behavior may challenge parents and decrease positive caregiving. Future research might investigate the complex ways in which adversity shapes children's self-regulation via biological, physiological, neurological, and social processes, in order to shed more light on socioeconomic differences in preschoolers' executive function and effortful control (Blair & Raver, 2012).

Though poverty may undermine optimal parenting, it is important to recognize that there is variability in the extent to which low-income parents support the development of preschoolers' self-regulation. Indeed, in low-income samples, higher levels of mother–child connectedness are associated with higher levels of preschoolers' effortful control (Li-Grining, 2007). Also, higher levels of maternal positive engagement are associated with elevated executive function skills in preschool children (Rhoades, Greenberg, Lanza, & Blair, 2011).

These findings are consistent with results from studies on families from a broader range of socioeconomic backgrounds, where more sensitivity, warmth, and limit setting have been related to young children's greater effortful control (Kochanska et al., 2000; Lengua, Honorado, & Bush, 2007; Spinrad et al., 2012) and executive function (Bernier, Carlson, & Whipple, 2010). Such positive interactions serve as a source of external regulation for children (Bernier et al., 2010). Taken together, emotional support appears to be a central mechanism that fosters preschoolers' self-regulation.

Parents' sensitivity tends to co-occur with another important mechanism that may shape children's self-regulation, which is cognitive stimulation (Bradley & Corwyn, 2005). As another form of external support, cognitive stimulation includes scaffolding, in which parents guide children's problem solving in ways that are tailored to children's existing skills levels (Bernier et al., 2010). Scaffolding has been linked to higher levels of children's executive function skill development and effortful control (Hammond, Mueller, Carpendale, Bibok, & Lieberman-Finestone, 2012; Lengua et al. 2007). Effective scaffolding also involves decreasing levels of parental support in response to increasing levels of children's competence on a given task. Children's higher executive function ratings are associated with such granting of autonomy, which provides children opportunities to practice executive function skills (Bernier et al., 2010). Additionally, parents may foster self-regulation when they use language to help children manage their emotions, behavior, and attention (e.g., teaching children how to label emotions, giving children reminders and explanations about rules, and talking with children about self-regulation strategies; Cole, Armstrong, & Pemberton, 2010).

Building on this nonexperimental literature, parenting intervention programs focused on enhancing children's executive function have begun to emerge (Bierman & Torres, in press; also see Welsh, Bierman, & Mathis, Chapter 11, this volume). A relatively large research base supports the power of parent-focused interventions to foster improved behavior in preschool children. However, to our knowledge, very few parent-focused programs specifically target improvement in effortful control.

PRESCHOOL INTERVENTIONS

Another key context for children's development includes their involvement in early childhood education programs. Indeed, researchers and practitioners are exploring the characteristics of programs that are most effective at improving self-regulation, and several different approaches are being evaluated, with some positive findings (Bierman & Torres, in press; Diamond & Lee, 2011). For example, the Tools of the Mind program focuses on teachers' scaffolding of sociodramatic play, including opportunities for children to talk through and enact play plans and activities that allow them to practice executive function skills (Bodrova & Leong, 2007; Diamond, & Lee, 2011). The Head Start Research-Based, Developmentally Informed (REDI) program centers on children's social-emotional learning and literacy skills (Bierman et al., 2008; also see Bierman, Domitrovich, Nix, Welsh, & Gest, Chapter 10, this volume). Teachers show children how to identify and talk about emotions, calm down when upset, and develop and choose plans to resolve conflict between peers, with the use of puppets, pictures, and stories, and with teachers coaching children throughout the day. Teachers also engage in activities that focus on building children's letter identification and vocabulary skills.

The CSRP Intervention Design

This chapter centers on the CSRP, which is a classroom-based, multicomponent mental health intervention (Raver et al., 2011). Like the Head Start REDI program, CSRP was a part of the Interagency School Readiness Consortium. Led by Cybele Raver (Principal Investigator) and Stephanie Jones (Co-Principal Investigator), a primary aim of CSRP was to enhance children's social behavior and academic skills by fostering their self-regulation in Head Start classrooms. CSRP research and the broader field have demonstrated that early childhood programs may significantly improve low-income children's adjustment. Thus, teachers who play central roles in such programs deserve attention.

Enhancing Teachers' Provision of Emotional Support

First, CSRP intended to enhance preschool teachers' provision of emotional support to children. In turn, the experience of greater emotional support in the classroom was expected to promote children's self-regulation. To reach this goal, CSRP involved both training of teachers in classroom behavior management strategies and coaching of teachers in how to implement these strategies in the classroom. The training component involved an adapted form of the Incredible Years Teacher Training program (Webster-Stratton, Reid, & Hammond, 2004; also see Raver et al., 2009). The CSRP model focused on the following five strategies to manage children's behavior in the classroom: (1) promoting positive behavior (e.g., giving praise and encouragement); (2) managing misbehavior (e.g., ignoring attention-seeking behavior, giving warnings); (3) redirection and limit setting (e.g., gentle reminders such as turning the lights on and off to get children's attention); (4) positive relationship building between teachers and children; and (5) problem solving (e.g., encouraging children to use words not hands; Li-Grining et al., 2010). A licensed clinical social worker and an experienced trainer led workshops on these strategies for teachers, and mental health consultants (MHCs) who were also licensed clinical social workers attended the workshops with teachers in order to foster collaboration with them. Each of the five trainings was 6 hours long and held on Saturdays from October through January.

Additionally, the MHCs visited teachers once a week from the fall through the spring of the preschool year. For the first 2.5 months of the intervention, the MHCs focused on following a set of manualized coaching steps, which included sharing and discussing feedback with teachers regarding their ability to foster children's behavioral and emotional development (see Raver et al., 2009, for more details). To account for the

MHCs increasing the teacher–student ratio in the treatment classrooms, teacher's aides, who held Child Development Associate degrees, visited each of the control classrooms for the same amount of time once a week.

Addressing Disruptions to Teachers' Provision of Emotional Support

Second, similar to the children in their classrooms, early childhood education teachers in low-income communities may face poverty-related stressors (Li-Grining et al., 2010). As such, CSRP strived to decrease stressors by offering teachers social support and discussing stress reduction techniques with them. It was hypothesized that, if they were less stressed, teachers would be in a better position to provide children with more emotional support, which would then foster children's self-regulation (Raver, Blair, & Li-Grining, 2012). In order to accomplish this aim, during the middle 2.5 months of the intervention, MHCs led a 1-day stress reduction workshop at each Head Start site in the winter of the preschool year. During classroom visits, MHCs provided teachers with social support, talked with teachers about their experience with stress, and discussed strategies for alleviating stress in the workplace, such as taking breaks and talking about concerns.

There is relatively little research on early childhood teachers' experiences, and particularly the stressors that early childhood teachers face in the workplace. The CSRP team set out to examine whether teachers in the treatment group reported changes in perceptions of their experiences in the workplace (Zhai, Raver, & Li-Grining, 2011). These experiences were captured using self-report measures of teachers' resources, control, demands at work, and confidence in classroom behavior management.

Directly Supporting Children's Self-Regulation

Recognizing that children's self-regulation may not improve via changes in teachers' practices and psychological well-being alone, CSRP also sought to support children's self-regulation directly. To meet this objective, in the spring of the preschool year, MHCs provided one-on-one services to children who displayed the highest levels of emotional and behavioral problems (Raver et al., 2009). As part of this process, MHCs worked collaboratively with parents, teachers, and social workers at each site to develop plans for this subgroup of children, which included three to four students per class. Across the last 2.5 months of the intervention, MHCs delivered direct services to these children, including individual and group behavior management plans to improve preschoolers' social, emotional, and behavioral competence.

The CSRP Evaluation

The CSRP was evaluated in the context of a randomized controlled design. The following research questions were addressed:

1. Did the CSRP set of intervention services significantly improve preschoolers' school readiness, defined in terms of better self-regulation, fewer behavior problems, and greater academic achievement?
2. Were improvements in preschoolers' academic achievement mediated by impacts on their self-regulation skills?

Participants

The CSRP was implemented across 2 years, serving one cohort of children during the 2004–2005 academic year, and another cohort during the 2005–2006 school year. A total of 543 children participated (with approximately 50% girls, 66% African Americans, 26% Latinos, 8% other race/ethnicity or biracial), although 34 of these children left their Head Start program before the end of the year. By the end of the spring, children were about 58-months-old on average (Raver et al., 2009, 2011). In addition, a total of 90 lead and assistant teachers participated across the two cohorts, with some teacher turnover during the course of the project (i.e., seven new teachers entering, and four teachers either moving or quitting). On average, teachers were 40 years old, nearly all female, and diverse in race/ethnicity (about 70% African American, 20% Latina, 10% European American; Li-Grining et al., 2010; Zhai et al, 2011).

Randomization

Consistent with recent school-based intervention models, CSRP used a cluster randomized design. Head Start sites with two or more full-day classrooms were selected from seven high-poverty neighborhoods in Chicago, which were on the south and west sides of the city, resulting in 18 participating centers (see Raver et al., 2008, for more details). Teachers and children were nested in 35 classrooms across these 18 sites, which were randomly assigned to intervention and control groups (see Raver et al., 2009, for more details). There were nine treatment sites, with a total of 18 intervention classrooms and 48 teachers who received the CSRP intervention. Also, there were nine control sites, with a total of 17 control classrooms and 42 teachers who continued with the "usual practice" teaching. Blind to treatment status, CSRP research staff recruited 83% of the children from these classrooms to join the project.

Data Collection Procedures

Data were collected longitudinally during the fall and spring of the intervention year (Raver et al., 2008, 2009, 2011; Zhai et al., 2011). Measures included direct observation of classroom quality and direct assessments of children's academic skills, peer interaction, and self-regulation, using the Preschool Self-Regulation Assessment (PSRA). Via the PSRA, self-regulation was assessed using tasks reflecting executive function, effortful control, and attention/impulse control. In addition, parents reported on their individual and family background characteristics (e.g., depressive symptoms), and on children's behavior problems, and teachers completed self-report measures on their background characteristics and work-related stressors. Teachers completed reports on children's behavior problems as well.

Impact of the CSRP on Classroom Management and Teacher Stress

In the logic model of the CSRP, the major strategy to improve children's self-regulation skills and school readiness was to enhance the quality of classrooms' emotional climate and behavioral management, and to reduce teacher stress. The teacher training addressed positive reinforcement, negative consequences, redirection, positive relationship building, and social problem solving. Collectively, these strategies were intended to improve the quality of the classroom climate and to foster more proactive versus reactive behavior management. The hypothesis was that classrooms that received training, visits, and the stress reduction workshop would demonstrate improvements in emotional climate and behavioral management, and decreases in teachers' stress.

Given the nested design of CSRP, in which children were embedded in classrooms, and classrooms were embedded in sites, testing of all hypotheses used hierarchical linear modeling (HLM). Furthermore, all analyses controlled for a host of child, family, classroom, and site characteristics. HLM analyses revealed that the first hypothesis was supported: Classrooms in the intervention group experienced increases in observational ratings of positive climate (e.g., warmth) and teacher sensitivity (e.g., responsiveness), and reductions in negative climate (e.g., harshness; Raver et al., 2008). Furthermore, teachers in intervention classrooms were also rated as using marginally more proactive and fewer reactive behavior management approaches than teachers in control classrooms. Across all outcomes, moderate to large effect sizes were detected, ranging from 0.52 to 0.89 (Cohen, 1992).

Additionally, CSRP yielded impacts on teachers' well-being, with effect sizes falling in the medium range (i.e., 0.51 to 0.74; Zhai et al.,

2011). In intervention classrooms, teachers reported feeling more control in the workplace and having access to better resources. Specifically, teachers' perceptions of work-related control improved substantially, and their perceived resources at work increased moderately. However, teachers also reported feeling less confident, with teachers' confidence in behavior management decreasing moderately. It could be that participating in CSRP heightened teachers' awareness of different behavior management strategies. As part of the process of learning how to improve their classroom management practices, teachers may have experienced self-doubt. In addition, teachers may have doubted that they could continue improving their practices without the help of the MHCs, who were scheduled to end their visits at the close of the school year. There were no significant changes in teachers' perceived job demands. Also, the impact of CSRP on teachers' stressors and confidence did not vary by teachers' race/ethnic background, education, teaching experience, or position as a head teacher, assistant teacher, or co-teacher.

With a focus on emotional climate, CSRP did not train teachers in instructional support, and thus did not test for impacts on the quality of teachers' instruction in the classroom. However, in another randomized study of Foundations of Learning, an early intervention program modeled after CSRP, but with slight modifications, there were positive impacts on children's engagement in learning activities (Morris, Raver, Lloyd, & Millenky, 2009). Future replications and expansions of CSRP might test for impacts on teachers' provision of both cognitive and emotional support. In the past, researchers have found that correlates of teachers' instructional support include markers of classrooms' emotional climate, suggesting some interdependency between the quality of emotional and instructional teacher–child interactions in the preschool classroom (Pianta, LaParo, Payne, Cox, & Bradley, 2002).

Impact of the CSRP on Preschoolers' School Readiness

The CSRP captured preschoolers' school readiness in areas of self-regulation (Raver et al., 2011), behavior problems (Raver et al., 2009), and academic skills (Raver et al., 2011; Zhai et al., 2010). The main focus of CSRP was to improve preschoolers' self-regulation and thereby reduce behavior problems and improve academic competence, and indeed CSRP significantly enhanced children's self-regulatory competence (Raver et al., 2011). Children's self-regulation scores were based on an executive function aggregate (e.g., Balance Beam; Pencil Tap tasks), an effortful control composite (based on four delay of gratification tasks), and an aggregate behavioral score based on assessors' ratings of preschoolers' attention and impulse control (see Raver et al., 2011, for details).

Compared to children who were randomly assigned to the control group in programs, children assigned to receive intervention services in programs performed better on the executive function assessments. Treatment status significantly predicted children's executive function scores in the spring of the preschool year, controlling for scores in the fall, with a moderate effect size of 0.37. Similar treatment effects were found for assessor reports of children's attention and impulse control, which were also medium in magnitude (effect size = 0.43). Furthermore, when teachers participated in a greater number of CSRP training sessions than their peers, the effect size on children's improvement in attention and impulse control was large (0.91; Zhai et al., 2010). However, there were no treatment effects on children's effortful control.

Children's behavior problems have been used as proxies for self-regulation, particularly when they include measures of hyperactivity and lack of impulse control (Duncan et al., 2007). The CSRP team examined the intervention's impact on children's externalizing (aggression) and internalizing (withdrawn) behavior problems (Raver et al., 2009). Children in CSRP intervention classrooms demonstrated significantly fewer behavior problems, as reported by teachers, than children in the "usual practice" control classrooms, including lower levels of aggression, hostility, withdrawal, and depression in the spring, relative to baseline levels in the fall. These results were consistent with findings based on observational ratings of externalizing behavior among a subsample of children. Across these outcomes, effect sizes were 0.64 to 0.89, which are considered moderate to large. Interestingly, some subgroups of children were more strongly affected by participation in the CSRP intervention than others, with greater benefits found for girls and Latino children. Among the subsample of children with observational ratings of externalizing behavior, there was also a higher impact for children facing fewer risk factors (i.e., children with family incomes above the poverty line, those whose mothers held more than a high school degree, and those whose mothers worked less than 10 hours a week).

Finally, the total effect of the intervention on children's academic competence was tested. Children in the CSRP intervention classrooms displayed significantly larger improvements on direct assessments of vocabulary, letter naming, and early math skills than children in the control classrooms (Raver et al., 2011). These findings emerged in models that predicted academic competence in the spring of the preschool year and controlled for academic performance in the fall of the preschool year. Effect sizes ranged from 0.34 to 0.63, which are considered moderate in size. Moreover, among children whose teachers attended more CSRP training sessions, effect sizes were large for vocabulary and math (i.e., ranging from 0.83 to 0.90; Zhai et al., 2010).

Mediation of the CSRP's Effects on Academic Skills by Self-Regulation

A central hypothesis of the CSRP study was that improving teacher classroom management and providing students with more positive behavioral and emotional support would enhance self-regulation skills and thereby improve academic learning. To test this link, the CSRP team examined whether intervention impacts on preschoolers' academic skills occurred via improvements in self-regulatory competence (Raver et al., 2011). The CSRP team detected treatment effects that were moderate in size (ranging from 0.34 to 0.63), in models that predicted preschoolers' academic and self-regulatory skills in the spring and controlled for baseline skills in the fall, and other child, family, classroom, and site characteristics. Measures of children's self-regulation were then added to the models as predictors of academic skills.

To yield estimates of the extent to which treatment effects were mediated by children's self-regulatory competence, treatment effects on children's self-regulation were multiplied by estimates of the association between self-regulation and academic skills, and standard errors were calculated. Estimates of mediated effects and their standard errors suggested that differences in children's executive function and attention/impulse control modestly explained the academic gap between children randomly assigned to the treatment versus the control group. Put another way, CSRP directly enhanced children's self-regulation, which was, in turn, correlated with their academic skills. The mediated effect size was 0.09 for executive function, and ranged from 0.08 to 0.11 for attention/impulse control.

Implications for Practice in Early Childhood Education

In response to concerns about the heightened risk faced by low-income preschoolers for poor school readiness (low academic skills; elevated behavior problems), the CSRP intervention program documents the potential for evidence-based preschool interventions to address successfully such gaps in school readiness. Children in sites randomized to receive the CSRP intervention package demonstrated greater self-regulation, better academic skills, and lower behavior problems at the end of the preschool year, in comparison to children in "usual practice" control classrooms. In reflecting on results from recent CSRP studies, implications emerge for the understanding and promotion of self-regulation skills among at-risk children, and for general preschool practice.

Improving Children's Executive Function

The impact of the CSRP intervention on preschoolers' academic skills at the end of the year was partially explained by its impact on children's executive function and attention/impulse control. Importantly, this may reflect the interwoven nature of preschoolers' self-regulatory and academic competence (Welsh, Nix, Blair, Bierman, & Nelson, 2010). Thus, programmatic efforts to improve low-income children's school readiness should be organized in ways that support the acquisition of both basic literacy and math skills, and the acquisition of preschoolers' higher-order cognitive skills, including attention control, inhibitory control, and working memory.

The logic model of the CSRP intervention was based upon a theoretical conceptualization that emphasizes the role of sensitive–responsive adult–child relationships and positive behavioral and emotional supports in the development of self-regulation skills (Bernier et al., 2010). Theory and research suggests that classrooms providing low-income children with predictable routines, warm and responsive teacher–student interactions, clear (nonpunitive) limit setting to reduce aggression, and positive supports to increase time on-task in learning activities will enhance their self-regulation skills. This may occur because children are not diverting cognitive resources to cope with perceived threats and stress, and instead may focus those cognitive resources on learning (Ursache et al., 2012). Additionally, it may reflect the utility of positive external regulation (consistent, contingent teacher limit setting and specific praise), in promoting behavioral self-control, which allows children to follow classroom rules and engage effectively in learning (Webster-Stratton, Reid, & Hammond, 2004). It may also reflect the improved quality of instructional presentations of which teachers are capable when their positive behavioral management skills are more extensive and effective, and when teacher–child relationships are more supportive (Driscoll & Pianta, 2010). Although the CSRP findings do not illuminate the specific mechanisms underlying the effects, they do document higher levels of children's executive function and attention/impulse control in classrooms that offered more emotional support and more positive behavior management than the control classrooms.

Notably, results from CSRP research also highlight the malleability of classroom emotional climate in preschool programs for low-income children, and the capacity of an evidence-based intervention to increase levels of positive behavior management. Teachers in sites randomly assigned to receive CSRP intervention services were observed to be significantly warmer, less harsh and more sensitive, and marginally more proactive in their management of children's behavior in the classroom. Certainly, professional development focused on instructional support is central to teaching children how to develop basic reading and math skills (see, in this volume, Starkey, Klein, & DeFlorio, Chapter 8; Bierman et al., Chapter 10; and Santos, Chapter 14). However, the CSRP findings suggest that professional development opportunities for early childhood teachers should also include components that strive to enhance teachers' provision of emotional support to children. Such efforts could help bolster teachers' efforts to foster directly children's academic performance.

Furthermore, it appears important to expand the view of the classroom emotional climate to include not only the emotional support that teachers provide to children but also the support they receive themselves. Similar to children, teachers' own executive function may get pulled in different directions and shift away from providing emotional support to children when they feel overwhelmed by stressors they experience in the workplace or at home (Raver et al., 2012). It is important to note that CSRP intervention services were also found to be successful at reducing teachers' perceived experience with stress at work. Teachers' own receipt of emotional support may have helped to facilitate their ability to demonstrate more warmth, greater sensitivity, and less harshness toward children.

Improving Classroom Practice

Together with other classroom-based intervention programs (e.g., Bierman et al., 2008; Diamond & Lee, 2011), CSRP documents the promise of improving low-income children's school readiness through classroom-based programs. For some children with the highest levels of behavior problems, ongoing, one-on-one services may be necessary, as the CSRP model recognizes. However, at a time when economic resources are tight, classroom-based programs may provide an efficient way of addressing various levels of behavior problems across children. Furthermore, the lessons learned during the preschool year of the CSRP intervention program might be applied to intervention efforts focused on kindergarten and elementary school. Additional CSRP studies are currently investigating older children's executive function and the school climate. This new set of studies will help shed light on how the CSRP intervention program might be expanded into upper grades, in order to support the development of low-income children's executive function skills beyond preschool.

The CSRP and other recent randomized interventions provide an important complement to the nonexperimental literature in providing guidance on how best to improve the quality of early education and its impact on children's outcomes. Randomized studies can make stronger claims regarding the causal impact of intervention strategies on children's school readiness in domains of both behavioral and academic competence. When designed well, as illustrated by the CSRP, randomized studies also allow the examination of program impact and processes at the classroom level, analyses of intervention participation and dosage, and exploration of mediation and moderation of intervention impact. Although these latter analyses are exploratory (because teachers and children are not randomly assigned to different participation levels or to different levels of mediation or moderation variables), they provide a basis for generating hypotheses about the mechanisms by which classroom-based intervention programs might affect children's individual outcomes. These hypotheses support the ongoing development of improved intervention approaches.

In general, as lessons from CSRP and other research-based programs are put into practice, early childhood programs might focus on not only the delivery of intervention services but also the support and tracking of the implementation of those services. As discussed earlier, attendance at more teacher training sessions was related to even higher benefits for children's school readiness (Zhai et al., 2010). These results suggest that we should devote effort to increasing participation in classroom-based intervention services made available to teachers in low-income communities. By doing so, early childhood programs may increase the likelihood of yielding a larger return from investments made in intervention services, classroom improvement, and children's school readiness in the context of poverty.

Acknowledgments

The project described in this chapter was supported by Award No. R01HD046160 from the Eunice Kennedy Shriver National Institute of Child Health and Human Development, and was supported by the Spencer Foundation as well. The content is solely the responsibility of the authors and does not necessarily represent the official views of the Eunice Kennedy Shriver National Institute of Child Health and Human Development, the National Institutes of Health, or the Spencer Foundation. We express our thanks to Cybele Raver, Stephanie Jones, Fuhua Zhai, and the rest of the CSRP team. Thanks also to Sophie Mir, Jessie Duncan, Donna Flores, and Sarah Pekoc for their research assistance. We are grateful to policy professionals, such as Anthony Raden, Karen Carradine, Mary Ellen Caron, and Vanessa Rich, who very generously supported CSRP's collaboration with Chicago Head Start programs. Last, we extend our deepest thanks to the children, parents, and teachers who made this research possible.

References

Allan, N. P., & Lonigan, C. J. (2011). Examining the dimensionality of effortful control in preschool children and its relation to academic and socioemotional indicators. *Developmental Psychology, 47*(4), 905–915.

Bernier, A., Carlson, S. M., & Whipple, N. (2010). From external regulation to self-regulation: Early parenting precursors of young children's executive function. *Child Development, 81*(1), 326–339.

Bierman, K. L., Domitrovich, C. E., Nix, R. L., Gest, S. D., Welsh, J. A., Greenberg, M. T., et al. (2008). Promoting academic and social-emotional school readiness: The Head Start REDI program. *Child Development, 79*(6), 1802–1817.

Bierman, K. L., & Torres, M. (in press). Promoting the development of executive functions through early education and prevention programs. In J. A. Griffin, L. S. Freund, & P. McCardle (Eds.), *Executive function in preschool age children*. Washington, DC: American Psychological Association.

Blair, C., & Raver, C. C. (2012). Child development in the context of adversity: Experiential canalization of brain and behavior. *American Psychologist, 67*(4), 309–318.

Blair, C., & Razza, R. P. (2007). Relating effortful control, executive function, and false belief understanding to emerging math and literacy ability in kindergarten. *Child Development, 78*(2), 647–663.

Bodrova, E., & Leong, D. J. (2007). *Tools of the Mind: The Vygotskian approach to early childhood education* (2nd ed.). Upper Saddle River, NJ: Prentice Hall.

Bradley, R. H., & Corwyn, R. F. (2005). Productive activity and the prevention of behavior problems. *Developmental Psychology, 41*(1), 89–98.

Clark, C. A. C., Pritchard, V. E., & Woodward, L. J. (2010). Preschool executive function abilities predict early mathematics achievement. *Developmental Psychology, 46*(5), 1176–1191.

Cohen, J. (1992). A power primer. *Psychological Bulletin, 112*(1), 155–159.

Cole, P. M., Armstrong, L. M., & Pemberton, C. K. (2010). The role of language in the development of emotion regulation. In S. D. Calkins & M. A. Bell (Eds.), *Child development at the intersection of emotion and cognition* (pp. 59–77). Washington, DC: American Psychological Association.

Diamond, A., & Lee, K. (2011). Interventions shown to aid executive function development in children 4 to 12 years old. *Science, 333*(6045), 959–964.

Driscoll, K. C., & Pianta, R. C. (2010). Banking time in Head Start: Early efficacy of an intervention designed to promote supportive teacher–child relationships. *Early Education and Development, 21*(1), 38–64.

Duncan, G. J., Dowsett, C. J., Claessens, A., Magnuson, K., Huston, A. C., Klebanov, P., et al. (2007). School readiness and later achievement. *Developmental Psychology, 43*(6), 1428–1446.

Espy, K. A., Sheffield, T. D., Wiebe, S. A., Clark, C. A. C., & Moehr, M. J. (2011). Executive control and dimensions of problem behaviors in preschool children. *Journal of Child Psychology and Psychiatry, 52*(1), 33–46.

Hammond, S. I., Mueller, U., Carpendale, J. I. M., Bibok, M. B., &

Libermann-Finestone, D. P. (2012). The effects of parental scaffolding on preschoolers' executive function. *Developmental Psychology, 48*(1), 271–281.

Jacobson, L. A., Williford, A. P., & Pianta, R. C. (2011). The role of executive function in children's competent adjustment to middle school. *Child Neuropsychology, 17*(3), 255–280.

Kochanska, G., & Knaack, A. (2003). Effortful control as a personality characteristic of young children: Antecedents, correlates, and consequences. *Journal of Personality, 71*(6), 1087–1112.

Kochanska, G., Murray, K. T., & Harlan, E. T. (2000). Effortful control in early childhood: Continuity and change, antecedents, and implications for social development. *Developmental Psychology, 36*(2), 220–232.

Lengua, L. J., Honorado, E., & Bush, N. R. (2007). Contextual risk and parenting as predictors of effortful control and social competence in preschool children. *Journal of Applied Developmental Psychology, 28*(1), 40–55.

Li-Grining, C. P. (2007). Effortful control among low-income preschoolers in three cities: Stability, change, and individual differences. *Developmental Psychology, 43*(1), 208–221.

Li-Grining, C. P., Raver, C. C., Champion, K. M., Sardin, L., Metzger, M. W., & Jones, S. M. (2010). Understanding and improving classroom emotional climate and behavioral management in the "real world." *Early Education and Development, 21*(1), 65–94.

Li-Grining, C. P., Votruba-Drzal, E., Bachman, H. J., & Chase-Lansdale, P. L. (2006). Are certain preschoolers at risk in the era of welfare reform?: The moderating role of children's temperament. *Children and Youth Services Review, 28*(9), 1102–1123.

Lonigan, C. J. (2006). Development, assessment, and promotion of preliteracy skills. *Early Education and Development, 17*(1), 91–114.

Marcovitch, S., & Zelazo, P. D. (2009). A hierarchical competing systems model of the emergence and early development of executive function. *Developmental Science, 12*(1), 1–18.

McClelland, M. M., Cameron, C. E., Connor, C. M., Farris, C. L., Jewkes, A. M., & Morrison, F. J. (2007). Links between behavioral regulation and preschoolers' literacy, vocabulary, and math skills. *Developmental Psychology, 43*(4), 947–959.

Morris, P., Raver, C., Lloyd, C. M., & Millenky, M. (2009). *Can teacher training in classroom management make a difference for children's experiences in preschool?: A preview of findings from the Foundations of Learning demonstration.* New York: MDRC.

National Center for Children in Poverty. (2012, June 3). Young child risk calculator. Retrieved from *www.nccp.org/tools/risk/?state=us&age-level=5&income-level=poor&ids[]=77&submit=calculate.*

Pears, K. C., Fisher, P. A., Bruce, J., Kim, H. K., & Yoerger, K. (2010). Early elementary school adjustment of maltreated children in foster care. *Child Development, 81*(5), 1550–1564.

Pianta, R. C., LaParo, K., Payne, C., Cox, M., & Bradley, R. (2002). The relation of kindergarten classroom environment to teacher, family, and school characteristics and child outcomes. *Elementary School Journal, 102*(3), 225–238.

Raver, C. C. (2012). Low-income children's self-regulation in the classroom: Scientific inquiry for social change. *American Psychologist, 67*(8), 681–689.

Raver, C. C., Blair, C., & Li-Grining, C. P. (2012). Extending models of emotional self- regulation to classroom settings: Implications for professional development. In C. Howes, B. K. Hamre, & R. C. Pianta (Eds.), *Effective early childhood professional development: Improving teacher practice and child outcomes* (pp. 113–130). Baltimore: Brookes.

Raver, C. C., Jones, S. M., Li-Grining, C. P., Metzger, M., Champion, K. M., & Sardin, L. (2008). Improving preschool classroom processes: Preliminary findings from a randomized trial implemented in Head Start settings. *Early Childhood Research Quarterly, 23*(1), 10–26.

Raver, C. C., Jones, S. M., Li-Grining, C., Zhai, F., Bub, K., & Pressler, E. (2011). CSRP's impact on low-income preschoolers' preacademic skills: Self-regulation as a mediating mechanism. *Child Development, 82*(1), 362–378.

Raver, C. C., Jones, S. M., Li-Grining, C., Zhai, F., Metzger, M. W., & Solomon, B. (2009). Targeting children's behavior problems in preschool classrooms: A cluster-randomized controlled trial. *Journal of Consulting and Clinical Psychology, 77*(2), 302–316.

Rhoades, B. L., Greenberg, M. T., Lanza, S. T., & Blair, C. (2011). Demographic and familial predictors of early executive function development: Contribution of a person-centered perspective. *Journal of Experimental Child Psychology, 108*(3), 638–662.

Rothbart, M. K., Sheese, B. E., & Posner, M. I. (2007). Executive attention and effortful control: Linking temperament, brain networks and genes. *Child Development Perspectives, 1*(1), 2–7.

Spinrad, T. L., Eisenberg, N., Silva, K. M., Eggum, N. D., Reiser, M., Edwards, A., et al. (2012). Longitudinal relations among maternal behaviors, effortful control and young children's committed compliance. *Developmental Psychology, 48*(2), 552–566.

Ursache, A., Blair, C., & Raver, C. (2012). The promotion of self-regulation as a means of enhancing school readiness and early achievement in children at risk for school failure. *Child Development Perspectives, 6*(2), 122–128.

Webster-Stratton, C., Reid, M. J., & Hammond, M. (2004). Treating children with early-onset conduct problems: Intervention outcomes for parent, child, and teacher training. *Journal of Clinical Child and Adolescent Psychology, 33*(1), 105–124.

Welsh, J. A., Nix, R. L., Blair, C., Bierman, K. L., & Nelson, K. E. (2010). The development of cognitive skills and gains in academic school readiness for children from low income families. *Journal of Educational Psychology, 102*(1), 43–53.

Wiebe, S. A., Sheffield, T., Nelson, J. M., Clark, C. A. C., Chevalier, N., & Espy, K. A. (2011). The structure of executive function in 3-year-olds. *Journal of Experimental Child Psychology, 108*(3), 436–452.

Zhai, F., Raver, C. C., Jones, S. M., Li-Grining, C. P., Pressler, E., & Gao, Q. (2010). Dosage effects on school readiness: Evidence from a randomized classroom-based intervention. *Social Service Review, 84*(4), 615–654.

Zhai, F., Raver, C. C., & Li-Grining, C. (2011). Classroom-based interventions and teachers' perceived job stressors and confidence: Evidence from a randomized trial in Head Start settings. *Early Childhood Research Quarterly, 26*(4), 442–452.

Zhou, Q., Hofer, C., Eisenberg, N., Reiser, M., Spinrad, T. L., & Fabes, R. A. (2007). The developmental trajectories of attention focusing, attentional and behavioral persistence, and externalizing problems during school-age years. *Developmental Psychology, 43*(2), 369–385.

CHAPTER 10

Integrating Evidence-Based Preschool Programs to Support Social-Emotional and Cognitive Development

Karen L. Bierman, Celene E. Domitrovich, Robert L. Nix, Janet A. Welsh, and Scott D. Gest

As children move through preschool and into kindergarten, they face a host of new social, emotional, and learning demands. School requires them to function effectively in a group context, establish positive relationships with peers and teachers, follow classroom rules, and involve themselves actively in the learning process (McClelland, Acock, & Morrison, 2006). Children's school readiness is embedded in the acquisition of the social-emotional and cognitive skills that underlie their capacity to meet these demands, and thereby to adjust socially and succeed academically in school.

A substantial number of children (up to 20–30% of children living in poverty) start school without the social-emotional and cognitive skills that foster this school readiness, contributing to delays in school progress and disparities in school attainment (McClelland et al., 2006; Ryan, Fauth, & Brooks-Gunn, 2006). Children who begin school unprepared for these learning and behavioral demands typically remain low achievers throughout elementary school and are more likely than their more advantaged peers to experience learning disabilities, conflictual relationships with teachers and peers, grade retention, early school dropout, and long-term underemployment (Ryan et al., 2006).

One important goal of early schooling efforts for at-risk children is to remediate delays in emergent literacy and math skills in order to close the achievement gap within the first few years of schooling (see Starkey, Klein, & DeFlorio, Chapter 8, and Li-Grining, Lennon, Marcus, Flores, and Haas, Chapter 9, this volume). A second goal is to promote the development of the social-emotional competencies and self-regulation skills that support motivated and goal-oriented classroom engagement and learning (Blair, 2002).

This chapter provides a brief review of the developmental research that documents the importance of focusing on both social-emotional and cognitive development during the preschool and early elementary years. We review evidence-based interventions that improve social-emotional school readiness. We then describe the implementation and outcomes of the Head Start REDI (Research-Based, Developmentally Informed) project, a preschool enrichment program that integrates evidence-based curriculum components targeting social-emotional and language–literacy skills, embracing this dual focus to improve the school readiness of socioeconomically disadvantaged children. Implications for professional development and classroom practice are discussed.

Social-Emotional Skills That Support School Success

The preschool and early elementary school years represent a watershed for social-emotional development (Eisenberg & Fabes, 1998). Attention and memory skills show rapid development, transforming the child's capacity for classroom learning (Raver, 2002). Skills associated with behavioral inhibition and impulse control mature, facilitating the child's ability to sustain effort and persist at tasks, as well as to learn on demand through listening and observation (McClelland et al., 2006). These skills reflect the growth of the prefrontal cortex and executive function skills, which support attention control and problem solving, fueling more independent and goal-oriented learning (Blair, 2002) and facilitating the acquisition of emergent literacy and numeracy skills (Blair & Razza, 2007; Welsh, Nix, Blair, Bierman, & Nelson, 2010).

Developmental transformations are also evident in children's social interactions during the preschool years as the parallel play that characterizes the peer interactions of young 3-year-olds gives way to the more complex, thematic, and coordinated peer play evident among 5- and 6-year-olds (Bierman & Erath, 2006). These emerging social abilities benefit from developing language and executive function skills, and also likely play a central role in promoting the development of those skills (Blair & Diamond, 2008; Coolahan, Fantuzzo, Mendez, & McDermott, 2000).

That is, children who are highly engaged socially with others have more opportunities to practice coordinated and thematic play than children who are isolated or excluded, and they face more frequent demands to communicate clearly and resolve conflicts in the context of that play, thereby enhancing their skill acquisition (Coolahan et al., 2000).

Corresponding to growth in the complexity of social interaction, children show dramatic gains in the area of emotional understanding during the preschool and early elementary years. Normatively, empathy and altruism emerge in preschool as children recognize and differentiate a broader array of emotions and begin to understand that their actions can cause feelings in other people that are different from their own (Eisenberg & Fabes, 1998). Children become more able to regulate their emotions, fostering their capacity to tolerate frustration and manage conflicts peacefully (Izard et al., 2001). These emotional skills are positively linked with academic performance (Garner & Waajid, 2008; Trentacosta & Izard, 2007) and positive peer relationships (Eisenberg & Fabes, 1998).

Recognizing that delays in social-emotional and self-regulation skills are common among children who adjust poorly to elementary school, a number of different interventions have been designed to promote the development of these skills and improve children's school readiness (Bierman & Erath, 2006; Blair & Diamond, 2008). In the next section, we describe several different intervention approaches that have proven effective at promoting social-emotional school readiness. We focus, in particular, on programs that have undergone rigorous randomized controlled evaluations.

Specific Interventions That Promote Social-Emotional School Readiness

Although they share a similar set of goals, school-based interventions targeting improvements in child social-emotional school readiness take different approaches, reflected in different logic models. The *logic model* of an intervention refers to the way that the program conceptualizes the change process. Logic models guide intervention design and implementation by identifying mechanisms of action and indicating how the intervention activities are expected to promote improvements in specific child outcomes. In the area of school readiness interventions, efforts to improve child outcomes typically focus on one or two kinds of change mechanisms, either (1) promoting new teacher skills/practices (e.g., affecting how teaching is being done; how teachers are interacting with students, and managing children's emotions and conflicts in the classroom) and/or (2) changing/enriching the curriculum content (e.g., modifying what is being taught and which learning activities are being used). Interventions designed to improve social-emotional school readiness also vary in the content domains or child skills that are a central focus of the intervention, demonstrating different levels of emphasis devoted to reducing problem behaviors, improving prosocial behaviors and social competence, enhancing attention skills and learning behaviors, or promoting social-cognitive skills that may provide a foundation for effective school adaptation, such as emotional understanding or social problem-solving skills. Examples of effective programs that reflect different logic models are reviewed briefly in the following sections.

The Incredible Years Teacher Training Program

Focused on teachers, the Incredible Years Teacher Training Program systematically strengthens teacher classroom management strategies to promote children's prosocial behavior and aggression control (Webster-Stratton, Reid, & Hammond, 2001). As proximal targets for change, the program focuses on the following teaching skills: (1) using specific, contingent attention, encouragement, and praise to support positive child behavior; (2) using incentives to motivate learning effort and engagement; (3) preventing behavior problems by structuring the classroom effectively, particularly planning for transitions; (4) decreasing inappropriate behavior with the use of nonpunitive consequences; and (5) building positive relationships with students. Based primarily on social learning theory, this intervention focuses on changing the contingencies and reinforcement for desired and undesired behaviors, in order to provide support for positive student development. Observational research suggests that teacher attention is often focused selectively on the behaviors that disrupt lessons, creating a situation in which a majority of positive student behaviors receive no teacher response (Martens, Hiralall, & Bradley, 1997). Incredible Years seeks to reorient teacher attention and affect, in order to provide children with a warm and supportive classroom environment in which the sensitive and contingent responding of teachers reinforces desired child behaviors, while the use of nonpunitive discipline strategies, such as planned ignoring, natural consequences, and time-out, reduces undesired behaviors (Webster-Stratton et al., 2001). The intervention is delivered via monthly workshops with teachers that involve review of modeling videotapes, group discussion, practice assignments, and consultation in response to the ongoing program experiences of the participating teachers.

In a randomized controlled study of the Incredible Years teacher and parent training programs, Webster-Stratton et al. (2001) examined differences between intervention teachers (i.e., teachers who followed the

Incredible Years program) and teachers engaging in their "usual practice" teaching in Head Start classrooms serving low-income children. Postintervention observations indicated that intervention teachers used more praise, more effective discipline techniques, and fewer harsh and critical techniques. In the Webster-Stratton et al. study, the children in the intervention classrooms also exhibited greater learning engagement and on-task behavior, increased prosocial behavior, and reduced aggression compared with their peers in the "usual practice" control condition classrooms.

In an independent evaluation, Raver and colleagues (2008) incorporated the Incredible Years Teacher Training Program into their Chicago School Readiness Project (CSRP), providing Head Start teachers with five 6-hour training sessions. In addition, CSRP provided a mental health consultant, who met with teachers weekly to support their implementation of the Incredible Years classroom management skills, and also to provide emotional support for their own stress reduction. Mental health consultants also implemented individualized management plans for children displaying high levels of disruptive behavior in the classroom. At the end of the year, observations documented significantly higher levels of positive climate, teacher sensitivity, and positive behavior management in intervention classrooms compared with the "usual practice" Head Start classrooms. Observations also documented lower levels of aggressive and disruptive behavior among children in the CSRP intervention classrooms compared with children in the control classrooms (Raver et al., 2009). Furthermore, significant benefits for children emerged in areas of preacademic skills, such as vocabulary, letter naming, math, and attention control (Raver et al., 2011). The investigators postulate that improvements in teacher classroom management skills led to increases in instructional time and child learning engagement, thereby promoting gains in academic as well as social-emotional skills.

Tools of the Mind

Taking a very different approach to the promotion of social-emotional school readiness is the Tools of the Mind program (Bodrova & Leong, 2007). Tools focuses on promoting child self-regulatory skills and aims to reduce child dependence on the external control provided by teachers. For this reason, Tools eschews the use of token or point reward systems in the classroom, although it supports teacher's use of praise and attention to reinforce positive child behaviors. To enhance child self-regulation, Tools restructures learning activities to reduce large-group activities and passive waiting time and increase small-group and peer-pairing activities that keep children more actively engaged in the learning process. Tools also places a special emphasis on sociodramatic play as a critical context for the development of self-regulatory skills. Teachers are taught how to introduce and support complex dramatic play themes in the classroom, and children spend time each day in planning and enacting sustained, collaborative sociodramatic peer play in prepared play centers. From a theoretical standpoint, reflecting Vygotsky, pretend sociodramatic play requires children to exercise executive function skills, as well as to regulate their social behavior (Blair & Diamond, 2008; Bodrova & Leong, 2007). Specifically, role playing requires children to (1) hold their own character role and those of others in mind, exercising working memory; (2) inhibit behavioral impulses to act out of character, exercising inhibitory control; and (3) flexibly adapt to unexpected changes in play scenarios, exercising attentional set-shifting skills. In the Tools program, teachers also lead games that involve turn taking, inhibitory control, and remembering to enact preplanned rather than impulsive behaviors, which are specifically designed to reinforce executive function skills. Tools represents a curriculum-based preschool intervention, but one that emphasizes the central role of the teacher in supporting and scaffolding child opportunities for engagement in the sorts of play and learning activities that foster the development of self-regulation skills.

Tools has been evaluated in a randomized controlled trial in which teachers and preschool children (ages 3 and 4 years old) were assigned to classrooms using the Tools curriculum or a curriculum developed by the school district (Barnett et al., 2008). Intervention teachers received 4 full days of training before classes began, along with additional training and discussion sessions scheduled during the school year. In addition, a Tools trainer provided ongoing coaching, making weekly, 30-minute classroom visits throughout the year, and meeting individually with teachers on an as-needed basis to clarify the curriculum and address implementation challenges. Observation documented a significant impact of the Tools curriculum on the quality of teaching in the classrooms, including measures assessing classroom structure and time use, quality of the literacy environment and instruction, and the use of scaffolding techniques by teachers in their interactions with children (Barnett et al., 2008). Observations were also conducted using the Classroom Assessment Scoring System (LaParo & Pianta, 2003), which focuses on the quality of teacher–student interactions, but these did not show a significant effect of the intervention. In terms of child outcomes, Barnett et al. (2008) found that intervention teachers rated children in their classrooms as having fewer behavior problems, and children also showed test gains in vocabulary but not in emergent literacy or math skills. Another assessment conducted a year later, after children had been exposed to the program for 2 years, also showed significant effects on children's executive function skills (Diamond, Barnett, Thomas, & Munro, 2007). However, these latter assessments were made after teachers and children were allowed to change programs if desired, thus compromising the original randomization and warranting confirmation in additional studies. Additional trials evaluating this program are currently under way.

In addition to the intervention approaches represented by the Incredible Years and Tools programs, a number of curriculum-based interventions have used explicit lessons and coaching to promote specific social-emotional skills.

SOCIAL-EMOTIONAL LEARNING CURRICULA AND CHILDREN'S SCHOOL READINESS

A rapidly growing research base suggests that social-emotional skills development can be enhanced using such systematic instructional approaches in the classroom, generally referred to as social-emotional learning (SEL) curricula (Consortium on the School-Based Promotion of Social Competence, 1994). SEL programs are informed, in part, by social learning theory and emphasize the acquisition of behavioral skills. They also emphasize the central role of children's social cognitions and social information-processing skills in fostering adaptive social-emotional functioning. Reflecting their social learning theory roots, SEL programs include presentations that help children understand targeted skills concepts using a combination of modeling, instruction, and discussion. They include opportunities for children to practice those skills and receive feedback and support from teachers. SEL programs also emphasize the importance of covert thinking processes in fostering skillful social interaction and self-regulatory control. For example, children's cognitive capacities to recognize and accurately assess social problems, to differentiate feelings and behaviors, to generate and evaluate multiple potential responses, to set goals, and to self-monitor their behavioral performance in light of those goals are considered critical building blocks for flexible and adaptive social behavior (for more detail, see Greenberg, 2006).

In SEL programs designed for young children, teachers use lessons, typically with modeling stories, puppets, and pictures to illustrate concepts and explain, demonstrate, and discuss the skills. These lessons also include practice activities, such as role plays, games, and cooperative activities that allow children to experience success enacting the skill. Finally, teachers provide support during the day to help children generalize the use of the skills in their everyday interactions in the classroom. This teacher role is important, because teachers model, prompt, and praise children for using the skills, thereby strengthening children's comfort and competence. There are several examples of preschool programs that utilize SEL curricula and have evidence of effectiveness based on randomized controlled evaluations.

The I Can Problem Solve (ICPS) program was one of the first such social-emotional learning programs designed specifically for preschool children (Shure, 1992; Shure & Spivack, 1982). In this program, children learn word concepts to help them describe social sequences (e.g., some vs. all, if–then, same–different). The next set of lessons focuses on helping children identify their own feelings and recognize the feelings of others. In subsequent lessons, teachers promote social problem-solving skills by introducing hypothetical preschool problem situations and asking children to generate and act out possible solutions. A randomized controlled trial showed that the ICPS program promoted gains in children's social problem-solving abilities and led to teacher-rated improvements in frustration tolerance, impulsivity, and task engagement (Shure & Spivack, 1982).

Al's Pals: Kids Making Healthy Choices is another example of a social-emotional learning program designed for preschool, kindergarten, and first-grade children. The program includes 46 lessons that focus on a hand puppet named Al, who, along with his puppet friends, demonstrate a set of social-emotional skills in role plays, discussions, original songs, and books. In a randomized controlled evaluation of Al's Pals, participating children showed improved social skills and problem-solving abilities, as assessed by teacher ratings, compared to children in "usual practice" classrooms (Dubas, Lynch, Gallano, Geller, & Hunt, 1998). Similarly, a second randomized controlled trial of this curriculum conducted in Head Start classrooms produced significant positive effects on teacher-rated behavior problems and independent functioning (Lynch, Geller, & Schmidt, 2004).

Similarly, the Incredible Years Dinosaur School Social Skills and Problem Solving curriculum is a social-emotional learning program designed to decrease aggression and promote social skills in young children ages 3–8 (Webster-Stratton, 2005). Findings from a randomized controlled group intervention study in 153 classrooms (including Head Start, kindergarten, and first-grade classes) with over 1,700 children indicated that teachers in classrooms offering the Dinosaur School program were significantly more nurturing and consistent with discipline, focused more on promoting social and emotional behaviors, and were less harsh and critical in their interactions with children. Compared with children in the "usual practice" classrooms, children in intervention classrooms were more cooperative with teachers and peers, and showed enhanced problem-solving skills (Webster-Stratton, Reid, & Stoolmiller, 2008).

The PATHS (Promoting Alternative Thinking Strategies) curriculum (Kusche & Greenberg, 1994) is one of the most comprehensive, evidence-based, social-emotional learning programs available. A number of randomized trials conducted with students in the early elementary grades have shown that the use of PATHS is associated with improved social cognitions, more socially competent behaviors, and reduced aggression (Conduct Problems Prevention Research Group, 1999, 2010), as well as improved executive function skills (Riggs, Greenberg, Kusche, & Pentz, 2006).

More recently, a downward extension of this curriculum was created to address school readiness by improving young children's emotional understanding and social problem-solving skills, and increasing their capacity to use language effectively in the service of emotion regulation (Domitrovich, Greenberg, Cortes, & Kusche, 1999). Preschool PATHS targets skills in four social-emotional domains: (1) friendship skills and prosocial behaviors (e.g., helping, sharing, taking turns); (2) emotional knowledge (e.g., recognizing and labeling core feelings); (3) self-control (e.g., using the "Turtle Technique" to stop, self-calm, and identify the feeling and problem); and (4) social problem solving (e.g., identifying the problem, generating solutions, considering consequences, and choosing the best plan). There are 33 brief lessons with stories, pictures, and puppets that provide skills instruction. Each lesson also includes ideas for formal and informal extension activities that teachers and preschool staff members can use throughout the day to generalize key concepts. Teachers are encouraged to provide emotion coaching throughout the day, modeling feeling statements themselves when appropriate, helping children notice the feelings of peers, and prompting children to describe their own feelings. Teachers are also encouraged to watch for naturally occurring "teachable moments," such as peer disagreements or conflicts. At these times, teachers are taught to help children stop and calm down, then talk through the problem-solving steps of defining the problem and their feelings, listening to their friend's feelings, and generating ideas for how to solve the problem. A randomized controlled trial compared the development of children in 10 Head Start classrooms using Preschool PATHS with children in 10 "usual practice" Head Start classrooms; 287 children were followed for 1 year. Children who received Preschool PATHS showed higher levels of emotional understanding and were rated as more socially competent by both teachers and parents than children in the control classrooms (Domitrovich, Cortes, & Greenberg, 2007).

Summary

The studies reviewed in this section demonstrate the substantial impact that preschool and early elementary school practices and programs can have on child social-emotional development and school readiness.

Effective interventions vary in their approach, alternatively placing a major emphasis on improving teacher classroom management skills, restructuring learning activities and investing in scaffolded sociodramatic play, or providing children with explicit lessons and coaching in social-emotional skills. Intervention programs using each of these approaches have proven effective in reducing child behavior problems and promoting child social competencies. Academic outcomes were not measured in all of the studies reviewed, but some showed evidence of the "crossover" impact of social-emotional intervention on child vocabulary (Barnett et al., 2008) and emergent literacy and math skills (Raver et al., 2011), suggesting that promoting social-emotional and self-regulation skills can foster cognitive as well as social-emotional school readiness (see also Durlak, Weissberg, Dymnicki, Taylor, & Shellinger, 2011). However, such "crossover" effects may not be sufficient by themselves to reduce the substantial gap in cognitive school readiness, including the emergent literacy and math skills associated with poverty and early adversity.

THE NEED FOR PRESCHOOL ACADEMIC ENRICHMENT

The relative importance of addressing the delays in cognitive versus social-emotional school readiness among children growing up in poverty has been a topic of considerable debate (see Barnett et al., 2008). Fueling the argument that instruction focused on promoting emergent literacy skills should begin during the preschool years are data demonstrating that skills such as knowledge of print (e.g., letter names), phonological awareness (e.g., being able to rhyme), and writing (e.g., being able to print one's name) are strong predictors of reading success well into elementary school (Whitehurst, 2001) and, furthermore, that prekindergarten instruction in these skills has a significant impact on promoting rapid skills acquisition, facilitating cognitive school readiness (Lonigan, 2006).

In contrast, other investigators have expressed concerns about the early push toward teacher-directed instruction and academic attainment during the preschool years (Elkind, 2001; Parker & Neuharth-Pritchett, 2006). They cite a lack of evidence showing long-term academic gains associated with preschool academic acceleration and note that academically focused preschool programs do not address the behavioral and social-emotional needs of at-risk children. Reflecting this concern, the longitudinal follow-up of a study that compared a highly academic preschool program, Direct Instruction, with a balanced curriculum that emphasized teacher-scaffolded, child-centered learning, High/Scope, found that the former failed to produce the long-term gains in child social competence and the reductions in child antisocial behavior produced by the latter (Schweinhart, Weikart, & Larner, 1986).

Clearly, given that children growing up under conditions of adversity often show delays in both cognitive and social-emotional school readiness, enhancing skills in both domains is important. Ideally, one would not choose between cognitive and social-emotional approaches in promoting school readiness, but rather combine intervention approaches to maximize gains in both domains. The Head Start REDI project was designed with this goal in mind.

The Head Start REDI Project

Head Start REDI was designed to provide an enrichment intervention that could be integrated into the existing framework of Head Start programs (Bierman, Domitrovich, et al., 2008). The goal was to demonstrate that evidence-based curricular enhancements targeting social-emotional learning and emergent literacy skills could complement the broad educational programming provided by High/Scope or Creative Curriculum, increasing the systematic emphasis teachers placed on target skills and improving child outcomes in areas of both social-emotional and cognitive school readiness. The REDI intervention was delivered by classroom teachers and integrated into their ongoing classroom programs. It included curriculum-based lessons, center-based extension activities, and training in teaching strategies to use throughout the day. These skills were selected because they are important predictors of grade school adjustment and achievement, and are associated with socioeconomic disparities in school readiness (Blair, 2002; Lonigan, 2006). In addition, prior efficacy studies had demonstrated that these instructional approaches used in isolation produced improvements in child skills and school readiness. A key question was whether teachers could implement these multiple approaches at the same time, so that children would show positive outcomes across domains, or alternatively, whether the combined approach would overburden teachers and therefore lead to a dilution of program effects.

REDI Intervention Components

In REDI, the Preschool PATHS curriculum (Domitrovich et al., 1999) was used to promote children's social-emotional skills. The 33 lessons that comprise this curriculum were delivered by teachers during circle time, supporting child understanding of prosocial friendship skills, emotional understanding and emotional expression skills, self-control, and social problem-solving skills. In addition to teaching one lesson per week, teachers conducted a weekly extension activity, leading a cooperative game or project that provided children with opportunities to practice the PATHS skills with teacher support. Teachers received mentoring that encouraged them to use PATHS compliments and positive classroom management strategies daily, and to support generalized skills development with ongoing emotion coaching and support for student use of the self-control technique (called the "Turtle Technique") and social problem-solving steps. The goal was to help students apply PATHS skills in their everyday interactions in the classroom.

Three program components were used to support the development of language and emergent literacy skills in REDI, including an interactive reading program, a set of sound games, and print center activities. The interactive reading program was based on the shared reading program developed by Wasik, Bond, and Hindman, 2006; see also Wasik & Hindman, Chapter 7, this volume, which in turn was an adaptation of the dialogic reading program (Whitehurst et al., 1994). The curriculum included two books per week, which were scripted with interactive questions. Each book had a list of targeted vocabulary words, presented with the aid of physical props and illustrations. In addition to presenting these materials in a systematic way during the week, teachers received mentoring in the use of language coaching strategies, such as expansions and grammatical recasts, to provide a general scaffold for language development in the classroom (Dickinson & Smith, 1994). The overall goal was to improve teachers' strategic use of language in ways that would increase child oral language skills, including vocabulary, narrative, and syntax. To enhance synergy across the social-emotional and cognitive curriculum components of REDI, the PATHS themes were linked systematically with the interactive reading program. Many of the interactive reading books teachers used featured the PATHS theme of the week, thereby serving as a second PATHS extension activity and tying together the reading and social-emotional learning programs. Conversely, language and literacy skills also were incorporated into many of the PATHS extension activities.

In addition, REDI provided teachers with curricular materials to promote phonological awareness and print knowledge. A set of sound games was based primarily upon the work of Adams, Foorman, Lundberg, and Beeler (1998). The games were organized developmentally, moving from easier to more difficult skills during the course of the year (e.g., listening, rhyming, alliteration, words and sentences, syllables, and phonemes). Teachers were asked to use a 10- to 15-minute sound game activity at least three times per week. Teachers also were provided with a developmentally sequenced set of activities and materials to be used in their alphabet centers, including letter stickers, a letter bucket, materials to create a letter wall, and craft materials for various letter-learning activities. Teachers were asked to make sure that each child visited the alphabet center several times per week, and they were given materials to track the children's acquisition of letter names.

The interactive reading program and emphasis on language use, as well as the emotion coaching and social problem-solving strategies that were central to the REDI program were philosophically compatible with the strategic, child-centered teaching approach used in High/Scope and Creative Curriculum. In contrast, the sound games and print center activities utilized more direct teacher instruction, about which some early childhood educators have worried because of the possibility of failing to engage motivated learning in young children (Elkind, 2001). These curriculum components were included in REDI based upon research documenting the essential nature of emergent literacy skills for school success and evidence of the effectiveness of these approaches in promoting emergent literacy skills in disadvantaged preschool children (Lonigan, 2006). In addition, it was anticipated that the previously limited effects of a direct instruction approach (Schweinhart et al., 1986) could be circumvented by integrating these strategies into a more comprehensive educational approach that included specific supports for social-emotional skills development.

Finally, to strengthen home–school connections, three take-home packets were mailed to parents during the course of the year, each containing a modeling videotape, with parenting tips and learning activities to use at home. In addition, the PATHS curriculum included handouts for parents, with suggestions for home activities. Children also took home letter stickers and compliment pages to prompt their parents to ask them about their school day and provide positive support at home.

The REDI Professional Development Model

To support teachers in their implementation of the multifaceted REDI model, they received detailed manuals and kits containing all materials needed to implement the intervention. A 3-day professional training was conducted in August, prior to initiating the intervention, and a 1-day booster training session was conducted midyear. Teachers also received weekly mentoring support provided by local educational consultants called REDI trainers, who were experienced master teachers supervised by two project-based, senior educational specialists. The weekly consultations were intended to enhance the quality of implementation through modeling, coaching, and providing ongoing feedback regarding program delivery. REDI trainers spent an average of 3 hours per week in each classroom observing, demonstrating, or team-teaching lessons. They also met with the head and assistant teachers for 1 hour each week outside of class. REDI trainers provided teachers with suggestions in the area of effective classroom management, such as establishing clear and appropriate rules and directions, providing positive and corrective feedback for appropriate behavior, applying natural response cost procedures to reduce problem behaviors, and strengthening positive relationships with children and parents.

REDI Research Evaluation Design

To evaluate its effectiveness, the REDI project employed a randomized controlled trial design, assigning 44 Head Start classrooms serving low-income children to intervention or usual practice conditions. Although classrooms contained 3- and 4- year-old children, only 4-year-olds participated in this evaluation. Teachers were studied as they implemented the intervention for the first time, and 4-year-old children in the intervention condition were assessed after receiving 1 year of REDI. Teachers in the comparison classrooms continued to implement High/Scope or Creative Curriculum as usual.

Study participants included 356 children (17% Hispanic, 25% African American, 42% European American; 54% girls), who represented a majority (86%) of the 4-year-old children in the participating classrooms. At the beginning of the Head Start year, these children were, on average, 4.49 years old (*SD* = 0.31, range = 3.72–5.65). On the Block Design scale of the Wechsler Preschool and Primary Scale of Intelligence—Third Edition (WPPSI-III), a measure of nonverbal cognitive ability that is highly correlated with Full Scale IQ (*r* = .72; Wechsler, 2002), children received an average standard score of 7.98 (*SD* = 2.88), approximately two-thirds of a standard deviation below the national mean of 10 and comparable to similar samples of children growing up in poverty.

At the beginning and end of the year, research assistants visited schools and conducted individual assessments with all child participants. In addition, teachers and parents provided ratings on each child in the study, and each child was observed during two 12- to 15-minute play sessions. Teachers were also observed to assess the quality of student–teacher interactions and quality of language use in the classroom.

Intervention Implementation

An important initial question was whether teachers were able to implement the multiple components of the REDI intervention effectively. Based on teacher reports, it appeared that most teachers were able to complete a majority of the REDI lessons and activities. On average, teachers reported conducting 1.77 PATHS lessons and extension activities, 6.08 dialogic reading activities, 2.57 sound game activities, and 3.56 alphabet center activities each week.

Rating 10 questions regarding the quality of their implementation, teachers gave an average quality rating of 2.78 on a 3-point scale, reflecting their feelings that the lessons were relatively easy to implement as written, children were engaged, and children seemed to understand the skills being taught. REDI trainers also observed and rated the fidelity and quality of the teachers' implementation of program components, using a 6-point Likert scale with response options ranging from poor to exemplary. REDI trainer ratings indicated "4 = adequate" to "5 = strong" implementation across intervention components. On average, teachers received a score of 4.61 (*SD* = 0.74) in their implementation of PATHS, a score of 4.39 (*SD* = 0.57) in their implementation of dialogic reading, a score of 4.70 (*SD* = 0.55) in their implementation of alphabet center activities, a score of 4.52 (*SD* = 0.72) in their implementation of sound games, and an overall score of 4.55 (*SD* = 0.67). In general, these data suggest that, with the manuals, materials, and professional development support teachers were given, they were able to implement the multiple components of REDI effectively in both emergent literacy and social-emotional learning domains.

Impact on Teaching Quality

The second question we addressed was the degree to which the REDI program improved the quality of teacher behavioral management, teacher–student interactions, and language use in the classroom. Research assistants who were blind to the teachers' intervention status visited classrooms in the spring of the year, and used the Classroom Assessment Scoring System (CLASS; LaParo & Pianta, 2003) to assess the quality of emotional support and instructional support evident in classrooms. In addition, observers rated teachers on teaching practices targeted specifically by the PATHS curriculum, and they assessed the quality of language used in the classroom.

On the CLASS Emotional Support subscales, REDI produced significant or near-significant increases in positive climate ($p < .04$) and teacher sensitivity ($p < .07$). REDI also produced a nearly significant effect on the CLASS Instructional Support scale ($p < .08$), indicating improvements in teachers use of instructional time and student productivity and engagement. Reflecting the specific teaching strategies that were a target of the intervention, observers also scored REDI teachers as significantly or nearly significantly higher than teachers in comparison classrooms on rating scales reflecting positive emotional climate ($p < .05$), which includes items reflecting emotion expression, support for emotion regulation, and emotion modeling, and classroom management skills ($p < .001$), which include items on setting clear expectations, consistent limit setting, and proactive/preventive management. Finally, positive changes were observed in teachers' language use in the classroom: REDI teachers made more statements ($p < .001$), asked more questions ($p < .001$), used more decontextualized talk ($p < .005$), and engaged in richer and more sensitive talk with children ($p < .004$) than teachers in the usual practice control group. The magnitude of these effects was in the small-to-moderate range for the ratings reflecting teacher social-emotional support, with effect sizes ranging from $d = 0.39$ to 0.61, and in the moderate-to-large range for the language use scales, with effect sizes ranging from $d = 0.67$ to 0.89 (see Domitrovich et al., 2009, for details). Overall, these findings indicate that the REDI intervention helped teachers establish a more positive classroom climate, use more preventive behavior management strategies, and talk with children more frequently and in more cognitively complex ways.

Impact on Child Outcomes

REDI intervention effects on child outcomes were evaluated using hierarchical linear models that accounted for the nesting of children within classrooms and controlled for child sex, race, and cohort (see Bierman, Domitrovich, et al., 2008; Bierman, Nix, Greenberg, Blair, & Domitrovich, 2008, for a full description). In the domain of language/emergent literacy skills, positive effects for REDI were found on children's growth in vocabulary skills ($d = 0.15$, $p < .05$), phonemic awareness ($d = 0.35$–0.39, $p < .001$), and print awareness ($d = 0.16$, $p < .10$). In the domain of social-cognitive skills and emotional understanding, children who received REDI, compared to those in the usual practice control classrooms, gained more in their ability to identify and recognize emotions in photographs ($d = 0.21$, $p < .06$) and stories ($d = 0.23$, $p < .05$). They also showed more ability to generate competent and nonaggressive solutions to hypothetical social problems ($d = 0.21$–0.35, $p < .05$). Teachers rated children who received REDI as more socially competent ($d = 0.24$, $p < .10$) and less aggressive ($d = 0.28$, $p < .05$) than children in the comparison classrooms, and observers who were blind to condition also rated children who received REDI as more socially competent ($d = 0.26$, $p < .10$). Finally, assessments of children's executive function skills revealed that REDI produced gains in children's attention regulation skills, reflected in their performance on the Dimensional Change Card Sort (Frye, Zelazo, & Palfai, 1995) a task measuring working memory, attention control, response inhibition, and set-shifting. Moreover, assessors rated REDI children higher on items reflecting their task persistence, ability to sustain concentration, frustration tolerance, and motivated engagement during the testing session (see Bierman, Nix, et al., 2008, for more details).

Summary and Future Directions

Interventions that promote school readiness represent a critical effort toward reducing the achievement gap associated with growing up in poverty. Developmental research documents delays in both cognitive and social-emotional school readiness associated with early adversity. As a result, interventions may be most effective when they take a dual focus on promoting cognitive and social-emotional competencies. Research conducted in the context of rigorous randomized controlled trials demonstrates that interventions targeting positive classroom management and supportive teacher–student relationships, and those that promote children's acquisition of emotional awareness, empathy, social interaction skills, and social problem-solving skills are effective at reducing problem behaviors and enhancing children's learning engagement in the classroom. A critical goal for the future is the broad dissemination of these evidence-based practices in order to improve the impact of preschool and early elementary school on child skills acquisition and social-emotional adjustment.

The REDI program was designed as an enrichment program that could be integrated into more comprehensive core programs, such as High/Scope or Creative Curriculum, to strengthen program impact on key school readiness skills. To make the integration of research-based practices easier, REDI provided teachers with manualized enrichment curricula that included brief lessons, hands-on extension activities, and specific instructional strategies, all arranged strategically to address a scope and sequence of social-emotional and language/emergent literacy skills. The value of this sort of specific curriculum is that it not only reduces the burden on teachers but it also provides the guidance and support necessary for easy incorporation of evidence-based practice into everyday classroom planning.

In addition, REDI provided mentoring to support teacher understanding and effective use of these instructional strategies. Increasingly, education research is documenting the value of ongoing professional development in the form of mentoring or coaching to foster teacher implementation of evidence-based practice and positive teaching strategies. Developing strategies to support the availability of this kind of professional development is an ongoing goal, and promising approaches are emerging. For example, a recent study documented the value of a web-based platform to deliver professional development support (Pianta, Mashburn, Downer, Hamre, & Justice, 2008). The online coaching program, My TeachingPartner, facilitated teacher implementation of a social-emotional learning program (Preschool PATHS) by providing an array of web-based professional development resources, including video exemplars and lesson plans. Teachers met regularly with an online coach, sharing videotaped excerpts of their classroom lessons, and receiving positive support and individualized feedback and suggestions. This kind of strategy offers hope for making teacher coaching widely accessible. Future research may contribute additional knowledge regarding optimal and efficient strategies to provide teachers with the professional development and curriculum resources they need to close the achievement gap associated with poverty and promote positive school outcomes for all children.

Acknowledgments

The REDI project was supported by National Institute of Child Health and Human Development Grant Nos. HD046064 and HD43763. Appreciation is expressed to the teachers, students, parents, and program personnel who served as partners in this project in the Huntingdon, Blair, and York County Head Start Programs of Pennsylvania. In addition, this work reflects the particular efforts and talents of Gloria Rhule, Harriet Darling, Julia Gest, the REDI intervention staff, and the entire REDI research team.

References

Adams, M. J., Foorman, B. R., Lundberg, I., & Beeler, T. (1998). *Phonological sensitivity in young children: A classroom curriculum*. Baltimore: Brookes.

Barnett, W. S., Jung, K., Yarosz, D., Thomas, J., Hornbeck, A., Stechuk, R., et al. (2008). Educational effects of the Tools of the Mind curriculum: A randomized trial. *Early Childhood Research Quarterly, 23*(3), 299–313.

Bierman, K. L, Domitrovich, C. E., Nix, R. L., Gest, S. D., Welsh, J. A., Greenberg, M. T., et al. (2008). Promoting academic and social-emotional school readiness: The Head Start REDI Program. *Child Development, 79*, 1802–1817.

Bierman, K. L., & Erath, S. A. (2006). Promoting social competence in early childhood: Classroom curricula and social skills coaching programs. In K. McCartney & D. Phillips (Eds.), *Blackwell handbook on early childhood development* (pp. 595–615). Malden, MA: Blackwell.

Bierman, K. L., Nix, R. L., Greenberg, M. T., Blair, C., & Domitrovich, C. E. (2008). Executive functions and school readiness intervention: Impact, moderation, and mediation in the Head Start REDI Program. *Development and Psychopathology, 20*, 821–843.

Blair, C. (2002). School readiness: Integrating cognition and emotion in a neurobiological conceptualization of child functioning at school entry. *American Psychologist, 57,* 111–127.

Blair, C., & Diamond, A. (2008). Biological processes in prevention and intervention: The promotion of self-regulation as a means of preventing school failure. *Development and Psychopathology, 20,* 899–911.

Blair, C., & Razza, R. P. (2007). Relating effortful control, executive function, and false belief understanding to emerging math and literacy ability in kindergarten. *Child Development, 78,* 647–680.

Bodrova, E., & Leong, D. J. (2007). *Tools of the Mind: The Vygotskian approach to early childhood education* (2nd ed.). Upper Saddle River, NJ: Prentice Hall.

Conduct Problems Prevention Research Group. (1999). Initial impact of the Fast Track prevention trial for conduct problems: 2. Classroom effects. *Journal of Consulting and Clinical Psychology, 67,* 648–657.

Conduct Problems Prevention Research Group. (2010). The effects of a multiyear universal social-emotional program: The role of student and school characteristics. *Journal of Consulting and Clinical Psychology, 78,* 156–168.

Consortium on the School-Based Promotion of Social Competence. (1994). The school-based promotion of social competence: Theory, research, practice, and policy. In R. J. Haggerty, L. R. Sherrod, N. Garmezy, & M. Rutter (Eds.), *Stress, risk, and resilience in children and adolescents: Processes, mechanisms, and interventions* (pp. 268–316). New York: Cambridge University Press.

Coolahan, K., Fantuzzo, J., Mendez, J., & McDermott, P. (2000). Preschool peer interactions and readiness to learn: Relationships between classroom peer play and learning behaviors and conduct. *Journal of Educational Psychology, 92,* 458–465.

Diamond, A., Barnett, W. S., Thomas, J., & Munro, S. (2007). Preschool program improves cognitive control. *Science, 318,* 1387–1388.

Dickinson, D. K., & Smith, M. W. (1994). Long-term effects of preschool teachers' book readings on low-income children's vocabulary and story comprehension. *Reading Research Quarterly, 29,* 104–122.

Domitrovich, C. E., Cortes, R., & Greenberg, M. T. (2007). Improving young children's social and emotional competence: A randomized trial of the preschool PATHS curriculum. *Journal of Primary Prevention, 28,* 67–91.

Domitrovich, C. E., Gest, S. D., Gill, S., Bierman, K. L., Welsh, J., & Jones, D. (2009). Fostering high quality teaching in Head Start classrooms: Experimental evaluation of an integrated curriculum. *American Education Research Journal, 46,* 567–597.

Domitrovich, C. E., Greenberg, M. T., Cortes, R., & Kusche, C. (1999). *Manual for the Preschool PATHS Curriculum.* University Park: The Pennsylvania State University.

Dubas, J. S., Lynch, K. B., Gallano, J., Geller, S., & Hunt, D. (1998). Preliminary evaluation of a resiliency-based preschool substance abuse and violence prevention project. *Journal of Drug Education, 28,* 235–255.

Durlak, J. A., Weissberg, R. P., Dymnicki, A. B., Taylor, R. D., & Shellinger, K. B. (2011). The impact of enhancing students' social and emotional learning: A meta-analysis of school-based universal interventions. *Child Development, 82*, 405–432.

Eisenberg, N., & Fabes, R.A. (1998). Prosocial behavior and development. In B. Damon (Ed.), *Handbook of child psychology* (pp. 701–778). New York: Academic Press.

Elkind, D. (2001). Much too early. *Education Next, 1*, 9–15.

Frye, D., Zelazo, P. D., & Palfai, T. (1995). Theory of mind and rule-based reasoning. *Cognitive Development, 10*, 483–527.

Garner, P.W., & Waajid, B. (2008). The associations of emotion knowledge and teacher–child relationships to preschool children's school-related developmental competence. *Journal of Applied Developmental Psychology, 29*, 89–100.

Greenberg, M. T. (2006). Promoting resilience in children and youth: Preventive interventions and their interface with neuroscience. *Annals of the New York Academy of Science, 1094*, 139–150.

Izard, C. E., Fine, S., Schultz, D., Mostow, A., Ackerman, B., & Youngstrom, E. (2001). Emotion knowledge as a predictor of social behavior and academic competence in children at risk. *Psychological Science, 12*, 18–23.

Kusche, C. A., & Greenberg, M. T. (1994). *The PATHS curriculum*. Seattle, WA: Developmental Research and Programs.

LaParo, K. M., & Pianta, R. C. (2003). *CLASS: Classroom Assessment Scoring System*. Charlottesville: University of Virginia.

Lonigan, C. J. (2006). Development, assessment, and promotion of preliteracy skills. *Early Education and Development, 17*, 91–114.

Lynch, K. B., Geller, S. R., & Schmidt, M. G. (2004). Multi-year evaluation of the effectiveness of a resilience-based prevention program for young children. *Journal of Primary Prevention, 24*, 335–353.

Martens, B. K., Hiralall, A. S., & Bradley, T. A. (1997). A note to teacher: Improving student behavior through goal setting and feedback. *School Psychology Quarterly, 12*, 33–41.

McClelland, M. M., Acock, A. C., & Morrison, F. J. (2006). The impact of kindergarten learning-related skills on academic trajectories at the end of elementary school. *Early Childhood Research Quarterly, 21*, 471–490.

Parker, A., & Neuharth-Pritchett, S. (2006). Developmentally appropriate practice in kindergarten: Factors shaping teacher beliefs and practice. *Journal of Research in Childhood Education, 21*, 63–76.

Pianta, R. C., Mashburn, A. J., Downer, J. T., Hamre, B. K., & Justice, L. M. (2008). Effects of web-mediated professional development resources on teacher–child interactions in pre-kindergarten classrooms. *Early Childhood Research Quarterly, 23*, 431–451.

Raver, C. (2002). Emotions matter: Making the case for the role of young children's emotional development for early school readiness. *Social Policy Report of the Society for Research in Child Development, 16*, 1–20.

Raver, C. C., Jones, S. M., Li-Grining, C. P., Metzger, M., Smallwood, K., & Sardin, L. (2008). Improving preschool classroom processes: Preliminary findings from a randomized trial implemented in Head Start settings. *Early Childhood Research Quarterly, 23*, 10–26.

Raver, C. C., Jones, S. M., Li-Grining, C., Zhai, F., Bub, K., & Pressler, E. (2011). CSRP's impact on low-income preschoolers' preacademic skills: Self-regulation as a mediating mechanism. *Child Development, 82*, 362–378.

Raver, C. C., Jones, S. M., Li-Grining, C., Zhai, F., Metzger, M. W., & Solomon, B. (2009). Targeting children's behavior problems in preschool classrooms: A cluster-randomized controlled trial. *Journal of Consulting and Clinical Psychology, 77*, 302–316.

Riggs, N. R., Greeenberg, M. T., Kusche, C. A., & Pentz, M. A. (2006). The meditational role of neurocognition in the behavioral outcomes of a social-emotional prevention program in elementary school students: Effects of the PATHS Curriculum. *Prevention Science, 7*, 91–102.

Ryan, R. M., Fauth, R. C., & Brooks-Gunn, J. (2006). Childhood poverty: Implications for school readiness and early childhood education. In B. Spodek & O. N. Saracho (Eds.), *Handbook of research on the education of children* (2nd ed., pp. 323–346). Mahwah, NJ: Erlbaum.

Schweinhart, L. J., Weikart, D. P., & Larner, M. B. (1986). Consequences of three preschool curriculum models through age 15. *Early Childhood Research Quarterly, 1*, 15–45.

Shure, M. B. (1992). *I Can Problem Solve: An interpersonal cognitive problem-solving program: Kindergarten and primary grades.* Champaign, IL: Research Press.

Shure, M. B., & Spivack, G. (1982). Interpersonal problem-solving in young children: A cognitive approach to prevention. *American Journal of Community Psychology, 10*(3), 341–355.

Trentacosta, C. J., & Izard, C. E. (2007). Kindergarten children's emotion competence as a predictor of their academic competence in first grade. *Emotion, 7*, 77–88.

Wasik, B. A., Bond, M. A., & Hindman, A. (2006). The effects of a language and literacy intervention on Head Start children and teachers. *Journal of Educational Psychology, 98*, 63–74.

Webster-Stratton, C. (2005). *Dina Dinosaur's Social, Emotional, Academic and Problem-Solving Curriculum for Young Children.* Seattle, WA: Incredible Years.

Webster-Stratton, C., Mihalic, S., Fagan, A., Arnold, D., Taylor, T., & Tingley, C. (2001). *Blueprints for violence prevention, book eleven: The incredible years: Parent, teacher and child training series.* Boulder, CO: Center for the Study and Prevention of Violence.

Webster-Stratton, C., Reid, J., & Hammond, M. (2001). Social skills and problem-solving training for children with early-onset conduct problems: Who benefits? *Journal of Child Psychology and Psychiatry and Allied Disciplines, 42*, 943–952.

Webster-Stratton, C., Reid, M. J., & Stoolmiller, M. (2008). Preventing conduct problems and improving school readiness: Evaluation of the Incredible Years teacher and child training programs in high-risk schools. *Journal of Child Psychology and Psychiatry, 49*, 471–488.

Wechsler, D. (2002). *Wechsler Primary and Preschool Scale of Intelligence (WPPSI™ III)* (3rd ed.). San Antonio, TX: Harcourt Assessment.

Welsh, J. A., Nix, R. L., Blair, C., Bierman, K. L., & Nelson, K. E. (2010). The development of cognitive skills and gains in academic school readiness for children from low income families. *Journal of Educational Psychology*, 102, 43–53.

Whitehurst, G. (2001). Much too late. Much too early. *Education Next, 1*, 9–16.

Whitehurst, G. J., Arnold, D., Epstein, J. N., Angell, A. L., Smith, M., & Fischel, J. E. (1994). A picture book reading intervention in daycare and home for children from low-income families. *Developmental Psychology, 30*, 679–689.

CHAPTER 11

Parenting Programs That Promote School Readiness

JANET A. WELSH, KAREN L. BIERMAN, and ERIN T. MATHIS

When attempting to understand the multitude of factors that contribute to children's school readiness, the role of family characteristics and parenting behaviors figures prominently. Researchers and practitioners in the fields of education and child development have long been aware of the potential impact of family-related variables on children's development in general, and on child school readiness in particular. School readiness includes cognitive (e.g., academic skills, language development) and social-emotional (e.g., self-control, peer competence) components that are interrelated and consistently relate to the quality of parent–child interactions. In this chapter, we describe developmental research that documents links between parenting and children's cognitive and social-emotional school readiness. We review evidence-based interventions that target parenting behaviors as a means of improving children's school readiness. Finally, we discuss emerging research on parenting interventions to promote school readiness and identify future directions for research and practice.

OVERVIEW OF EVIDENCE-BASED PARENTING PROGRAMS TO ENHANCE CHILD SCHOOL READINESS

Recognizing the consistent relationship between parenting variables and children's school readiness (Chazan-Cohen, Raikes, Brooks-Gunn, Ayoub,

& Pan, 2009), many interventions designed to boost school readiness target parents and parenting skills. Although some parenting programs are "universal" and target all parents, a majority of the interventions we review here are "selective" or "indicated" programs, designed to reach parents whose children are at risk for school readiness delays. Based on robust research that links family socioeconomic disadvantage with child school readiness delays (Farkas & Hibel, 2008; Zill & Collins, 1995), many programs target families with low socioeconomic status (SES). Poverty often compromises parenting by creating conditions of heightened stress, exposure to violence, and social isolation. Poverty is also associated with elevated levels of parent psychopathology (particularly depression) and low levels of parent education, which are in turn associated with deficits in the development of child self-control and self-regulation (Goldsmith & Rogoff, 1997; Li-Grining, 2007). The hope is that by focusing on low-SES families and intervening in ways that strengthen parenting and improve child school readiness, parenting programs might reduce the disparities in school adjustment and long-term academic attainment that are associated with economic disadvantage (McLoyd, 1998). This logic is supported by a number of studies indicating that parenting behaviors, particularly language stimulation and lack of harsh, inconsistent discipline, appear to mediate the impact of economic adversity on child outcomes (Hart & Risley, 1995; McLoyd, 1998). Children with constitutional risks (e.g., low birthweight) are also often targeted for parenting interventions, based on research identifying parent support as a source of resilience (Landry, Smith, Swank, & Guttentag, 2008).

The parenting interventions we review here vary in terms of the developmental period they target (e.g., infancy, toddlerhood, preschool or early elementary school years). Some have a broad focus, targeting multiple aspects of parent and child functioning; others target a more specific set of parent and child skills. A majority of the evidence-based school readiness interventions deliver services via home visits, although center-based group meetings or combined formats (e.g., some home visiting combined with parent group training) are also utilized.

In selecting intervention programs to highlight in this review, we used several selection criteria, focusing on programs (1) that are characterized by a strong logic model based on developmental research that helps to guide inferences and hypotheses regarding the relations among variables, (2) that specifically target and measure child outcomes in school readiness skill domains, and (3) that have been evaluated for efficacy with rigorous randomized trials. Although some might argue conceptually that any program that strengthens parenting in the early years should enhance child school readiness, the reality is that parenting interventions that have demonstrated benefits in the area of improved parenting (e.g., increasing parent sensitivity and decreasing harsh discipline) often show only weak or no effects on child school readiness outcomes (Brooks-Gunn, Berlin, & Fuligni, 2002). Several comprehensive reviews suggest that, overall, parenting interventions have significant effects and add to the value of school-based programs (e.g., Head Start), but the effects are relatively small and inconsistent across studies (Barnett & Escobar, 2002; Sweet & Applebaum, 2004). A critical assessment of the ways in which various approaches are (or are not) producing consistent effects is important, in order to fuel hypotheses about key mechanisms of action and barriers to success, thereby informing future program development and refinement. In the following sections, we organize the review of programs by their developmental foundations and primary areas of focus.

PROGRAMS THAT FOCUS ON PARENT WELL-BEING AND EMPOWERMENT

Under conditions of economic disadvantage, parents are often stressed, depressed, and demoralized, suffering from social isolation and distress that impairs their capacity fully to support their children's development (Liaw & Brooks-Gunn, 1994). Poverty, and the factors associated with it, including low levels of maternal education, high levels of maternal depression and social isolation, as well as exposure to violence and stress, is related to impaired parenting practices (Lengua, Honorado, & Bush, 2007; Goldsmith & Rogoff, 1997). For example, compared to nondepressed parents, depressed parents are often more negative, intrusive, critical, and disengaged in their interactions with their infants and toddlers, as well as more likely to engage in coercive and abusive interactions with their children (Cummings & Davies, 1994). Children of depressed mothers often demonstrate low levels of social-emotional competence and elevated rates insecure attachment, along with externalizing behavioral problems that may interfere with their subsequent school adjustment (Goodman, Brogan, Lynch, & Fielding, 1993; Spieker & Booth, 1988). Similarly, Chazan-Cohen and colleagues (2009) found that when mothers reported high rates of parenting stress during the toddler years, children showed low levels of emotion regulation and school readiness when they were 5 years old. When parents report high levels of stressful daily hassles and negative life events, children often exhibit heightened cortisol levels (Brennan, Pargas, Walker, Green, & Newport, 2008; Essex, Klein, Cho, & Kalin, 2002), suggesting a spillover effect of parental stress that may impede child prefrontal cortex development and reduce attention control (Blair, 2002).

Recognizing the relations between parental well-being and mental health, and child development, some parenting interventions focus broadly on supporting and empowering parents in order to promote parental efficacy and problem-solving skills, and thereby enhance the overall quality of parenting. The goals of these programs are often quite broad and emphasize the importance of helping parents help themselves, by providing them with the information and support they need to access educational and social service resources. Often, these programs begin during pregnancy or infancy and target parenting behaviors that are related to multiple domains of child functioning, including children's physical health and safety, as well as their cognitive and behavioral development.

The Nurse–Family Partnership Program

Perhaps the best known and most extensively researched parent-focused intervention approach, the Nurse–Family Partnership Program (NFP; Olds, Kitzman, Cole, & Robinson, 1997) targets young, low-income, first-time mothers. Home visitation by nurses begins during the second trimester of pregnancy and continues across the first 2 years of the child's life. The emphasis of the program shifts over time, with a preliminary focus on a healthy pregnancy outcome and maternal well-being, followed by an emphasis on child health and safety, positive mother–infant interactions, appropriate cognitive stimulation, and positive child management techniques. Evaluations of this program indicate multiple positive effects for some mothers, with mothers with fewer resources experiencing more benefits (Kitzman et al., 2010; Olds, 2002). An initial randomized trial of this program that included follow-up through the preschool period found no statistically significant effects on children's cognitive and language development or parent reports of child behavior problems at age 4 (Olds et al., 1994). However, positive effects were evident for children of a subgroup of mothers with the highest levels of need (e.g., young, single, and with limited social support or psychological resources) (Olds et al., 2004). Within this subgroup of mothers, the program promoted more stimulating home environments for children, and these children had statistically significantly higher scores on tests of language development and executive functioning at age 4 than children of similar mothers who were randomly assigned to a control group (Olds et al., 2004). A second randomized trial of NFP with young, single, African American mothers in Memphis revealed statistically significant elevations favoring the treatment group in intellectual functioning and language skills when children were in first grade (Olds et al., 2004). Within a subgroup of mothers with low psychological resources, nurse visitations also promoted elevated math achievement scores for children in first grade. These findings suggest that the NFP approach has the capacity to improve child outcomes several years after intervention. However, the effects on children's intellectual and language functioning were relatively small (*SD* = 0.17 to 0.25), and somewhat inconsistent across studies, emerging as a main effect in the Memphis study, as a subgroup effect in the Denver study, and not emerging in the Elmira study of NFP.

Early Start

Early Start (Fergusson, Grant, Horwood, & Ridder, 2005) is a home visitation program developed in New Zealand to serve high-risk families of infants and toddlers. Early Start is similar to NFP in its scope, targeting multiple factors related to child and family well-being, although it begins after birth and home visitors are not nurses. Additionally, Early Start continues throughout the child's preschool years, unlike NFP which ends at age 2, although the average program duration is similar (about 24 months). Families are eligible for Early Start if they have two or more risk factors in areas of parenting and family functioning (e.g., low levels of social support, unplanned pregnancy, parent substance use, family financial difficulties, domestic violence). During an initial set of weekly visits, family support workers strive to develop positive partnerships with parents and conduct individualized assessment of family needs, issues, challenges, strengths, and resources. In subsequent sessions, family support workers use collaborative problem solving to devise solutions to family challenges, and provide mentoring and advice to help families mobilize their strengths and resources. Additionally, the program targets parent and family outcomes, including improvements in parent mental and physical health, increased workforce participation, and reductions in domestic violence (Fergusson et al., 2005). A randomized, controlled trial of Early Start conducted in New Zealand revealed significant positive effects on children's outcomes at 6, 12, 24, and 36 months postbaseline. These included better child behavioral adjustment, according to parent report (significantly reduced internalizing and marginally reduced externalizing behaviors), higher rates of well-child medical and dental visits and preschool enrollment, and reductions in hospitalizations associated with accidents. Parent outcomes included reductions in self-reports of abuse and harsh discipline, and increases in positive parenting (Fergusson et al., 2005). No cognitive outcomes for children were assessed in the Early Start evaluation, and follow-up studies of children's subsequent school adjustment have not been conducted.

Summary

These program results suggest that providing parents a broad scope of intervention support over a 2-year period when the child is young benefits the parents, which sometimes (and for some subgroups) confers school readiness benefits for children. Given the relatively small and inconsistent findings on child school readiness, however, the evidence suggests that this approach to parent intervention, if used alone, will not produce effects on child skills acquisition that are substantial enough to reduce the socioeconomic gap in school readiness or school attainment in a meaningful way.

Programs That Focus on Enhancing Parent Sensitivity and Responsiveness

Parent–child interaction patterns established in infancy and toddlerhood are related to the development of cognitive skills and self-regulatory capacities, both of which figure prominently in school readiness. An element of parenting associated with optimal development for infants and toddlers is *sensitive responsiveness*, which is defined as parents' emotional warmth and availability, as well as appropriate and contingent responses to children's signals (Calkins, & Hill, 2007; Dennis, 2006; Landry, Smith, & Swank, 2006). Sensitive responsiveness appears to be particularly critical for the development of emotional self-regulation (McCabe, Clark, & Barnett, 1999), and has been linked with the development of attention control and executive function in early childhood as well (Bernier, Carlson, Deschenes, & Matte-Gagne, 2012; Hughes, 2011; Hughes & Ensor, 2009).

Conversely, parents who use harsh, coercive, or inconsistent discipline strategies often have children who are less cognitively and behaviorally ready for school than parents who provide positive rule structures and contingent positive support for compliance (McCabe et al., 1999; Kilgore, Snyder, & Lentz, 2000). Developmental theorists speculate that exposure to parent anger and dysregulation may both deprive children of positive role models for emotional expression and impair their ability to regulate their own emotions and control impulses, both important aspects of school readiness (Blair, 2002). Bidirectional influences may also operate, such that children who are more impulsive and irritable evoke more negative parental control. Negative transactions between parents and children may cascade over time, increasing rates of parent–child conflict and reducing opportunities for parent–child conversation and joint attention, thereby impeding the development of child oral language and attention skills.

Given the critical role of sensitiveresponsive parenting in fostering child social-emotional and cognitive development, a number of parent intervention programs focus on promoting sensitive responsive parenting as a central goal. Some also aim to reduce restrictive, critical parenting and the use of harsh punishment.

Playing and Learning Strategies

Playing and Learning Strategies (PALS; Landry et al., 2006) is a home visiting intervention designed to teach low-income parents to interact with their infants in a sensitive responsive manner. The 10-session program utilizes coaching and videotaped modeling to teach parents techniques for maintaining children's attention, responding contingently, showing warmth, and providing rich verbal input. Randomized trials of PALS using an attention control condition (where parents were provided with general child development information but no specific coaching in parent–child interaction) resulted in large increases in sensitive responsiveness in parents who received the intervention (Landry et al., 2006). PALS also had positive effects on infants, increasing their use of words and tending to increase their levels of social cooperation in play interactions (Landry et al., 2006). In an attempt to understand better the relations between developmental timing of the intervention and children's outcomes, as well as the longer term effects of this early intervention, a subsequent trial of PALS extended the intervention past infancy into the early preschool period (Landry et al., 2008). Recognizing the challenges associated with remaining sensitive and responsive in the face of young children's increasing demands for autonomy, the PALS-II intervention included a component designed to help parents avoid conflicts and power struggles with their children. Child outcomes included receptive vocabulary, cooperativeness, and coordination of language and joint attention. Interestingly, while the PALS-I (Infant) program had its largest effects on children's positive social engagement, the toddler/preschool intervention produced gains in both positive social engagement and children's use of complex language. Although children were not followed through school entry in the PALS studies, the outcomes involving children's receptive vocabulary and communicative and social competence in the preschool period suggest that this intervention may effectively lay important groundwork for school readiness. In this study, effects were generally greater for parents than for children, especially for some outcomes. For example, strong effects were found for PALS at increasing mothers' use of verbal scaffolding, contingent responsiveness, and labeling, and reducing mothers' use of redirection (Landry et al., 2006). Effects on child outcomes were fewer and generally more often in the small-to-moderate range, although strong effects were found for children's increase in word use and decreases in negative affect.

Child and Family Interagency Resource, Support, and Training

Child and Family Interagency Resource, Support, and Training (Child FIRST; Lowell et al., 2011) is a program for high-risk families of children ages 6–36 months. It includes two major components: (1) a system of care designed to boost and coordinate access to social services (e.g., housing assistance, early intervention), and (2) a parent–child relationship enhancement component that seeks to improve children's social-emotional competence through increases in sensitive, responsive parenting. The program is delivered to parents at home by mental health clinicians, who provide dyadic psychotherapeutic intervention, and care coordinators, who connect families with community-based services. A randomized controlled trial of this intervention involving 157 families revealed significant positive effects for children whose parents completed 12 months of intervention, including reductions in externalizing behavior and improved language competence. Effect sizes of this intervention were significant and large for reductions in parental stress and in children's externalizing behavior problems, and moderate for improvements in children's language. However, dropout rates for this program were quite high, with a 25% attrition by the end of the 1-year program (Lowell et al., 2011).

Incredible Years

The Incredible Years parenting program (Webster-Stratton, 1998) targets parents of preschool children at risk for poor school adjustment due to externalizing behavior problems. Originally designed as a clinical intervention for parents of children with conduct problems, Incredible Years has recently been evaluated as a selective school readiness intervention for low-income parents. Utilizing a weekly, 2-hour, group training format, the 12-session program teaches parents to use child-directed play skills, positive and consistent discipline strategies, strategies for coping with stress, and methods that strengthen children's social skills. In the first randomized trial with Head Start parents, Incredible Years promoted improved parenting practices and child behavior observed at home. There were also significant treatment effects on Head Start teachers' reports of children's social competence at school (Webster-Stratton,

1998). Because teachers also received the intervention, it is not clear how much the parenting program played a role in promoting improved behavior at school. A second randomized trial of Incredible Years with Head Start families found that the intervention promoted significant gains in positive parenting practices, decreases in negative parenting practices, and reductions in children's conduct problems at home and at Head Start (Webster-Stratton, Reid, & Hammond, 2001). A later analysis suggested moderated effects, with the impact on disruptive behavior problems primarily evident for children who had high rates of problem behaviors prior to the intervention–approximately 28% of the Head Start sample (Reid, Webster-Stratton, & Baydar, 2004).

Summary

These studies provide evidence that parent sensitivity and responsiveness can be improved, and negative parenting can be decreased with focused, skills-building interventions. These interventions each provided parents with instructions, videotaped models, practice opportunities, and feedback, in order to improve the quality of their interactions with their young children. For infants, sensitive, responsive parenting was the primary goal, whereas for older toddlers and preschool children, an additional goal was to reduce coercive parenting and harsh punishment, as well as to support positive parent–child interactions. In all three studies, improved parenting was associated with improvements in child functioning in areas of relevance for school functioning (e.g., enhanced social competence, reduced behavior problems). However, program impact on children's preschool functioning was not assessed for PALS or Child FIRST, and only teacher ratings of child behavior were collected in the Incredible Years trials. Hence, further research is needed to estimate the degree of impact these parent programs may have on closing the school readiness gap associated with socioeconomic disadvantage.

Programs That Enrich Parent–Child Communication and Increase Parent Support for Learning

School readiness research has identified language competence in the preschool years as a powerful predictor of both academic and behavioral school readiness and later adjustment. In the cognitive realm, early language is closely linked to later reading ability. Children's vocabulary scores at school entry are predictive of later reading comprehension skills (Dickinson & McCabe, 2001). Additionally, language skills are key for the development of self-control and social competence (Mendez, Fantuzzo, & Cicchetti, 2002). As children develop the capacity to label and describe their feelings, they are better able to manage negative emotions and interpersonal conflicts (Cole, Michel, & Teti, 1994). Conversely, low language and low levels of emotional understanding are related to poor interpersonal skills in interactions with peers and adults (Botting & Conti-Ramsden, 2000). Because language development is highly dependent on the quality of the linguistic environment to which young children are exposed, it is no surprise that parent–child verbal interactions during infancy and the preschool years are strongly associated with children's school readiness. Families vary widely in both the quality and quantity of language input provided to young children, and SES is a powerful predictor of this variability. Children in middle- and upper-income families are exposed to far more words, more syntactically complex utterances, and more conversational exchanges than children from disadvantaged homes (Hart & Risley, 1995).

Beyond the simple volume of speech, specific conversational strategies are associated with increased linguistic competence in children. First, parents who utilize high rates of *conversational recasting* with their preschoolers have children with higher levels of both expressive and receptive language competence. Recasting involves restating a child's utterances in a way that maintains the child's topic and focus of interest but includes a new linguistic challenge unfamiliar to the child (Nelson, Welsh, Camarata, Tjus, & Heimann, 2001). Conversational recasting promotes language growth through repeated exposure to both novel words and challenging and complex grammatical structures (e.g., the "ing" ending) and also provides motivation for children to engage in conversation with competent speakers (by talking about things that children find interesting) (Nelson et al., 2001). Recasting can be regarded as a form of *verbal scaffolding* that reflects parents' ability to match the content and complexity of their utterances to children's interests and developmental level (Landry et al., 2008).

The content of parents' language when speaking to children may contribute significantly to both cognitive and social-emotional aspects of school readiness. *Mind-mindedness* refers to parents' tendency to make ongoing comments on children's emotions and mental states, which offers children the opportunity to reflect upon and verbally mediate their own experiences. Parents' use of these techniques in toddlerhood has been found to predict children's later executive function development (Bernier, Carlson, & Whipple, 2010). Conversely, when parents talk with their children using brief statements, limited vocabulary, and focus primarily on directives and prohibitions, children are more likely to show low levels of readiness at school entry. Low-income mothers, especially those experiencing multiple risk factors (e.g., depression and low education level) are disproportionately likely to engage in these types of linguistic exchanges with their children (Hart & Risley, 1995).

In addition to variations in their language use in the home, parents vary considerably regarding their beliefs about the need and value of structuring learning opportunities for their children and the degree to which they provide learning materials, such as books, puzzles, drawing supplies, and educational toys. Cheadle (2008) found that higher SES families structure more learning opportunities for their children, engage them in more conversations, and have more involvement in schooling, including interactions with teachers and other school personnel, whereas lower SES parents are more likely to endorse a philosophy of "natural development," which involves fewer structured learning experiences and less adult involvement in children's lives. The pattern of "concerted cultivation" that is more common among higher SES families is associated with higher child reading and math scores in elementary school (Cheadle, 2008). Building upon this developmental research, a number of parent interventions have been developed to improve the quality of parent's communication and language use with children, and increase levels of cognitive stimulation and learning support in the home.

The Parent–Child Home Program

Originally developed in 1965 as the Mother–Child Home Program (Levenstein & Sunley, 1968), this intensive intervention involves 46 biweekly home visits, spread over 2 years (usually when the child is 2–3 years of age). The program is designed for children at risk for delayed school readiness due to family risk factors such as poverty, low levels of parental education, isolation, teen parent or single-parent status, and immigrant status. The overall program goal is to improve support for the child's learning within the home and to empower the parents to feel effective and involved in supporting the child's development and education, with a particular emphasis on verbal communication. Paraprofessionals conduct home visits, bringing parents new toys and books each visit, and coaching parents in how to use these materials as platforms for language enrichment. Home visitors are trained to use modeling and reinforcement to encourage positive parent–child interaction but to avoid didactic instruction. In addition, home visitors facilitate referrals to other social and educational services, as needed.

The program has undergone multiple evaluations over the years, using both quasi-experimental and randomized controlled designs. The initial, quasi-experimental evaluations indicated that children who received the intervention had significantly higher IQ's than the comparison group children (Levenstein, 1970), and these results were sustained at follow-up for children who received the full two year program (Madden, Levenstein, & Levenstein, 1976). This original sample was followed for many years, with program effects detectable at fifth grade (Lazar & Darlington, 1982) and seventh grade (Royce, Darlington, & Murray, 1983). A much more recent study, also employing a quasi-experimental design, compared the outcomes of program participants in rural North Carolina with the state norms for low-income children's school readiness and found similar, positive effects for the intervention, with program recipients scoring significantly better on measures of school readiness in first grade (Levenstein, Levenstein, & Oliver, 2002).

However, more rigorous designs have resulted in less consistent findings. An early evaluation conducted not long after the original trial utilized a randomized controlled design and found robust impacts on parenting behavior but much smaller effects on child IQ, achievement, and social adjustment, and no child effects were detectable at the first-grade follow-up. Interestingly, this study also found that parenting behaviors and child outcomes were uncorrelated, suggesting that treatment effects were not mediated by parenting (Madden, O'Hara, & Levenstein, 1984). Similarly, on the one hand, a randomized controlled trial in Bermuda found no effects of this program (Scarr & McCartney, 1988). On the other hand, a longitudinal follow-up of students randomly assigned to intervention and control conditions found a small but positive effect for high school completion among program participants (Levenstein, Levenstein, Shiminski, & Stolzberg (1998). The lack of findings in these trials may highlight problems in the comparison samples of the quasi-experimental evaluations. They also may reflect socioeconomic and cultural differences in the populations studied or the more common use of child care in the more recent studies, which may have washed out the effects of improved parental involvement seen in the initial studies. For example, in the Bermuda study, all children in both conditions were enrolled in preschool, which may have washed out the effects of the parent program.

The Home Instruction Program for Preschool Youngsters

The Home Instruction Program for Preschool Youngsters (HIPPY; Lombard, 1981) is a home visitation program for parents of low-income 4-year-olds that includes the transition to kindergarten. It was developed in Israel in 1969 and has been broadly disseminated to other countries, including the United States and Canada. Guided by a curriculum, trained paraprofessionals meet bimonthly with parents over a 2-year period, providing books and activities designed to promote language, motor, sensory, perceptual, and problem-solving skills. Parents receive coaching in the use of these materials with their children, including instruction, modeling, and role-play practice with feedback. They are asked to work with children on the activities for 15–20 minutes per day. Like the Parent–Child Home Program, much of the research on its effects is qualitative or quasi-experimental. Two quasi-experimental evaluations suggested that family participation in this home visiting program enhanced child academic performance in grade school, promoting higher grades, improved achievement scores, and more favorable teacher ratings of social adjustment (Bradley & Gilkey, 2002; Nievar, Jacobson, Chen, Johnson, & Dier, 2011). However, these studies were subject to selection biases, in which the parents who participated in the program were not directly comparable to parents who did not. The only randomized control trial of HIPPY showed equivocal results, with meaningful effects for children in one cohort at the end of kindergarten and first grade, but no effects for children in a second cohort (Baker, Piotrkowski, & Brooks-Gunn, 1998). For children in the first cohort, intervention was associated with higher scores on a test of general cognitive ability and more positive teacher ratings of classroom adaptation—gains that were sustained at 1-year follow-up. However, no differences emerged between intervention and control group children in the second cohort (Baker et al., 1998).

Getting Ready

Getting Ready (Sheridan, Marvin, Knoche, & Edwards, 2008) is a program for Head Start children that spans the transition to kindergarten and has the goal of improving school readiness. The intervention involves a series of approximately eight, 1-hour home visits between the parent and the child's Head Start teacher that occur over a 2-year period. Specific targets of the intervention include (1) increasing parental warmth and sensitivity, (2) increasing parents' support for children's autonomy, and (3) boosting parents' participation in children's learning, through both greater engagement in home learning activities and a more active home–school partnership. Teachers receive extensive training in how to engage parents in conversations about children's strengths and needs, their goals and expectations for their child, and brainstorming any developmental issues (Sheridan, Knoche, Kupzyk, Edwards, & Marvin, 2011). Additionally, teachers implement some of the strategies taught to parents in the classroom. Finally, the program is designed to strengthen the parent–teacher relationship and to promote more active parent participation in children's schooling. A recent randomized controlled trial of the Getting Ready program included 217 three-year-olds from diverse backgrounds enrolled in Head Start. Because the intervention targeted teachers, randomization was done at the level of the school building. Teacher ratings collected over the course of the 18-month intervention revealed that children who received the Getting Ready intervention, relative to controls, showed accelerated growth in teacher-rated oral language use, reading, and writing, as well as improvements in teacher-reported social-emotional competencies such as attachment to adults and reductions in anxiety and withdrawal (Sheridan, Knoche, Edwards, Bovaird, & Kupzyk, 2010). However, no significant impacts were noted relative to children's aggression or self-control (Sheridan et al., 2010). When the impact of potential moderators was examined, children for whom there were developmental concerns at the outset of the study, and those who did not speak English, showed significantly greater intervention-related gains, while those whose parents had low education levels or high rates of health problems experienced significantly fewer benefits (Sheridan et al., 2011). Although this study had a strong, randomized control group design and suggests that the Getting Ready intervention accelerated children's development during the Head Start years, its effects on elementary school adjustment are not yet known. Additionally, the evaluation sample had a very high attrition rate, although the attrition affected control and intervention groups equally and was largely related to families' departure from Head Start rather than from the Getting Ready program itself, with nearly half of the families discontinuing, which compromises the strength of the findings. Further research on the effects of Getting Ready on children's school readiness is clearly warranted.

Parents as Teachers Program

Parents as Teachers (PAT; Pfannenstiel & Seltzer, 1989) utilizes a curriculum, Born to Learn, to provide parents with child development knowledge and parenting support during the early years of parenting (primarily ages 0–3). The PAT model includes one-on-one home visits, monthly group meetings, developmental screenings, and a resource network for families. In the first randomized controlled trial of the Born to Learn curriculum delivered in the PAT model, Drotar, Robinson, Jeavons, and Kirchner (2009) randomly assigned 532 eligible families to receive PAT or a control experience that involved access to informational handouts and groups. The PAT Born to Learn model included two home visits in the first month, with monthly visits thereafter, delivered by trained parent educators who provided handouts and videos to review key developmental principles. Parents also attended group meetings. Using a conservative analytic approach that retained participants in their assigned groups whether or not they actually completed the intervention or withdrew from the study, no overall group differences emerged on child cognitive or language development, or adaptive behavior at 12, 24, or 36 months.

However, moderation analyses showed that the low-SES families showed some benefits, with children from low-SES families showing higher cognitive development scores and higher motivational approach at 24 months than comparable families in the control group. Two additional randomized trails evaluated the impact of PAT on Latino parents and teen parents, respectively, producing small and inconsistent positive effects on parent knowledge, attitudes, and behavior, but no overall gains in child development (Wagner & Clayton, 1999). However, additional analyses suggested significant gains for children in some subgroups (e.g., children in primarily Spanish-speaking Latino families) and under some circumstances (e.g., when families received more intensive services.)

Dialogic Reading Programs for Parents

Dialogic reading programs focus specifically on promoting parent reading practices and high-quality language use (Lonigan & Whitehurst, 1998; Whitehurst & Lonigan, 1998; Arnold & Whitehurst, 1994; Whitehurst, Arnold, Epstein, Angell, & Smith, 1994). *Dialogic reading* is a form of joint book reading that involves conversational engagement, modeling of novel vocabulary, and the use of complex questions (Arnold & Whitehurst, 1994). When utilized by preschool teachers, this technique results in improved vocabulary, comprehension, and oral language skills (Wasik & Bond, 2001; Arnold & Whitehurst, 1994; Whitehurst et al., 1994).

Utilizing a group training format, Whitehurst and colleagues (Arnold & Whitehurst, 1994; Whitehurst et al., 1994) adapted this technique for parents. During two 1-hour training sessions (an initial training session and a later "booster" session), the trainer teaches dialogic reading techniques by showing a modeling videotape and engaging parents in role playing. Parents are taught to ask thought-provoking questions, engage in active listening, elaborate on child utterances, and reinforce children's attention and participation (Lonigan & Whitehurst, 1998). Parents are then expected to read to their child 10–15 minutes a day, three to five times a week. Home interventions vary in length from 4 to 8 weeks, while school and home combination interventions may last up to 30 weeks.

Parents' consistent ability to use dialogic reading at home has been shown to significantly improve language skills in preschool children from both middle- and low-income backgrounds (Arnold & Whitehurst, 1994). Additionally, this intervention has improved emergent literacy skills in preschoolers who performed significantly below average on tests of expressive and receptive vocabulary (Lonigan & Whitehurst, 1998). What has yet to be evaluated is whether dialogic reading programs facilitate behavioral or emotional aspects of school readiness through their impact on language and cognitive capacities.

Parents as Tutors

Some interventions have used parents as tutors, setting them up with curriculum materials and support that allows them to offer children instruction in specific academic skills. An additional goal is to facilitate parents' engagement in their children's schooling. Parents have been successfully taught to implement remedial reading tutoring programs, resulting in significant improvements in kindergarten children's reading skills (Mehran & White, 1988). In this study, children who had been identified as being at risk for reading difficulties were randomly assigned to receive "usual services" (Title I tutoring at school) or Title I plus parent tutoring. Parents of children in the intervention were successfully trained to tutor their children at home using the Reading Made Easy curriculum, and were assisted and supervised by teachers and classroom aides who had been trained by the researchers. Children in the intervention group showed improvements on direct assessments of reading proficiency compared to controls, and the effects were moderated by dosage of tutoring, with children whose parents reported attending more sessions showing the strongest benefits. This study was somewhat atypical, as it required parents to be trained to a specific criterion; this may have strengthened its impact relative to similar programs.

In addition, several meta-analyses of parent tutoring interventions have indicated that, overall, these interventions are effective at increasing children's academic skills. Erion (2006) reviewed 37 studies examining the impact of parent tutoring programs and found moderate effect sizes across a number of content areas, including reading, math, spelling, and writing. A second meta-analysis also examined multiple academic outcomes (math, reading, science), as well as multiple parent teaching strategies (direct instruction and practice, use of positive rewards), and found a significant positive effect for parent involvement in children's reading but not math (Nye, Turner, & Schwartz, 2006). Interestingly, in this meta-analysis, parents' use of positive rewards was more strongly associated with children's academic outcomes than other aspects of involvement.

Summary

On the basis of the positive findings from initial quasi-experimental evaluations, several of these home visiting programs have been widely disseminated (e.g., Parent–Child Home Program, PAT). Yet the results from the randomized trials of those programs are disappointing, and suggest that the programs are underperforming (see Gomby, 2005). More research is critically needed, in order to understand better the circumstances under which these types of parenting interventions have significant effects on children's school readiness outcomes. Based upon the available evidence, programs that focus on coaching parents in specific behaviors linked closely with their children's academic progress (e.g., the dialogic reading and parents as tutor programs) appear more consistent in promoting gains in child cognitive skills than programs that have broader goals and are more focused on educating parents about developmental issues. However, social-emotional outcomes and motivational aspects of school readiness have not been well studied for either kind of program. In addition, without more direct comparisons, one cannot tell whether the differences in the findings among programs reflect differences in the populations being served, the quality of the implementation, or the intervention approach itself. As research moves forward, it will be most useful if study designs are expanded to compare more clearly the effects of different intervention components and/or test hypothesized mechanisms of action. In the next section, we consider critical issues for future research and program development. One factor that remains unclear from the research reviewed is the level of intensity and dosage of intervention required to impact school readiness meaningfully. While some programs advocate brief, "light touch" interventions (e.g., Positive Parenting Program [Triple P], Family Check-Up), others argue in favor of more intensive and sustained programs (e.g., NFP, Parent–Child Home Program). Because this is an important issue with significant implications for education and child development, it should be the explicit focus of future studies of school readiness.

Future Considerations for Research and Practice

Enriching Intervention Approaches with Recent Developmental Research

Many of the parenting programs included in this chapter were not designed specifically to enhance child school readiness but rather to target multiple needs of the parents. Although this approach may produce programs that are beneficial to parents and children in important ways (e.g., improving parent well-being, reducing child abuse), it appears unlikely to provide sufficient targeted support to reduce the socioeconomic gap in child school readiness to a meaningful extent. If improvements in child school readiness are a central goal of an early childhood parenting intervention, the approach likely needs to focus more on building the specific child competencies that are important to school readiness. For example, skills developed during the toddler and preschool years that contribute directly to children's learning capacity when they enter school include phonological sensitivity (ability to discriminate sounds), narrative understanding (ability to recognize beginning, middle, and end in stories and events; understanding of cause and effect), and emotion knowledge (being able to recognize and label one's own and others' feelings), as well as oral language skills. This may be why parenting programs that utilize parents as tutors and provide specific learning activities and materials to help parents build these foundational skills (e.g., dialogic reading) have shown stronger effects on child academic readiness than programs with more diffuse goals (e.g., Parent–Child Home Program, HIPPY, PAT). In addition, recent developmental research points to the critical importance of the development of the prefrontal cortex and executive functions during early childhood, along with language skills, as neural foundations for effective learning (Blair & Diamond, 2008). Because so many of the children who lag behind in the acquisition of language skills and executive functioning skills also have problems with emotional and behavioral regulation, it is critical to consider academic and behavioral school readiness in tandem (Blair, 2002).

Some parenting processes appear to play a central role in promoting several of these foundational skills, contributing to multiple aspects of child school readiness. For example, sensitive, responsive parent–child interactions that scaffold child attention and support sustained problem-solving efforts simultaneously may promote attachment security, language learning, attention control, and child social cooperation and competence (Dickinson & McCabe, 2001; Landry, Smith, Swank, & Miller-Loncar, 2000; Nelson et al., 2001). This may be why parenting programs that target sensitive, responsive parenting in an intensive and focused way also show promise for promoting school readiness (e.g., PALS). Conceptually, enriching some of the current parent intervention approaches focused on improving parent–child interaction quality with more specific learning activities designed to promote child acquisition of executive function and emergent literacy and math skills may be effective in strengthening program impact.

Engaging Parents in Intervention

A common struggle for parent interventions involves eliciting and sustaining high-quality parental engagement (Kaminski, Stormshak, Good, & Goodman, 2002; see also Nix, Bierman, McMahon, & the Conduct Problems Prevention Research Group, 2009). For example, several of the programs reviewed in this chapter struggled to engage and retain parents in the intervention. Both the Incredible Years and Getting Ready programs showed positive effects but also had high attrition rates—20–24% in the Head Start evaluation of Incredible Years and nearly half the families in the Getting Ready program (Reid, Webster-Stratton, & Baydar, 2004;

Sheridan et al., 2008). It may be difficult to engage parents for several reasons, including both the burden of intervention and parent's perception that the services are not needed, or instability in the living situation or preschool placement of the children. Indeed, given the frequency with which moderated effects emerge for parent interventions, with only subgroups benefiting, it may be the case that parents need more differentiated or flexible intervention options. Two programs warrant mention as examples of service delivery systems that offer parents more autonomy and choice in navigating the services—possibly enhancing program engagement and impact.

In the Family Check-Up program (FCU; Dishion & Stormshak, 2007), parents participate in an initial three-session ecological assessment of the child's and family's strengths and weaknesses; receive feedback, with a focus on the parents' own goals and priorities; then are presented options that allow them to make choices about any additional services they receive. FCU also provides annual check-ups, providing families with long-term follow-up as they navigate key developmental transitions. A recent randomized controlled evaluation of FCU implemented with high-risk families of 2-year-old children revealed that the program had significant impacts on positive parenting, including parental involvement, use of positive reinforcement, parent–child engagement, and scaffolding problems (Gardner, Shaw, Dishion, Burton, & Supplee, 2007; Dishion et al., 2008). A follow-up assessment when children were age 4 found a marginally significant effect on children's inhibitory control but no significant effect on language skills (Lunkenheimer et al., 2008). Although these are not strong effects on school readiness skills, the approach warrants ongoing exploration given its potential to reduce intervention cost and burden on parents, while promoting positive parenting change.

A second example of a more flexible and adaptive intervention delivery system is seen in the organization of the Triple P (Positive Parenting Program) design (Sanders, 1999). Triple P utilizes tiered interventions designed to provide a graduated set of services that differ in intensity depending upon parental need. The Level 1 Triple P programs are typically low-intensity and universal, and include suggestions and information regarding positive management of behaviors that many children demonstrate (e.g., bedtime issues), while the higher-level interventions are more intensive and selectively target families experiencing more serious problems (e.g., effective management of aggressive–disruptive behavior problems). Triple P is wide ranging, with different versions of the program available for parents of children with disabilities, children at risk for maltreatment, and those experiencing significant family dysfunction (e.g., marital conflict). School readiness components have been developed for Triple P but have not yet been subjected to a randomized trial.

Stronger Research Designs

Finally, it is important to strengthen the research designs used to evaluate parent interventions in early childhood, to provide a stronger basis for bootstrapping and improving program impact. Currently, the research supporting many of the parent-focused programs, particularly home visiting, can be criticized for weak research designs that lack robust controls for selection effects. Without a randomized control group, there is a significant danger that only subgroups of parents who are highly motivated to invest in their children's education participate in the intervention—an effect of parent investment that is not controlled in many of the quasi-experimental control groups. Hence, it becomes difficult to know whether the positive effects are due to the characteristics of the parents who decided to participate or to the program itself. For this reason, the use of more rigorous, randomized trials is important.

In addition, research designs should examine different facets of the program, in order to understand better the factors underlying success or failure to make an impact. Assessing the process of program implementation is important, in order to understand barriers to implementation and to determine how well the intervention was implemented and what features of the program created implementation challenges. Assessing proximal variables, such as changes in parenting skills targeted by the program, and their impact as mediators of improvements in child school readiness skills will help strengthen theoretical models of critical change processes. Factors that may serve as predictors of intervention impact also deserve further study, such as the impact of the experience, credentials, and training of home visitors. In addition, ongoing exploration of factors that might moderate program effectiveness is important. For example, programs might vary in impact depending upon the age or developmental status of the child (Landry et al., 2008), the ethnicity or cultural beliefs of the parents (Brooks-Gunn & Markman, 2005), or the risk status of the parents (Olds et al., 2004).

Summary

Early childhood interventions appear critical in order to reduce the delays in school readiness associated with poverty and to prevent the growing gap in achievement that results in lifelong educational, economic, and health disparities for children growing up in adverse circumstances. On the one hand, early childhood parenting interventions have considerable potential to reduce this gap given research documenting the important role that parents play in the development of school readiness skills. The current findings from parent interventions might best be viewed as a promissory note—evidence of "proof of concept" that parenting can be improved with benefits for children. On the other hand, when evaluated in the context of rigorous randomized controlled trials, the effects of early parenting interventions on school readiness outcomes are small and inconsistent. In the coming years, the challenge for researchers and practitioners is to strengthen and refine parenting interventions, in order to increase their impact on child school readiness and academic attainment.

Acknowledgment

This work was supported in part by the National Institute of Child Health and Human Development Grant Nos. HD057908 and HD046064.

References

Arnold, D. S., & Whitehurst, G. J. (1994). Accelerating language development through picture book reading: A summary of dialogic reading and its effect. In D. Dickinson (Ed.), *Bridges to literacy: Children, families, and schools* (pp. 103–128). Malden, MA: Blackwell.

Baker, A. J., Piotrkowski, C. S., & Brooks-Gunn, J. (1998). The effects of the Home Instruction Program for Preschool Youngsters (HIPPY) on children's school performance at the end of the program and one year later. *Early Childhood Research Quarterly, 13*, 571–588.

Barnett, W. S., & Escobar, C.M. (2002). Research on the cost effectiveness of early educational intervention: Implications for research and policy. In T. A. Revenson, A. R. D'Augelli, S. E. French, D. L. Hughes, D. Livert, E. Seidman, M. Shinn, & H. Yoshikawa (Eds.), *Ecological research to promote social change: Methodological advances from community psychology* (pp. 63–92). New York: Kluwer Academic/Plenum.

Bernier, A., Carlson, S. M., Deschenes, M., & Matte-Gagne, C. (2012). Social factors in the development of early executive functioning: A closer look at the caregiving environment. *Developmental Science, 15*(1), 12–24.

Bernier, A., Carlson, S. M., & Whipple, N. (2010). From external regulation to self-regulation: Early parenting precursors of young children's executive functioning. *Child Development, 81*, 326–339.

Blair, C. (2002). School readiness: Integrating cognition and emotion in a neurobiological conceptualization of children's functioning at school entry. *American Psychologist, 57*, 111–127.

Blair, C., & Diamond, A. (2008). Biological processes in prevention and intervention: The promotion of self-regulation as a means of preventing school failure. *Development and Psychopathology, 20*, 899–911.

Botting, N., & Conti-Ramsden, G. (2000). Social and behavioural difficulties in children with language impairment. *Child Language Teaching and Therapy, 16*, 105–120.

Bradley, R. H., & Gilkey, B. (2002). The impact of the Home Instructional Program for preschool youngsters (HIPPY) on school performance in 3rd and 6th grades. *Early Education and Development,13*, 301–311.

Brennan, P. A., Pargas, R., Walker, E. F., Green, P., & Newport, D. J. (2008). Maternal depression and infant cortisol: Influences of timing, comorbidity and treatment. *Journal of Child Psychology and Psychiatry,49*, 1099–1107.

Brooks-Gunn, J., Berlin, L. J., & Fuligni, A. S. (2002). Early childhood intervention programs: What about the family? In J. P. Shonkoff & S. J. Meisels (Eds.), *Handbook of early childhood intervention* (2nd ed., pp. 549–588). New York: Cambridge University Press.

Brooks-Gunn, J., & Markman, L. B. (2005). The contribution of parenting to ethnic and racial gaps in school readiness. *The Future of Children, 15*, 139–168.

Calkins, S. D., & Hill, A. (2007). Caregiver influences on emerging emotion regulation: Biological and environmental transactions in early development. In J. J. Gross, (Ed.), *Handbook of emotion regulation* (pp. 229–248). New York: Guilford Press.

Chazan-Cohen, R., Raikes, H., Brooks-Gunn, J., Ayoub, C., & Pan, B. A. (2009). Low-income children's school readiness: Parent contributions over the first five years. *Early Education and Development, 20*, 958–977.

Cheadle, J. E. (2008). Educational investment, family context, and children's math and reading growth from kindergarten through the third grade. *Sociology of Education, 81*, 1–31.

Cole, P. M., Michel, M. K., & Teti, L. O. (1994). The development of emotion regulation and dysregulation: A clinical perspective. *Monographs of the Society for Research in Child Development, 59*, 250–283.

Cummings, E. M., & Davies, P. T. (1994). Maternal depression and child development. *Journal of Child Psychology and Psychiatry, 35*, 73–112.

Dennis, T. (2006). Emotional self-regulation in preschoolers: The interplay of child approach reactivity. *Developmental Psychology, 42*, 84–97.

Dickinson, D. K., & McCabe, A. (2001). Bringing it all together: The multiple skills, origins, and environmental supports of early literacy. *Learning Disabilities Research and Practice, 16*, 186–202.

Dishion, T. J., Shaw, D. S., Connell, A., Gardner, F., Weaver, C., & Wilson, M. (2008). The Family Check Up with high risk indigent families: Preventing problem behavior by increasing parents' positive behavior support in early childhood. *Child Development, 79*, 1395–1414.

Dishion, T. J., & Stormshak, E. (2007). *Intervening in children's lives: An ecological, family centered approach to mental health care.* Washington, DC: American Psychological Association.

Drotar, D., Robinson, J., Jeavons, L., & Kirchner, L. (2009). A randomized, controlled evaluation of early intervention: The Born to Learn curriculum. *Child Care, Health and Development, 35*, 643–649.

Erion, J. (2006). Parent tutoring: A meta-analysis. *Education and Treatment of Children, 29*, 79–106.

Essex, M. J., Klein, M. H., Cho, E., & Kalin, N. H. (2002). Maternal stress beginning in infancy may sensitize children to later stress exposure: Effects on cortisol and behavior. *Biological Psychiatry, 52*, 776–784.

Farkas, G., & Hibel, J. (2008). Being unready for school: Factors affecting risk and resilience. In A. Booth & A. Crouter (Eds.), *Disparities in school readiness* (pp. 3–30). New York: Erlbaum.

Fergusson, D. M., Grant, H., Horwood, L. J., & Ridder, E. M. (2005). Randomized trial of the Early Start Program of home visitation: Parent and family outcomes. *Pediatrics, 116*(6), 803–809.

Gardner, F., Shaw, D. S., Dishion, T. J., Burton, J., & Supplee, L. (2007). Randomized trial of a family centered approach to preventing conduct problems: Linking changes in proactive parenting to boys' disruptive behavior in early childhood. *Journal of Family Psychology, 21*, 398–406.

Goldsmith, D. F., & Rogoff, B. (1997). Mothers' and toddlers' coordinated joint focus of attention: Variations with maternal dysphoric symptoms. *Developmental Psychology, 33*, 113–119.

Gomby, D. (2005). *Home visitation in 2005: Outcomes for children and parents.* Committee for Economic Development: Invest in Kids Working Group. Available online at *www.ced.org/projects/kids.shtml.*

Goodman, S. H., Brogan, D., Lynch, M. E., & Fielding, B. (1993). Social and emotional competence in children of depressed mothers. *Child Development, 64*, 516–531.

Hart, B., & Risley, T. R. (1995). *Meaningful differences in the everyday experience of young American children.* Baltimore: Brookes.

Hughes, C. (2011). *Social understanding and social lives: From toddlerhood through to the transition to school.* New York: Psychology Press.

Hughes, C., & Ensor, R. (2009). Independence and interplay between maternal and child risk factors for preschool problem behaviors? *International Journal of Behavioral Development, 33*, 312–322.

Kaminski, R. A., Stormshak, E. A., Good, R. H., & Goodman, M. R. (2002). Prevention of substance abuse with rural head start children and families: Results of project STAR. *Psychology of Addictive Behaviors, 16*, S11–S26.

Kilgore, K., Snyder, J., & Lentz, C. (2000). The contribution of parental discipline: Parental monitoring and school risk to early onset conduct problems in African-American boys and girls. *Developmental Psychology, 36*, 835–845.

Kitzman, H., Olds, D. L., Cole, R., Hanks, C., Anson, E., Sidora-Arcoleo, K., et al. (2010). Enduring effects of prenatal and infancy home visiting by nurses on children: Age-12 follow-up of a randomized trial. *Archives of Pediatric and Adolescent Medicine, 164*, 412–418.

Landry, S. H., Smith, K. E., & Swank, P. R. (2006). Responsive parenting: Establishing early foundations for social, communication, and independent problem-solving skills. *Developmental Psychology, 42*, 627–642.

Landry, S., Smith, K. E., Swank, P. R., & Guttentag, C. (2008). A responsive parenting intervention: The optimal timing across early childhood for impacting maternal behaviors and child outcomes. *Developmental Psychology, 44*, 1333–1353.

Landry, S. H., Smith, K. E., Swank, P. R., & Miller-Loncar, C. L. (2000). Early maternal and child influences on children's later independent cognitive and social functioning. *Child Development, 71*, 358–375.

Lazar, I., & Darlington, R. (1982). Lasting effects of early education: A report from the Consortium for Longitudinal Studies. *Monographs of the Society for Research in Child Development, 47*(2–3, Serial No. 195).

Lengua, L. J., Honorado, E., & Bush, N. R. (2007). Contextual risk and parenting as predictors of effortful control and social competence in preschool children. *Journal of Applied Developmental Psychology, 28*, 40–55.

Levenstein, P. (1970). Cognitive growth in preschoolers through verbal interaction with mothers. *American Journal of Orthopsychiatry, 40*, 426–432.

Levenstein, P., Levenstein, S., & Oliver, D. (2002). First grade school readiness of former child participants in a South Carolina replication of the Parent–Child Home Program. *Journal of Applied Developmental Psychology, 23*, 331–353.

Levenstein, P., Levenstein, S., Shiminski, J. A., & Stolzberg, J. E. (1998). Long-term impact of a verbal interaction program for at-risk toddlers: An exploratory study of high school outcomes in a replication of the Mother–Child Home Program. *Journal of Applied Developmental Psychology, 19*, 267–286.

Levenstein, P., & Sunley, R. (1968). Stimulation of verbal interaction between disadvantaged mothers and children. *American Journal of Orthopsychiatry, 38*, 116–121.

Liaw, F., & Brooks-Gunn, J. (1994). Cumulative familial risks and low-birthweight children's cognitive and behavioral development. *Journal of Clinical Child Psychology, 23*, 360–372.

Li-Grining, C. P. (2007). Effortful control among low income preschoolers in three cities: Stability, change and individual differences. *Developmental Psychology, 43*, 208–221.

Lombard, A. (1981). *Success begins at home*. Lexington, VA: Lexington Books.

Lonigan, C. J., & Whitehurst, G. J. (1998). Relative efficacy of parent and teacher involvement in shared-reading intervention for preschool children from low-income backgrounds. *Early Childhood Research Quarterly, 13*, 263–290.

Lowell, D. I., Carter, A. S., Godoy, L., Paulicin, B., & Briggs-Gowan, M. J. (2011). A randomized controlled trial of Child FIRST: A comprehensive home-based intervention translating research into early childhood practice. *Child Development, 82*, 193–208.

Lunkenheimer, E. S., Dishion, T. J., Shaw, D. S., Connell, A. M., Gardner, F., Wilson, M. N., et al. (2008). Collateral benefits of the Family Check Up on early childhood school readiness: Indirect effects of parents' positive behavior support. *Developmental Psychology, 44*, 1737–1752.

Madden, J., Levenstein, P., & Levenstein, S. (1976). Longitudinal IQ outcomes of the Mother-Child Home Program. *Child Development, 47*, 1015–1025.

Madden, J., O'Hara, J., & Levenstein, P. (1984). Home again: Effects of the Mother–Child Home Program on mother and child. *Child Development, 55*, 636–647.

McCabe, K. M., Clark, R., & Barnett, D. (1999). Family protective factors among urban African American youth. *Journal of Clinical Child Psychology, 28*, 137–150.

McLoyd, V. C. (1998). Socioeconomic disadvantage and child development. *American Psychologist, 53*, 185–204.

Mehran, M., & White, K. R. (1988). Parent tutoring as a supplement to compensatory education for first-grade children. *Remedial and Special Education, 9*, 35–41.

Mendez, J. L., Fantuzzo, J., & Cicchetti, D. (2002). Profiles of social competence among low-income African American preschool children. *Child Development, 73*, 1085–1100.

Nelson, K. E., Welsh, J. A., Camarata, S. M., Tjus, T., & Heimann, M. (2001). A rare event transactional model of tricky mix conditions contributing to language acquisition and varied communicative delays. In K. E. Nelson, A. Aksu-Koc, & C. Johnson (Eds.), *International Congress of the International Association for the Study of Child Language (IASCL)* (pp. 165–195). Mahwah, NJ: Erlbaum.

Nievar, M. A., Jacobson, A., Chen, O., Johnson, U., & Dier, S. (2011). Impact of HIPPY on home learning environments of Latino families. *Early Childhood Research Quarterly, 26*, 268–277.

Nix, R. L., Bierman, K. L., McMahon, R., & the Conduct Problems Prevention Research Group. (2009). How attendance and quality of participation affect treatment response in parent behavior management training. *Journal of Consulting and Clinical Psychology, 77*, 429–438.

Nye, C., Turner, H., & Schwartz, J. (2006). Approaches to parent involvement for improving the academic performance of elementary school age children [Campbell Systematic Reviews]. Oslo, Norway: Campbell Collaboration.

Olds, D. L. (2002). Prenatal and infancy home visiting by nurses: From randomized trials to community replication. *Prevention Science, 3*, 153–172.

Olds, D. L., Kitzman, H., Cole, R., & Robinson, J. (1997). Theoretical foundations of a program of home visitation for pregnant women and parents of young children. *Journal of Community Psychology, 25*, 9–25.

Olds, D. L., Robinson, J., Pettitt, L., Luckey, D. W., Holmberg, J., Ng, R. K., et al. (2004). Effects of home visits by paraprofessionals and by nurses: Age-four follow-up of a randomized trial. *Pediatrics, 114*, 1560–1568.

Pfannenstiel, J., & Seltzer, D. A. (1989). New parents as teachers: Evaluation of an early parent education program. *Early Childhood Research Quarterly, 4*, 1–18.

Reid, M. J., Webster-Stratton, C., & Baydar, N. (2004). Halting the development of conduct problems in Head Start children: The effects of parent training. *Journal of Clinical Child and Adolescent Psychology, 33*, 279–291.

Royce, J., Darlington, R., & Murray, H. (1983). Pooled analyses: Findings across studies. In the Consortium for Longitudinal Studies (Ed.), *As the twig is bent: Lasting effects of preschool programs* (pp. 411–459). Hillsdale, NJ: Erlbaum.

Sanders, M. R. (1999). Triple P–Positive Parenting Program: Towards an empirically validated multilevel parenting and family support strategy for the prevention of behavior and emotional problems in children. *Clinical Child and Family Psychology Review, 2*, 71–90.

Scarr, S., & McCartney, K. (1988). Far from home: An experimental evaluation of the Mother–Child Home Program in Bermuda. *Child Development, 59*, 531–543.

Sheridan, S. M., Knoche, L. L., Edwards, C. P., Bovaird, J. A., & Kupzyk, K. A. (2010). Parent engagement and school readiness: Effects of the Getting

Ready intervention on preschool children's social-emotional competencies. *Early Education and Development, 21,* 125–156.

Sheridan, S. M., Knoche, L. L., Kupzyk, K. A., Edwards, C. P., & Marvin, C. A. (2011). A randomized trial examining the effects of parent engagement on early language and literacy: the Getting Ready intervention. *Journal of School Psychology, 49,* 361–383.

Sheridan, S. M., Marvin, C. A., Knoche, L. L., & Edwards, C. P. (2008). Getting ready: Promoting school readiness through a relationship-based partnership model. *Early Childhood Services, 3,* 149–172.

Spieker, S. J., & Booth, C. (1988). Family risk typologies and patters of insecure attachment. In J. Belsky & T. Nezworski (Eds.), *Clinical implications of attachment* (pp. 95–135). Hillsdale, NJ: Erlbaum.

Sweet, M., & Appelbaum, M. (2004). Is home visiting an effective strategy?: A meta-analysis of home visiting programs for families with young children. *Child Development, 74,* 1435–1456.

Wagner, M. M., & Clayton, S. L. (1999). The Parents as Teachers Program: Results from two demonstrations. *The Future of Children, 9,* 91–115.

Wasik, B. A., & Bond, M. A. (2001). Beyond the pages of a book: Interactive book reading and language development in preschool classrooms. *Journal of Educational Psychology, 93,* 243–250.

Webster-Stratton, C. (1998). Preventing conduct problems in Head Start children: Strengthening parenting competencies. *Journal of Consulting and Clinical Psychology, 66,* 715–730.

Webster-Stratton, C., Reid, M. J., & Hammond, M. (2001). Preventing conduct problems, promoting social competence: A parent and teacher training partnership in Head Start. *Journal of Clinical Child Psychology, 30,* 283–302.

Whitehurst, G. J., Arnold, D. S., Epstein, J. N., Angell, A. L., & Smith, M. (1994). A picture book reading intervention in day care and home for children from low-income families. *Developmental Psychology, 30,* 679–689.

Whitehurst, G. J., & Lonigan, C. J. (1998). Child development and emergent literacy. *Child Development, 69,* 848–872.

Zill, N., & Collins, M. (1995). *Approaching kindergarten: A look at preschoolers in the United States* (Statistical Analysis Report NCES 95-280). Washington, DC: U.S. Department of Education.

PART IV

GOING TO SCALE WITH EVIDENCE-BASED PROGRAMS

Sustaining High-Quality Practice

CHAPTER 12

Better Beginnings, Better Futures

A Comprehensive, Community-Based Early Child Development Project to Facilitate Transition to Primary School and Beyond

Ray DeV. Peters and Angela Howell-Moneta

When families face social and economic disadvantage, the learning and caregiving environments of children are often affected adversely, placing them at risk for school failure and social, emotional, and behavioral problems (Biglan, Flay, Embry, & Sandler, 2012; Engle, 2012). Recently, a proliferation of research has identified mediating processes through which social disadvantage works to undermine children's readiness for school. These studies have generally employed an ecological systems framework whereby individuals and their environments are viewed as malleable and influenced by multiple interacting levels of contextual systems (Bronfenbrenner, 1979; Schoon, 2012), such as the family, school, and community.

Some of the mediating processes that hinder children's school readiness operate at the level of parent–child relations, such as higher rates of media exposure and lower rates of caregiver–child verbal interactions (Mendelsohn et al., 2008), and less parental involvement in learning activities (Blutosky-Shearer, Wen, Faria, Hahs-Vaughn, & Korfmacher, 2012). Other processes operate within the family system, such as low levels of family literacy activities (Peifer & Perez, 2011). Recent research has also documented mediating processes that operate at the level of the neighborhood, such as a lack of safety and limited resources that reduce opportunities for children to go on outings (Kenney, 2012) and engage in outdoor play (Milteer, Ginsburg, the Council on Communications and Media Committee on Psychosocial Aspects of Child and Family Health, & Mulligan, 2012).

Various early childhood development programs have been designed to compensate for the risk factors and associated mediating processes that link family socioeconomic disadvantage with low levels of child school readiness. Early childhood development programs have typically focused on either directly influencing the child through a school or center-based educational curriculum or indirectly affecting the child through home-based interventions designed to improve parenting practices.

There is a growing recognition that effective intervention programs provide services across multiple developmental systems, including the parent–child relationship, family, child care settings, school and local neighborhood (Crosnoe, 2012). Despite a general consensus that community-level factors in school readiness intervention need to be incorporated into large-scale interventions, few projects have done this (Biglan et al., 2012). Recent community-based school readiness initiatives target limited child outcomes, such as improving literacy practices, rather than considering more broad-based outcomes (e.g., Peifer & Perez, 2011). Others have broader goals, but only include evaluations of limited outcomes such as academic achievement or health, failing to evaluate effects on children's behavior, family support, or psychological resources (Dobbie & Fryer, 2011).

A few recent broad-based community initiatives demonstrate significant potential to impact children and families, as well as the community overall, such as the Toronto First Duty Program (Corter & Pelletier, 2010). However, long-term evaluations have not yet been conducted. Finally, many intervention projects use evidence-based research to establish programs and exclude the active involvement of community members in the planning and implementation of intervention goals.

The Better Beginnings, Better Futures (BBBF) project (Peters, Bradshaw, et al., 2010) is among the few early childhood development projects to implement successfully a large-scale, community-based intervention approach based on an ecological model of human development. It has been operating in eight disadvantaged Ontario, Canada neighborhoods since 1991. BBBF is neither a service nor a program; it is a strategic initiative to mobilize disadvantaged neighborhoods and foster resilience by promoting positive functioning in young children, their families, and their neighborhoods. BBBF is funded by the Ontario government to evaluate the effectiveness of a community-based approach to programs that are locally operated jointly by community residents and professionals. Extensive longitudinal research has been conducted to determine the impact and costs of the BBBF program in the eight project sites. BBBF is the first large-scale, government-funded, community-based project of its kind in Canada.

In this chapter we review the current research literature on school readiness and early child development programs. Then we describe the BBBF project. The chapter concludes with a discussion of policy implications of the results of the research and evaluation of BBBF over the past 20 years.

Approaches to the Promotion of School Readiness

Since the initiation of BBBF in 1991, programs designed to promote early childhood development and school readiness have focused primarily on improving the quality of early preschool and elementary school programs for children or improving the quality of parenting. Most of these programs have employed standardized, curriculum-based interventions developed by experts. In this section, several of these expert-driven, "top-down" approaches are reviewed briefly then contrasted with the "bottom-up" community-based approach that provided the foundation for the BBBF project.

In a comprehensive review of effective early childhood interventions, Karoly, Kilburn, and Cannon (2005) categorized these programs as (1) home visiting/parent education interventions, (2) center-based early childhood education interventions combined with home visiting/parent education, or (3) center-based early childhood education only. Only one program (the Oklahoma Pre-K program) appeared in the third category, while there were eight programs in the first category and 10 in the second category.

Center-Based Early Childhood Interventions with Parenting Components

The Carolina Abecedarian Project is one of the earliest center-based programs designed to promote school readiness for very high-risk children growing up in poverty. Beginning in 1967, children received year-round, full-day educational day care beginning soon after birth through age 5 (Campbell et al., 2012; Campbell, Ramey, Pungello, Sparling, & Miller-Johnson, 2002). Family support services were also provided during biweekly home visits with parents. Unlike many early childhood development programs that found decreasing gains in cognitive skills over time, a follow-up of 54 children who participated in this program showed gains in reading and math achievement of 0.50 *SD* from ages 8 to 21, lower rates of special education and grade retention, and greater educational attainment by age 30 compared to a control group of 51 children (Campbell et al., 2012). The Abecedarian project demonstrated lasting effects that may be partly explained by an additional intensive educational program provided to participants from kindergarten to age 8 (Nelson, Westhues, & MacLeod, 2003). Also the cost of this very intensive program for a small sample of children was very high—$20,000 per child per year for 5 years, yielding a total cost of $100,000 per child (Barnett & Masse, 2007). Note that all project costs reported in this chapter have been converted to 2005 Canadian dollars.

The Perry Preschool Project, another well-known, center-based early childhood education program, targeted a small sample of 58 3- and 4-year old African American children living in poverty (Schweinhart et al., 2005). This program, initiated in 1967, included a half-day educational preschool curriculum and weekly home visits. Teachers in this program were highly educated, with at least a baccalaureate degree. Teacher-to-child ratios were small (5:1), enabling frequent highly individualized educational interactions and both teacher-directed and child-initiated activities. Longitudinal follow-up of 58 children in the project group and 61 in the control group showed significant gains for children receiving the intervention in reading and math tests to age 40 (Schweinhart et al., 2005). The costs of this 2-year intensive preschool program were quite high at $14,000 per child per year, for a total of $28,000 per child (Barnett, 1996).

Both the Perry Preschool program and the Abecedarian project were noteworthy for the high quality of the educational curriculum and the intensity of the "dosage" of treatment provided (Barnett, 2011). Significant long-term effects were demonstrated in these projects. However, the small sample sizes and high levels of education of teachers made these programs expensive to implement. It is therefore unclear how these program models would work for larger and more heterogeneous groups of participants.

The Chicago Child–Parent Centers program (CPC; Reynolds, 2000), operated in elementary schools in Chicago, providing 2.5 hours of educational programming daily for children ages 3 and 4 from neighborhoods with high rates of poverty. An individualized, child-focused curriculum was used, and parents were required to volunteer in their child's classroom one half-day per week. A longitudinal research cohort was recruited in 1983 and included a large sample of 1,150 children in the program intervention group, and 389 children in a quasi-experimental control group. Similar to the Abecedarian and Perry Preschool projects, longitudinal follow-up of children in the program was conducted throughout childhood until age 28 and showed positive effect sizes of 0.14–0.34 on math and language achievement tests throughout childhood (Reynolds, Temple, Ou, Arteaga, & White, 2011). Additional benefits were shown for children in the intervention group, who received an additional educational component from kindergarten to grade 3 (Reynolds, 2000). By age 28, young adults in the intervention group had higher educational attainment, higher income, and less involvement in the court system than adults in the control group (Reynolds et al., 2011). The average cost of the CPC was $7,500 per child per year for 2 years (ages 3 and 4; Reynolds, Temple, Robertson, & Mann, 2002), for a total cost of $15,000 per child.

Recent reviews have found that center- and school-based interventions can have positive short-term effects on children's cognitive development, with average effect sizes (ESs) of 0.23 reported, although these effects tend to diminish over time (Burger, 2010; Camilli, Vargas, Ryan, & Barnett, 2010; Karoly et al., 2005). More enduring but smaller effects have been found through elementary school for social and emotional functioning, (ES = 0.16), and grade retention and special education placement (ES = 0.14) (Karoly et al., 2005). These effect sizes are reported at a probability level of $p < .05$.

These reviews of center-based early childhood development programs also report qualities of the interventions that have the greatest influence on child outcomes. These characteristics include a smaller child-to-teacher ratio, more educated caregivers or teachers, and home visiting programs that involve a nurse versus a paraprofessional (Karoly et al., 2005). The majority of center-based programs that also included a home visiting/parental education component had stronger effects than programs that used an educational curriculum alone. Effects were strongest when teachers provided direct instruction in individualized (ES = 0.25) or small-group settings (ES = 0.16) (Camilli et al., 2010).

There is a general consensus that insufficient information is available from current early childhood development programs to determine the precise combination of curriculum, mode of delivery, and additional services that yield the strongest effects on child outcomes (Barnett, 2011; Burger, 2010; Camilli et al., 2010; Karoly et al., 2005). A common feature among programs that demonstrate long-term positive outcomes for children is the high quality of the care and instruction provided to children. Through the provision of cognitively stimulating interactions between teachers and children, and the incorporation of effective parental involvement in the learning process, children are more likely to achieve school readiness (Bulotsky-Shearer et al., 2012; Mashburn et al., 2008).

Home Visiting and Parent Education Programs

Recognition of the central role of parents in the creation of nurturing learning environments for their children has led to early childhood development programs that focus on empowering parents from low-income, low-education backgrounds. These programs provide an educational curriculum related to parenting practices, psychological support, and in some cases, referrals to community resources needed to enable parents to prepare their children for entry to school.

One well-researched parent-focused program is the Nurse–Family Partnership (NFP; Olds, 2008), a home visiting program focused on first-time mothers with low levels of education and income. Nurses with a minimum of a baccalaureate degree visit mothers weekly from the second trimester of pregnancy until the child's second birthday. Nurses provide education to mothers regarding maternal health (e.g., impact of smoking and alcohol on prenatal development), parenting strategies, and family functioning. Once a trusting relationship is established, nurses attempt to garner sources of support for the mother within the family system, particularly through inclusion of fathers in the home visit, and by connecting families with needed resources in the community. Nurses also try to help families formulate plans for future education or employment (Olds, 2008).

The NFP program has been found indirectly to influence children's school readiness by reducing maternal and family risk factors and helping families work toward economic self-sufficiency. The costs of the program, however, are quite high, averaging over $5,000 per family per year for 2-1/2 years of home visits (from 6 months prenatal to 2 years postnatal), for a total of over $12,000 per family.

Another parenting program that, like NFP, is being widely implemented internationally is the Positive Parenting Program (Triple P; Sanders, Markie-Dadds, & Turner, 2003). The goal of Triple P is to support parents in promoting nurturing family environments and preventing the behavioral and emotional problems of children from birth to age 16 through a behavioral family intervention based on social learning principles (e.g., Patterson, 1982). Parents participate in workshops designed to increase knowledge of child development, self-awareness, and self-regulation, and to decrease dysfunctional and coercive patterns of family interaction.

Multiple randomized controlled evaluations of Triple P revealed strong positive effects on children and parents (Prinz, Sanders, Shapiro, Whitaker, & Lutzker, 2009). For example, a meta-analysis of 55 trials of Triple P (34 trials in Australia, 21 trials in other countries) showed that Triple P had positive effects on parenting (ES = 0.38), reduced child problem behaviors (ES = 0.35), and improved parental well-being (ES = 0.17). Larger effects on child behavior problems (ES = 0.56) and parenting (ES = 0.49) were found for more distressed families that received more intensive interventions (Nowak & Heinrichs, 2008). A meta-analysis of parenting programs that provide therapeutic components similar to Triple P yielded slightly higher average effect sizes on parenting (ES = 0.43), and lower effect sizes on children's externalizing behaviors (ES = 0.25) compared to those reported in Triple P (Kaminski, Valle, Filene, & Boyle, 2008). There are no reports of improved academic or cognitive performance resulting from the Triple P program, and there is little available information on the costs of Triple P. In a recent implementation of Triple P in Switzerland, no positive effects on child or parent behaviors were found (Eisner, Nagin, Ribeaud, & Malti, 2012).

One limitation of many of the early childhood development programs reviewed here is that they focused on a limited number of the developmental contexts and settings included in Bronfenbrenner's (1979) ecological model. Most of the programs had a single focus, for example, on young children within a preschool setting, or parents in the home setting. Very few of the program evaluations investigated long-term impacts on family or parent outcomes, despite the inclusion of home visits or parent training components in most of the programs. None of the programs aimed to change the neighborhood or the broader social or cultural context that surrounded the children and their families, and none investigated neighborhood or community outcomes, such as parental community involvement or neighborhood satisfaction.

The programs reviewed offered few opportunities for local community members to become involved in the development and implementation of the programs. Researchers generally carried out program development and implementation with little or no input from parents or other local residents. For example, although the principal investigators of intervention programs may recognize that community engagement is critical for the long-term success of programs, they may nonetheless be "committed to a theoretical model that specified *a priori* the desired change targets, change agents, and change methods" (Conduct Problems Prevention Research Group, 2002, p. 2). Thus, the establishment of collaborative partnerships with schools and families may occur primarily within a highly prescriptive, top-down, researcher-led program model. A lack of community engagement is common among preventive interventions (St. Pierre & Layzer,

1998). Other than BBBF, only two multisite programs, the Comprehensive Child Development Project, (CCDP; St. Pierre, Layzer, Goodson, & Bernstein, 1997) and Early Head Start (Vogel, Xue, Moiduddin, Kisker, & Carlson, 2010), described in the next section, attempted to integrate with other local services or organizations. BBBF however, was designed to include local residents' involvement in all aspects of planning and implementation, and to form partnerships with other local service providers.

Integrated and Community-Based Interventions

There is a current focus on "scaling up" the qualities of small demonstration projects into larger-scale, publicly funded programs, so that larger segments of the population can benefit from the intervention (Barnett, 2011; Dodge, 2011). In this section, we describe three multisite, large-scale school readiness interventions that have adopted an integrated community-based approach.

Early Head Start is a large-scale, U.S. federal program that provides comprehensive, community-based services to children and toddlers (Vogel et al., 2010). Early Head Start provides child care and educational curriculum, parent and adult education, and activities in which parents and children can participate together. In randomized trials of 3,001 children attending 2 years of Early Head Start, effect sizes were small, ranging from 0.01 to 0.15 on cognition and social skills at ages 2 and 3 years. By age 5, the effects were no longer significant. However, children who participated in the intervention showed less aggression than children in the control group. By grade 5, however, no differences were found between the groups (Vogel et al., 2010). Early Head Start cost approximately $10,000 per child/family per year for 3 years (Ludwig & Phillips, 2007), for a total cost of $30,000 per child.

The CCDP (St. Pierre, Layzer, Goodson, & Bernstein, 1997), an early childhood development program, attempted to provide greater access to community services and more integrated services for low-income families through a combination of home visiting, center-based educational/life-skills training, case management, counseling, and referrals to existing community services. CCDP also aimed to increase family economic self-sufficiency by providing support for parents from pregnancy to children's transition to school.

Evaluations of the CCDP were conducted at the end of this 5-year intervention (St. Pierre et al., 1997). No short- or long-term positive effects were found on any child or parent outcomes despite the fact that the program annually cost $15,000 per family for 5 years. Numerous methodological problems with this study were noted, such as a lack of standardized curriculum, so that families differed significantly in the type and intensity of services they received. In addition, random assignment of participants to the control and intervention groups was done inconsistently across the 18 sites. Only participants in the control group received monetary remuneration for participating, possibly contributing to the high rates of attrition in the intervention group. It has been suggested that this program was more of a case management and parenting intervention than an early childhood educational intervention (Gilliam, Ripple, Zigler, & Leiter, 2000; Karoly et al., 2005).

The BBBF is among the few early childhood development projects that successfully implemented a large-scale, community-based intervention approach, with a longitudinal follow-up of children into late adolescence. The BBBF project model was unique in that it defined "high-risk" by the characteristics of neighborhoods rather than by characteristics of children or their parents. The neighborhoods selected for project implementation were characterized by socioeconomic disadvantage. However, all children in the designated age range and living in the neighborhood, as well as their families, were eligible for program involvement. Thus, the BBBF project was designed as a universal intervention to improve developmental outcomes among children and their families living in a high-risk environment. One of the key aims of the BBBF project was to enhance neighborhood capacity to support its families through the creation of voluntary leadership roles along with new participatory structures in the neighborhoods.

The BBBF Project

Project Overview

Beginning in 1991, the eight BBBF neighborhood projects began to develop and implement programs designed to incorporate components of an ecological model of human development (Bronfenbrenner, 1979). The BBBF project guidelines were ambitious. Each community was funded to develop a local prevention project designed (1) to reduce emotional and behavioral problems of young children; (2) to strengthen the capacity of parents, families, and the neighborhood to respond to the needs of their children; (3) to develop a local organization to provide programs for children ages 0 to 4 years or 4 to 8 years that responded effectively to local needs; (4) to encourage parents and neighbors to participate as equal partners with service providers to develop and carry out programs; and (5) to establish partnerships with existing and new service providers and schools, and to coordinate programs with these partners.

Project Implementation and Activities

Two variations of the BBBF project were implemented. In five *younger child* project sites, programs focused on children from birth to age 4 and their families. In three *older child* project sites, programs focused on children between ages 4 and 8 years and their families (see Table 12.1). Between 64 and 83% of the families in these neighborhoods fell below the Statistics Canada Low-Income Cutoff, and 37% were single-parent families.

The BBBF project model required each community to develop and deliver high-quality programs that were expected to produce positive child, family, and neighborhood outcomes. High-quality programs were defined as programs paying careful attention to (1) staff recruitment, training, adequate compensation, and participation in decision making; (2) favorable child-to-staff ratios; (3) curriculum development relating program activities to goals and objectives; and (4) provision of time for staff to develop close relations with families and the communities in which they work.

TABLE 12.1. BBBF Project Locations and Demographics of the Children Served

City	Neighborhood	Children in project age range in each site: 1996–1997
Younger child sites		
Guelph	Willow Road	500
Kingston	Northern Area	876
Ottawa	Albion–Hetherington social housing complexes	552
Toronto	Regent Park/Moss Park social housing complexes	900
Walpole Island First Nation		200
	All younger child sites	3,785
Older child sites		
Cornwall	4 Francophone primary schools	530
Rexdale	Highfield Junior School	517
Sudbury	Flour Mill/le Moulin à Fleur and Donovan	503
	All older child sites	1,549
	All sites	5,334

The five *younger child* sites focused on providing programs for children from birth to age 4 and their families. They were required by the government funder to provide home visiting programs plus supports to increase the quality of local child care (e.g., providing additional staff and resources to existing day care and preschool programs). The three *older child* sites focused programming on children ages 4 to 8 years and their families. These sites were required to provide in-classroom or in-school programs, plus support to increase the quality of local child care, through, for example, before- and afterschool and summer holiday care, homework support, and recreation programs. (Ontario provides half-day junior kindergarten or PreK for all 4-year-olds, and senior kindergarten for all 5-year-olds).

All sites provided a variety of programs tailored to local needs, either by themselves or through partnerships with other education and service providers. Examples included parent–child drop-in programs, toy-lending libraries, parent training and support groups, nutrition support, neighborhood safety initiatives, cultural awareness activities, recreation, and mentoring programs. The five *younger child* sites provided an average of 26 different programs, whereas the three *older child* sites provided an average of 16 different programs for the children, their families, and the local neighborhood. All sites attempted to adapt the programs to the needs and context of their neighborhoods.

In the *older child* sites, all children and most parents were involved in some of the BBBF programs, since they were offered before, during, and after school. In the *younger child* sites, some children and families were touched directly by the BBBF programs (e.g., home visitors, parent training, play groups). Some attended programs on a regular basis, others on a very random or part-time basis. Some did not attend any programs but may have been influenced indirectly, for example, by a neighbor who attended programs and offered support, or by safer streets and parks, or by increased community participation.

BBBF Evaluation: Research Methods

A team of multidisciplinary researchers from seven Ontario universities and field researchers in each local site were responsible for the research design, data collection, analysis, and reporting. The BBBF Research Coordination Unit coordinated all research activities with central offices at Queen's University in Kingston, Ontario.

Qualitative and Descriptive Research on Project Implementation

Local site researchers were trained to write descriptive reports on program development and implementation at each site using a common protocol. Steering committee members reviewed these local site reports to ensure that local contexts were accurately captured in this report. These individual site reports were also summarized in comprehensive "cross-site" reports on each topic. All reports are available on the BBBF website: *www.bbbf.ca.* These reports formed the basis for the "toolkit" on how to develop and implement the BBBF project that is described later in this chapter.

Quantitative Research Outcomes

Information about children, parents, families, and neighborhoods was collected in a variety of ways, including (1) annual, 2-hour in-home parent interviews and direct child measures carried out by local site researchers employed by the Research Coordination Unit; (2) annual teacher reports; and (3) federal and provincial databases (e.g., Statistics Canada Census data, Ontario Principals' Reports of Special Education Instruction). In 1992–1993, three comparison sites were selected, based on Statistics Canada Census data. Comparison sites were similar to the BBBF sites in terms of average annual family income, single-parent status, parent education and employment, and cultural identity.

For the first phase of the research (evaluation of the short-term findings; see section below for more details), 1,536 children and their families in the eight BBBF sites and three comparison neighborhoods agreed to participate in a longitudinal research group. The longitudinal research sample comprised children born in 1994 at the *younger child* sites and children who were 4 years or older at the *older child* sites. Data were gathered regularly over a 4-year period at the *younger child* sites and comparison sites when the children were 3, 18, 33, and 48 months of age. At the *older child* sites, data were collected annually from age 4, when the children were in publicly funded junior kindergarten, until they were 8 years old and in grade 2. The quasi-experimental control group design examined how changes in children and families in the BBBF neighborhoods over 4 years of programming differed from changes in those from the demographically similar comparison sites that did not receive BBBF funding.

Project Impact: Child, Family, and Neighborhood Outcomes

Short-Term Outcomes

The results presented in this section summarize data collected in 1998, when the BBBF children in our longitudinal research sample ended their 4 years of program eligibility. Note that effect sizes are reported at $p < .05$. For detailed reports of these data, see Peters et al. (2000) and Peters,

Petrunka, and Arnold (2003). A positive impact of the BBBF project on children's social-emotional functioning and physical health was found. Teachers rated children as having significantly fewer overanxious behavior problems (ES = 0.48) and greater self-control (ES = 0.46). Teachers also rated their relationships with parents of children in the BBBF study as having improved since the inception of the study, and teachers rated parents as more involved in their children's schooling (ES = 0.20). In grade 3, fewer special education services (ES = 0.23) were used by children at the three *older child* BBBF sites than children in the comparison sites. The impact of the study on children's school readiness was also evident at later follow-up periods.

Reduced smoking by mothers was found across all sites. This finding is encouraging, since smoking levels tend to be high in disadvantaged communities, and the long-term health effects of smoking are well known. The change in smoking rates in BBBF sites may be related to the fact that parents had increased opportunities to meet other parents, participate in support groups or committees, and volunteer in community activities, especially since meetings and events were often held in public locations where smoking is restricted or discouraged.

For neighborhood outcomes, in each *younger child* BBBF site, parents reported increased safety when walking at night. In the three *older child* sites, parents reported greater satisfaction with the general quality of their neighborhoods and housing. In all eight BBBF sites, parents perceived more improvement in the quality of life in their neighborhoods than did parents from the comparison sites.

In summary, both the *younger* and *older child* BBBF sites yielded similar positive short-term outcomes. Thus, there was little support for the prediction that programs starting earlier in children's development, in this case, immediately after birth, would be more effective than programs starting later in children's development.

Medium-Term Outcomes

The same measures of child, parent, and neighborhood outcomes were used to collect data 4 years after children and their families completed program participation. These data were collected when children from the *younger child* sites were in grade 3 and those from the *older child* sites were in grade 6. The BBBF research team has established the most extensive and intensive longitudinal database involving children and families from disadvantaged neighborhoods in Canada.

The analyses of these data yielded a picture in stark contrast to that of the short-term findings just described. At grade 3, children and families from the five BBBF *younger child* sites showed no positive outcomes relative to those from the comparison sites on any measures (Peters et al., 2006). In contrast, children in grade 6 from the three *older child* BBBF sites showed significantly positive outcomes relative to those from the comparison sites. Grade 6 teachers rated children in the BBBF group as demonstrating greater self-control in conflicts with peers (ES = 0.34), lower hyperactivity and inattention problems (ES = 0.23), and fewer school suspensions (ES = 0.21). Children also required fewer special education services (ES = 0.22) and obtained higher scores on a standardized math test (ES = 0.21) than youth in the comparison group. Also, parents from the three *older child* BBBF sites reported higher levels of social support (ES = 0.38), better family functioning (ES = 0.31), more community involvement (ES = 0.30), and greater neighborhood satisfaction (ES = 0.35) than parents from the comparison neighborhoods (Peters, Bradshaw, et al., 2010).

Long-Term Outcomes

Due to the positive findings in favor of the three *older child* BBBF sites when the children were in grade 6, subsequent longitudinal follow-up studies were completed on the children and their families when the children were in grades 9 and 12 (7 and 10 years after ending program involvement). These results, along with extensive descriptions of the BBBF project history and complete methodology, are presented in Peters, Bradshaw, et al. (2010), and in less technical publications (Roche, Petrunka, & Peters, 2008; Peters, Nelson, et al., 2010). Youth from the three *older child* BBBF neighborhoods continued to show superior school and academic performance relative to youth from the comparison neighborhoods. Grade 9 teachers rated youth from the BBBF sites as being better prepared for school (ES = 0.25), using fewer special education services (ES = 0.20), showing more adaptive functioning in school (ES = 0.22), repeating fewer grades (ES = 0.22), and displaying fewer emotional problems (ES = 0.22) and hyperactive/inattentive behaviors in the classroom (ES = 0.33). Also, parents from these BBBF neighborhoods were more satisfied with their marital relationship (ES = 0.26) and reported more positive family functioning (ES = 0.28) and greater social support (ES = 0.40). By grade 12, BBBF youth required significantly fewer special education services (ES = 0.18) and had higher average grades (ES = 0.18) relative to youth in the comparison group.

Economic Analysis

Program costs for BBBF were funded directly by the Ontario government and included staff salaries, facilities, equipment, materials, and any items necessary to implement the programs successfully at each BBBF site. Since the BBBF programs were available and potentially accessible to all children and their families in the respective site locations, the cost of the programs has been related to the *total* number of children in each of the BBBF neighborhoods who fall within the project range (i.e., 0–4 or 4–8 years of age). Therefore we calculated a "cost per capita" based on an "intent to treat" analysis. The average annual cost per child/family in the five *younger child* sites for 1996–1997 was $733, and that for the three *older child* sites was $748. This yields a 4-year average project cost of approximately $3,000 per child/family.

At grade 9, for the *older child* sites, a cost-savings analysis was carried out, contrasting the cost to the Ontario government of providing the BBBF programs for up to 4 years compared to the cost of providing government services to children and their families from both the project and comparison communities. The costs associated with government-provided health, educational, and social services provided to children and families from the three BBBF sites were approximately $4,000 less than the cost of those services provided to youth and families from the comparison sites. Thus, the $3,000 initial investment in the BBBF project by the Ontario government yielded savings of $4,000 per family when the youth were in grade 9 (Peters, Bradshaw, et al., 2010).

Results from a similar economic analysis carried out 3 years later when the youth were in grade 12 documented that cost savings to the Ontario government associated with BBBF program involvement increased substantially from the grade 9 analyses to over $7,500 per family. Compared to the $3,000 cost of providing the BBBF model for 4 years for each family, this represents a benefit–cost ratio of 2.5 or a return to the Ontario government of $2.50 for every $1 invested in the BBBF project. The largest cost savings at grades 9 and 12 resulted from lower special education costs for the BBBF youth, and less use of welfare and disability support services by BBBF families (Peters, Nelson, et al., 2010). Aos, Lieb, Mayfield, Miller, and Pennucci (2004) wrote:

> Does prevention pay? Can an ounce of prevention avoid (at least) an ounce of cure? More specifically for public policy purposes, is there credible scientific evidence that for each dollar a legislature spends on "research-based" prevention or early intervention programs for youth, more than a dollar's worth of benefits will be generated? If so, what are the policy options that offer taxpayers the best return on their dollar? (p. 1)

In the case of the BBBF projects at the *older child* sites, the answer is yes; more than a dollar's worth of benefits was generated. The limitations and challenges to the BBBF project model, as well as policy implications, are discussed in the following sections.

Limitations and Challenges of the BBBF Intervention Model

As described throughout this chapter, the BBBF project was an extremely ambitious initiative by the Ontario government. The project model required each site to involve local residents and parents, as well as other organizations that provided services in all aspects of project development, organization, and implementation. This community-based approach presented many challenges. In fact, it took each community 2 years to develop its organization and programs. The Ontario government provided funding for these 2 years of project development, in addition to the following 4 years of program implementation. Convincing funders to provide adequate resources to allow for 2 years of project development may constitute a serious limitation for any community considering implementing a BBBF-type project.

We recently developed training materials, including manuals and videos, for use by other disadvantaged neighborhoods when planning and implementing a BBBF-type model. This "toolbox" was developed in a manner that allowed the project to be tailored to widely varying local contexts (Hayward, Loomis, Nelson, Pancer, & Peters, 2011). The information in the toolkit is based on the extensive descriptive reports produced by our local researchers describing how each of the eight BBBF project sites developed, organized, and implemented the programs in their neighborhoods.

The toolkit contains information about (1) the history and overview of the BBBF project, (2) how to develop a community-based project model, (3) research and evaluation methods, (4) how to generate community resident participation, (5) how to engage and partner with local organizations, (6) how to establish a workable organizational structure, and (7) how to collaborate effectively with government and other funders. The specific challenges related to each of these topics (except the history and overview) are described.

The time and effort required to involve local residents actively in disadvantaged neighborhoods in project organization and management presented a major challenge to each local BBBF project, as did forming partnerships with existing organizations that provide services and schools. For example, in the toolkit unit dealing with community resident participation, the following challenges are described.

> Despite the many benefits from having local residents meaningfully and fully involved, each site experienced its own barriers, obstacles and challenges. These included *residents' apprehension and discomfort* (anxiety or shyness among those used to staying at home; distrust or fear of working with service providers); *conflicting commitments and difficulties juggling responsibilities* (residents living in poverty felt stressed and overwhelmed); *ethnic*

> *tensions, language barriers, and cultural differences; failed expectations and disappointments* (too much expected too soon and residents feeling undervalued for their work); *high rates of turnover*; and a *lack of resources* (for training volunteers or translating project materials). (Hayward et al., 2011, p. 18)

Each of these challenges is described in some detail, and discussion of possible solutions is based on the experiences of the local projects. Thus, the design of the toolkit enables the project model to be tailored to widely varying local contexts, and to identify potential challenges involved in the implementation of a BBBF project. It is hoped that the toolkit will decrease the amount of time required by local communities to develop and implement a BBBF project to less than the 2 years required by the original sites from 1991 to 1993.

Implications for Policy and Practice

Several social policy implications arise from the BBBF longitudinal evaluation study. First, the outcome data collected immediately after the program ended indicated positive effects on children, families, and neighborhoods in the BBBF sites relative to data collected from demographically matched comparison groups. This was true for both the *younger child* (0 to 4 years) and *older child* (4 to 8 years) projects.

Second, the longitudinal follow-up data collected from participants 4 years after the project ended (grade 3 for *younger child* programs, and grade 6 for *older child* programs) yielded no positive outcomes for the *younger child* sites, but a wide range of positive child, family, and neighborhood outcomes for the *older child* sites. Similar positive outcomes were found 3 and 6 years later when youth from the three *older child* BBBF sites were in grades 9 and 12, respectively. Findings related to children's school readiness, including their in-school behavior and academic functioning, were particularly positive for children from the *older child* BBBF sites. These differences between the *younger child* and *older child* project sites are inconsistent with a "starting younger is better" view of early child development programs designed to foster successful transition to primary school and beyond. How can these results, especially the lack of enduring effects from the *younger child* projects, be explained?

One possible reason for these differences is the greater amount of program participation that occurred in the *older child* BBBF sites. Since all children attended primary school during the 4 years of program implementation (junior kindergarten through grade 2), many of the BBBF child-focused programs were delivered either in the school or immediately before and after school. We found that 100% of the children in our research sample participated in BBBF programs. In two of three sites, 98% of children attended program sessions 80 times or more each year. For younger children ages 0 to 4 years, there was no universal early childhood learning system equivalent to the primary school system available or mandated for children or their parents. Consequently, it was more difficult to develop and implement prevention programs that had a high probability of reaching all infants and preschool children and their families; for example, in one BBBF *younger child* site only 15% of families participated in BBBF program sessions 80 times or more each year. The lower program exposure of children and their families in the *younger child* BBBF sites relative to those in the three *older child* sites may help to explain the absence of durable medium-term outcomes in the *younger child* sites. To maintain the advantage of children from the *younger child* BBBF sites through kindergarten and grade 1, they likely would have benefited from extra support, such as educational assistants in the classroom and coordinators working to involve parents in the child's education. These were activities used successfully in the *older child* BBBF sites.

The broad mandate for the BBBF programs (i.e., to improve all aspects of children's development, provide programs for parents and the neighborhood while involving community residents in all project activities, and to collaborate with other service providers) may have been asking too much of the *younger child* sites. As described earlier, the *older child* BBBF programs were organized in and around the neighborhood schools attended by all children. These schools are funded by the Ontario Ministry of Education at the level of approximately $7,000 per child annually. The *older child* BBBF programs were able to add their programs before, during, and after school, engaging virtually every child in ongoing programs during the school year for up to 4 years. The relatively modest BBBF program resources of approximately $3,000 over 4 years per child/family then represent "value added" to the well-financed primary school system. For children younger than 4 years of age, there exists no comparable universal, well-financed service system with which to connect. If a universal, high-quality, affordable, optional early learning and child care system existed, similar to what already exists in many other developed countries (Organization for Economic Development and Cooperation, 2006), BBBF programs could be organized in conjunction with such a system. This could possibly provide "value added" outcomes for children and their families, similar to those of the *older child* BBBF sites.

The major policy implications from this analysis are that in order for early child development initiatives funded at the level of BBBF to be effective, they may need to be added to a well-financed, universally available early childhood education system. Without such a system, currently unavailable in Canada and the United States, it is extremely expensive for public funders to implement effective "stand-alone" programs such as the Abecedarian, Perry Preschool, Chicago Child–Parent Centers, and the Nurse–Family Partnership, and these types of programs may simply be beyond their capability to provide on a large scale.

CONCLUSION

In a recent article entitled "Context Matters in Child and Family Policy," Dodge (2011) argues that the traditional way that basic research findings in the field of child development are "translated" into social policy has been woefully ineffective. He argues that most attempts to generalize research findings from highly controlled laboratory studies to real-world settings have failed precisely because researchers fail to appreciate the importance of contextual factors.

> The traditional model of translation from basic laboratory science to efficacy trials, to effectiveness trials to community dissemination has flaws that arise from false assumptions that context changes little or matters little. One of the most important findings in developmental science is that context matters, but this fact is not sufficiently taken into account in many translation efforts. (p. 433)

To rectify this situation, Dodge recommends that researchers initiate their research studies in community contexts in order to facilitate the translation of the research findings into social policy. That is exactly what the BBBF research study has done. Given the widely varying real-world neighborhood contexts in which the BBBF project model has been implemented and evaluated, this increases the confidence that these results may be applicable to many other disadvantaged neighborhoods across Canada. Further information about the BBBF project research findings and the toolkit is available on our website: *www.bbbf.ca.*

REFERENCES

Aos, S., Lieb, R., Mayfield, J., Miller, M., & Pennucci, A. (2004). *Benefits and costs of prevention and early intervention programs for youth.* Olympia: Washington State Institute for Public Policy.

Barnett, W. S. (2011). Effectiveness of early educational intervention. *Science, 333,* 975–978.

Barnett, W. S., & Masse, L. N. (2007). Comparative benefit-cost analysis of the Abecedarian program and its policy implications. *Economics of Education Review, 26,* 113–125.

Barnett, W. S. (1996). *Lives in the balance: Benefit–cost analysis of the Perry Preschool Program through age 27. Monographs of the High/Scope Educational Research Foundation.* Ypsilanti, MI: High/Scope Press.

Biglan, A., Flay, B. R., Embry, D. D., & Sandler, I. N. (2012). The critical role of nurturing environments for promoting human well-being. *American Psychologist, 67,* 257–271.

Blutosky-Shearer, R., Wen, X., Faria, A., Hahs-Vaughn, D. L., & Korfmacher, J. (2012). National profiles of classroom quality and family involvement: A multilevel examination of proximal influences on Head Start children's school readiness. *Early Childhood Research Quarterly, 27*(4), 627–639.

Bronfenbrenner, U. (1979). *The ecology of human development.* Cambridge, MA: Harvard University Press.

Burger, K. (2010). How does early childhood care and education affect cognitive development?: An international review of the effects of early interventions for children from different social backgrounds. *Early Childhood Research Quarterly, 25*(2), 140–165.

Camilli, G., Vargas, S., Ryan, S., & Barnett, S. W. (2010). Meta-analysis of the effects of early education interventions on cognitive and social development. *Teachers College Record, 112,* 579–620. Retrieved from *http://spot.colorado.edu/~camillig/papers/38_15440.pdf.*

Campbell, F. A., Pungello, E. P., Burchinal, M., Kainz, K., Pan, Y., Wasik, B. H., et al. (2012). Adult outcomes as a function of an early childhood educational program: An Abecedarian Project follow-up. *Developmental Psychology, 48,* 1033–1043.

Campbell, F. A., Ramey, C. T., Pungello, E., Sparling, J., & Miller-Johnson, S. (2002). Early childhood education: Young adult outcomes from the Abecedarian Project. *Applied Developmental Science, 6,* 42–57.

Conduct Problems Prevention Research Group. (2002). The implementation of the Fast Track Program: An example of a large-scale prevention science efficacy trial. *Journal of Abnormal Child Psychology, 30,* 1–17.

Corter, C., & Pelletier, J. (2010). Schools as integrated service hubs for young children and families: Policy implications of the Toronto First Duty Project. *International Journal of Child Care and Education Policy, 4*(2), 45–54. Retrieved from *www.kicce.re.kr/upload/info/5.carl_corter_canada_.pdf.*

Crosnoe, R. (2012). Family–school connections, early learning, and socioeconomic inequality in the US. *REMIE-Multidisciplinary Journal of Educational Research, 2*(1), 1–36.

Dobbie, W., & Fryer, R. G. (2011). Are high-quality schools enough to increase achievement among the poor?: Evidence from the Harlem Children's Zone. *American Economic Journal: Applied Economics, 3,* 158–187.

Dodge, K. A. (2011). Context matters in child and family policy. *Child Development, 82*(1), 433–442.

Eisner, M., Nagin, D., Ribeaud, D., & Malti, T. (2012). Effects of a universal parenting program for highly adherent parents: A propensity score matching approach. *Prevention Science, 15,* 252–266.

Engle, P. (2012). Poverty and developmental potential. In J. Boyden & M.

Bourdillon (Eds.), *Childhood poverty: Multidisciplinary approaches* (pp. 129–147). New York: Palgrave Macmillan.

Gilliam, W. S., Ripple, C. H., Zigler, E. F., & Leiter, V. (2000). Evaluating child and family demonstration initiatives: Lessons from the Comprehensive Child Development Program. *Early Childhood Research Quarterly, 15*, 41–59.

Hayward, K., Loomis, C., Nelson, G., Pancer, M., & Peters, R. (2011). A toolkit for Building Better Beginnings and Better Futures. Kingston, ON: Better Beginnings, Better Futures Research Coordination Unit. Retrieved from *www.bbbf.ca*.

Kaminski, J. W., Valle, L. A., Filene, J. H., & Boyle, C. L. (2008). A meta-analytic review of components associated with parent training program effectiveness. *Journal of Abnormal Child Psychology, 36*, 567–589.

Karoly, L. A., Kilburn, M. R., & Cannon, J. S. (2005). Early childhood interventions: Proven results, future promises. Santa Monica, CA: RAND Corporation. Retrieved from *www.rand.org/pubs/research_briefs/rb9145.html*.

Kenney, M. K. (2012). Child, family, and neighborhood associations with parent and peer interactive play during early childhood. *Maternal and Child Health Journal, 16*, S88–S101.

Ludwig, J., & Phillips, D. (2007). The benefits and costs of Head Start. *SRCD Social Policy Report: Giving Child and Youth Development Knowledge Away, 21*(3), 3–18. Retrieved from *www.srcd.org/documents/publications/spr/213_early_childhood_education.pdf*.

Mashburn, A., Pianta, R., Hamre, B., Downer, J., Barbarin, O., Bryant, D., et al. (2008). Measures of classroom quality in prekindergarten and children's development of academic, language and social skills. *Child Development, 79*, 732–749.

Mendelsohn, A. L., Berkule, S. B., Tomopoulos, S., Tamis-LeMonda, C. S., Huberman, H. S., Alvir, J., et al. (2008). Infant television and video exposure associated with limited parent–child verbal interactions in low socioeconomic status households. *Archives of Pediatric Adolescent Medicine, 162*, 411–417.

Milteer, R. M., Ginsburg, K. R., Council on Communications and Media Committee on Psychosocial Aspects of Child and Family Health, & Mulligan, D. A. (2012). The importance of play in promoting healthy child development and maintaining strong parent–child bonds: Focus on children in poverty. *Pediatrics, 129*, e204–e213.

Nelson, G., Westhues, A., & MacLeod, J. (2003). A meta-analysis of longitudinal research on preschool prevention programs for children. *Prevention and Treatment, 6*(1), 1–35.

Nowak, C., & Heinrichs, N. (2008). A comprehensive meta-analysis of Triple P–Positive Parent Program using hierarchical linear modelling: Effectiveness and moderating variables. *Clinical Child and Family Psychological Review, 11*, 114–144.

Olds, D. L. (2008). Preventing child maltreatment and crime with prenatal and infancy support of parents: The Nurse–Family Partnership . *Journal of Scandinavian Studies in Criminology and Crime Prevention, 9*(Suppl. 1), 2–24.

Organization for Economic Development and Cooperation. (2006). *Starting strong II: Early child education and care* (No. 9, 445 pp.). Retrieved from *www.oecd.org/education/preschoolandschool/37417240.pdf.*

Patterson, G. R. (1982). *Coercive family process.* Eugene, OR: Castalia.

Peifer, K., & Perez, L. (2011). Effectiveness of a coordinated community effort to promote early literacy behaviors. *Maternal and Child Health Journal, 15,* 765–771.

Peters, R. DeV., Arnold, R., Petrunka, K., Angus, D., Brophy, K., et al. (2000). Developing capacity and competence in the Better Beginnings, Better Futures communities: Short-term findings report [Technical Report]. Kingston, ON: Better Beginnings Research Coordination Unit. Retrieved from *www.bbbf.ca.*

Peters, R. DeV., Bradshaw, A. J., Petrunka, K., Nelson, G., Herry, Y., Craig, W. M., et al. (2010). The Better Beginnings, Better Futures project: Findings from grade 3 to grade 9. *Monographs of the Society for Research in Child Development, 75*(3), 1–176.

Peters, R. DeV., Nelson, G., Petrunka, K., Pancer, S. M., Loomis, C., Hasford, J., et al. (2010). Investing in our future: Highlights of Better Beginnings, Better Futures research findings at grade 12. Kingston, ON: Better Beginnings, Better Futures Research Coordination Unit, Queen's University. Retrieved from *www.bbbf.ca.*

Peters, R. DeV., Petrunka, K., & Arnold, R. (2003). The Better Beginnings, Better Futures Project. A universal, comprehensive, community-based prevention approach for primary school children and their families. *Journal of Clinical Child and Adolescent Psychology, 32,* 215–226.

Peters, R. DeV., Petrunka, K., Ridgeway, D., Arnold, R., Bélanger, J.-M., Boyce, W., et al. (2006). *Medium-term follow-up outcomes of the Better Beginnings, Better Futures Project for young children: Too little and too much?* [Technical report]. Kingston, ON: Better Beginnings, Better Futures Research Coordination Unit.

Prinz, R. J., Sanders, M. R., Shapiro, C. J., Whitaker, D. J., & Lutzker, J. R. (2009). Population-based prevention of child maltreatment: The U.S. Triple P system population trial. *Prevention Science, 10*(1), 1–12.

Reynolds, A. J. (2000). *Success in early intervention: The Chicago Child–Parent Centers program and youth through age 15.* Lincoln: University of Nebraska Press.

Reynolds, A., Temple, J., Ou., S., Arteaga, I., & White, B. A. B. (2011). School-based early childhood education and age-28 well-being: Effects by timing, dosage, and subgroups. *Science, 333,* 360–364.

Reynolds, A. J., Temple, J. A., Robertson, D. L., & Mann, E. A. (2002). Age 21 cost–benefit analysis of the Title I Chicago Child–Parent Centers. *Educational Evaluation and Policy Analysis, 24*(4), 267–303. Retrieved from *www.irp.wisc.edu/publications/dps/pdfs/dp124502.pdf?q=others.*

Roche, J., Petrunka, K., & Peters, R. DeV. (2008). *Investing in our future: Highlights of Better Beginnings, Better Futures research findings at grade 9.* Kingston, ON: Better Beginnings, Better Futures Research Coordination Unit. Retrieved from *www.bbbf.ca.*

Sanders, M. R., Markie-Dadds, C., & Turner, K. M. T. (2003). Theoretical, scientific and clinical foundations of the Triple P Positive Parenting Program: A population approach to the promotion of parenting competence. *Parenting Research and Practice Monograph No. 1,* 1–25. Retrieved from *www.triplep.net/files/pdf/parenting_research_and_practice_monograph_no.1.pdf.*

Schoon, I. (2012). Temporal and contextual dimensions to individual positive development: A developmental-contextual systems model of resilience. *The Social Ecology of Resilience, 3,* 143–156.

Schweinhart, L. J., Montie, J., Xiang, Z., Barnett, W. S., Belfield, C. R., & Nores, M. (2005). *Lifetime effects: The HighScope Perry Preschool study through age 40* (Monographs of the HighScope Educational Research Foundation, No. 14). Ypsilanti, MI: HighScope Press. Retrieved from *www.highscope.org/content.asp?contentid=219&referer=http%3a%2f%2fworks.bepress.com%2fwilliam_barnett%2f3%2f.*

St. Pierre, R. G., & Layzer, J. I. (1998). Improving the life chances of children living in poverty: Assumptions and what we have learned. *Society for Research in Child Development Social Policy Report, 12,* 1–25.

St. Pierre, R. G., Layzer, J. I., Goodson, B. D., & Bernstein, L. S. (1997). *National impact evaluation of the Comprehensive Child Development Program: Final report.* Cambridge, MA: Abt Associates.

Vogel, C. A., Xue, Y., Moiduddin, E. M., Kisker, E. E., & Carlson, B. L. (2010). *Early Head Start children in grade 5: Long-term follow-up of the Early Head Start Research and Evaluation Study Sample* (OPRE Report No. 2011-8). Washington, DC: Office of Planning, Research, and Evaluation, Administration for Children and Families, U.S. Department of Health and Human Services.

CHAPTER 13

Large-Scale Dissemination of an Evidence-Based Prevention Program for At-Risk Kindergartners

Lessons Learned from an Effectiveness Trial of the Fluppy Program

FRANÇOIS POULIN, FRANCE CAPUANO, FRANK VITARO, PIERRETTE VERLAAN, MONIQUE BRODEUR, and JACINTHE GIROUX

Disruptive behavior can take the form of hyperactivity, aggression, or oppositional behavior and can be physical or verbal. A high proportion of kindergarten students (9–15% according to the literature) are rated as frequently displaying these problems (Conseil Supérieur de l'Éducation, 2001; National Longitudinal Survey of Children and Youth; NLSCY, 1999). From the very start of their schooling, students with elevated disruptive behavior tend to struggle academically (Hinshaw, 1992). They often enter school without the necessary academic prerequisites, which, along with their high levels of disruptive classroom behavior, contributes to their failure at school (Vitaro, Brendgen, & Tremblay, Chapter 2, this volume). Many of these students also maintain a high rate of disruptive behavior throughout their schooling (Tremblay, 2004). These pupils are especially at risk of dropping out of school and failing to obtain a high school diploma (Vitaro, Brengden, Larose, & Tremblay, 2005). In addition, many of them display delinquency and violent behavior in adolescence (Hill &

Maughan, 2001). Together, the risks associated with elevated disruptive behaviors at school entry point to the need for preventive interventions in kindergarten. In addition to reducing the levels of disruptive behavior, these preventive interventions should also aim to improve the academic prerequisites of these children, since these two aspects of school readiness (behavioral and academic) independently predict later outcomes such as high school graduation (Vitaro et al., Chapter 2, this volume).

A multimodal prevention program for kindergarten students with a high levels of disruptive behavior, known as the "Fluppy program," has been widely implemented in the province of Québec over the past 20 years. Our goals in this chapter are to (1) provide a brief overview of the program's underlying conceptual model, (2) outline the history of the program's development, (3) describe its dissemination across Québec and document a number of implementation issues, and (4) report the findings of an effectiveness trial.

Risk and Protective Factors in the Development of Disruptive Behaviors

The intervention components of the Fluppy program are designed to decrease the harmful effects of risk factors and maximize the favorable effects of protective factors in the emergence, maintenance, or escalation of disruptive behaviors. The origin of disruptive behavior is complex and results from a series of biological, social-cognitive, and environmental factors that interact with one another in the course of development (Dodge, Coie, & Lynam, 2006; Tremblay, Hartup, & Archer, 2005). From a prevention perspective, social-cognitive and environmental factors (e.g., family, peers, and school) are of particular interest, because they tend to be relatively malleable.

With regard to social-cognitive characteristics, disruptive behavior is associated with certain deficiencies in social information processing (Dodge, 2006). Children who display disruptive behavior tend to attribute hostile intentions to others in ambiguous circumstances and have a very small repertoire of solutions when confronted with difficult interpersonal situations. In addition, these children also have deficiencies in emotion regulation and self-control (Lochman, Whidby, & FitzGerald, 2000). Social integration into the peer group can also be challenging in two respects for these children. First, students with disruptive behavior are likely to be rejected by their peers (Bierman, 2004). This negative status among peers in turn contributes to the maintenance and exacerbation of behavior problems and reduces academic motivation among highly disruptive children (Véronneau, Vitaro, Brendgen, Dishion, & Tremblay,

2010). Second, children with disruptive behavior tend to form friendships with each other as early as kindergarten (Boivin, Vitaro, & Poulin, 2005; Snyder et al., 2005). These friendships then contribute to an increase in behavior problems and to a decrease in both academic performance and school motivation in subsequent years, as they provide norms and responses that support antisocial activity and undermine school engagement (Véronneau, Vitaro, Pedersen, & Tremblay, 2008). Parent–child relationships are also a crucial factor in the development of disruptive behaviors. Parental practices characterized by inconsistent and ineffective discipline (Patterson, Reid, & Dishion, 1992) and by a lack of warmth and affection (DeKlyen & Speltz, 2001) contribute to the maintenance or aggravation of disruptive behavior, particularly when parents have a very limited support network. Finally, in the school context, teachers can also play an important role in maintaining and fostering disruptive behavior—particularly in the early stages of schooling—through a lack of both class management skills and positive personal ties to students and parents (Birsch & Ladd, 1997; Brendgen, Wanner, & Vitaro, 2006; Meehan, Hugues, & Cavell, 2003).

These risk and protective factors have implications for effective prevention design. To address the complex set of factors associated with disruptive behavior development, it is recommended that in addition to intervening directly with the child, interventions be implemented in the child's family, peer group, and school in order to make use of the child's main socialization agents, including his or her parents, peers, and teachers (Conduct Problems Prevention Research Group [CPPRG], 1992). Moreover, academic interventions should be introduced very early in these students' schooling to assist with learning. In line with the current literature on the most active elements of school readiness, such interventions should target emergent literacy and emergent numeracy skills, since the presence of these skills in kindergarten supports and predicts primary and secondary school success (Duncan et al., 2007; Ensminger & Slusarcick, 1992).

The History of the Fluppy Program and Its Large-Scale Dissemination in Québec

In 1984, a group of researchers headed by Richard E. Tremblay and Frank Vitaro launched the Montréal Experimental Longitudinal Study (MELS). Guided by the developmental model described earlier, the main goal of the MELS was to experiment with and evaluate a multimodal preventive intervention for boys identified by their kindergarten teachers as being highly disruptive. These boys were exposed to a 2-year multimodal preventive intervention in grades 2 and 3. In line with other evidence-based prevention programs implemented in the early 1980s, the MELS included three components: (1) a social skills and self-control skills training program in which the at-risk child participated in sessions with three children considered to have good social skills; (2) home visits over a 2-year period aimed at providing parents with the tools to understand their children's problems better and develop the means to change their disruptive behaviors; and (3) teacher support to promote positive child socialization and integration at school. To evaluate the impact of this prevention program, 250 disruptive boys were randomly assigned to the experimental condition (i.e., exposure to the three intervention components) or the control condition (i.e., usual practice). All the interventions were administered by members of the research team. At the end of elementary school, the results showed that the boys in the experimental prevention condition, compared to the controls, had fewer behavior problems, were less likely to repeat the school year, and were less often placed in specialized classes (Tremblay, Vitaro, Gagnon, Piché, & Royer, 1992; Tremblay, Pagani-Kurtz, Masse, Vitaro, & Pihl, 1995). A follow-up assessment in young adulthood showed that by age 24, these boys were also more likely to have completed a high school diploma (Boisjoly, Vitaro, Lacourse, Barker, & Tremblay, 2007).

These and other findings had a significant impact on the development of large-scale prevention programs in the 1990s. Encouraged by the success of MELS, a number of similar multicomponent prevention programs were initiated in the United States, including the Fast Track program (CPPRG, 2002), Metropolitan Area Child Study (Metropolitan Area Child Study Research Group, 2002), and Early Alliance (Dumas, Prinz, Smith, & Laughlin, 1999). Like the MELS, each of these programs was designed to promote the school readiness of aggressive–disruptive children by providing coordinated prevention services in the school and home. In Québec, following the publication of these promising results and in response to requests from the educational community, the conceptors of the MELS asked the Centre de Psychoéducation du Québec (CPEQ), a nonprofit organization, to adapt this multimodal program so that it could be implemented in kindergarten classrooms. The CPEQ works closely in partnership with research teams that want to disseminate promising programs. Adapting the MELS program required changing its content and its methods in a number of ways. For example, professionals in the school system rather than members of the research team became responsible for implementing the program in kindergarten classrooms. The number of sessions in each component also needed to be adjusted to accommodate the capacity of the schools to offer this type of preventive program to as many at-risk kindergarten students as possible. This is a common challenge for programs as they move from efficacy trials to dissemination (Durlak & DuPree, 2008; Dusenbury, Brannigan, Hansen, Walsh, & Falco, 2005; Elias, Graczyk, & Weissberg, 2003). Efficacy trials often use one format, but dissemination requires a different (usually less intense) format. The adaptation of the MELS program thus led to the creation of the Fluppy program (Fluppy is the name of a puppet, the character used in many program activities). The Fluppy program maintained many of the same goals as the MELS program. Both are targeted prevention programs for children who display disruptive behavior problems. Both programs are multimodal and include the same three components: (1) social skills and problem-solving training; (2) home visits; and (3) support for teachers.

The Fluppy program, however, integrated new elements and hence diverged from the MELS program in several ways. First, in the Fluppy program, the social skills and problem-solving training component is universal. Thus, all children in the at-risk child's classroom are exposed to this intervention. The goal of this whole-class administration is to promote positive changes in peer norms, so that the classroom peer group supports and promotes the target skills (see Vitaro & Tremblay, 2008). Second, unlike the MELS program, the Fluppy program is offered to both boys and girls. Third, the procedure for screening at-risk children was changed. In the MELS, boys were screened with a questionnaire completed by the kindergarten teacher. In the Fluppy program, screening is based on both teachers' and parents' assessments. There is empirical evidence showing that cross-setting consistency in child behavior problems is associated with elevated levels of adjustment problems during adolescence and beyond (Dishion, 2000). Moroever, it was thought that selecting children who were considered disruptive by their parents would facilitate parent engagement in the prevention program. Fourth, the MELS and the Fluppy programs differ in terms of the length of the intervention components provided to children and their families. The MELS program provided the boys and their families with interventions over a 2-year period while the Fluppy program offers interventions for 1 year only (i.e., kindergarten). The decision to shorten the program to 1 year was made solely on the basis of available resources in the education and health systems when the Fluppy program was created in 1990. Finally, in the MELS program, the family component was based on social learning theory (Patterson, 2002) whereas, in the Fluppy program, it is based equally on attachment theory and social learning (DeKlyen & Speltz, 2001). Similarly to MELS interventionists, Fluppy interventionists use principles from social learning theory in order to support the parents in modifying the child's disruptive behavior. However, in the Fluppy program parent–child play sessions were added with the aim of strengthening the parent–child relationship, promoting shared positive moments, and teaching the child nondisruptive ways to get parents' attention. Interventionists use principles from both social learning and attachment theory to organize these play sessions.

Since the Fluppy program was created in 1990, the CPEQ has successfully promoted its dissemination across Québec. The CPEQ requires that teachers and professionals who wish to implement the program participate in training and undergo supervision when administering the program. These requirements were established to ensure that the professionals who administer the program respect its philosophy and provide the recommended conditions for its implementation. Maintaning high fidelity in implementation quality is a critical challenge as programs move from efficacy trials to dissemination, and this CPEQ requirement was designed to safeguard implementation quality. In the early 2000s, the Fluppy program was recognized as a promising prevention program by the National Institute of Public Health (2003). As a result of this recognition, several health and social service agencies across Québec supported the establishment of the Fluppy program in their areas. A number of alliances were forged between the education and health and social services networks in order to administer the Fluppy program in accordance with the conditions set out by the CPEQ. Under most agencies that implemented the original three-component version of the Fluppy program, trained professionals were responsible for administering the family component, whereas teachers were mainly responsible for the classroom component.

A survey conducted across Québec by Capuano, Poulin, Vitaro, Verlaan, and Vinet (2010) revealed that, between 1990 and 2007, more than 2,725 teachers and professionals from all the 17 administrative regions of Québec were trained by the CPEQ to use the Fluppy program. Of these, 925 were surveyed in 2001 concerning implementation of the program in their area. Almost all the respondents reported that they had applied the universal social skills component in the classroom. Moreover, 84% had implemented at least half of the sessions prescribed by the program. Based on very conservative estimates, at least 200,000 kindergarten students have been exposed to the universal component of the program since it was created.

Unfortunately, the implementation of the family component was less successful. Indeed, this component was offered in only 33% of the classes with at least one child who met the screening criteria. In addition, when this component was implemented, its intensity was drastically reduced compared to the MELS program and the 20 sessions recommended by Fluppy promoters: On average, the family component included eight home visits per family.

To sum up, as the Fluppy program made the transition from efficacy trial to dissemination, several changes were made. Some of these were planned, based on research (e.g., changing to a universal delivery of the social problem-solving skills curriculum) or on feasibility considerations (e.g., moving from a 2-year to a 1-year program length.) In addition, unplanned changes also occurred, as in many cases only the universal component was actually administered (and the indicated home visits were not implemented). In other cases, although all three program components were applied, the intensity of their application was significantly lower than originally recommended. Such changes are typical—hence, the challenges faced in Fluppy are very representative of those faced by other prevention programs as they move from efficacy trial to dissemination (Durlak & DuPree, 2008; Dusenbury et al., 2005; Elias et al., 2003). Therefore, it was deemed important to examine the actual effectiveness of the Fluppy program as it was currently being implemented in the field.

An Effectiveness Trial of the Fluppy Program

Depending on the context in which it is carried out, the evaluation of a prevention program can be aimed at demonstrating its efficacy or its effectiveness (Brown et al., 2008; Dodge, 2001). Efficacy is evaluated in a context where the methodological controls are optimal. The MELS is an example of an efficacy study. An evaluation of effectiveness, on the other hand, is conducted in the field and aimed more at determining the impact of an intervention as applied "in real life." Although the Fluppy program was widely disseminated in Québec by 2007, its effectiveness had yet to be evaluated.

Thus, in line with past research (Evans et al., 2001; Henry, Farrell, & the Multisite Violence Prevention Project, 2003), a partnership involving various stakeholders was formed to evaluate the effectiveness of the Fluppy program. This partnership brought together (1) a team of university researchers; (2) the program's disseminator (CEPQ); (3) a large school board in which many professionals had been trained to use Fluppy; (4) a health and social services center; and (5) a health and social services development agency.

The trial evaluated the effectiveness of two versions of the Fluppy program. The first version corresponded to the original three-component Fluppy program disseminated across Québec since 1990. Its three components were universal social skills and problem-solving training, teacher support, and family intervention. The second version included two new components added to strengthen the impact of the Fluppy program based on recent research on school readiness and the role of peers in young children's lives (Boivin et al., 2005; Ladd & Dinella, 2009). These two new components were friendship skills and preacademic skills. The trial also tested whether extending the program by 1 year, that is, allowing the children to be exposed to the interventions in kindergarten with booster sessions in grade 1, would improve its effectiveness. The research design is illustrated in Figure 13.1. It was hypothesized that children exposed to either of the two kindergarten versions of the Fluppy program (e.g., three-component or five-component) would show fewer disruptive behaviors (in school and at home) than children in a comparison condition that included only the universal program component. It was also hypothesized that children exposed to the five-component version would show better preacademic skills (by the end of the kindergarten year) and better academic skills (by the end of grade 1) than children in the comparison condition. Finally, it was hypothesized that the addition of booster sessions in grade 1 would be more effective in terms of its impact on the various outcomes than the kindergarten intervention alone.

Participants

Recruitment of a sufficient number of participants spanned 3 consecutive years and involved over 40 schools in a large urban school board. The following steps and criteria were used to screen and recruit students who displayed a high level of disruptive behavior problems. At the beginning of October, the teachers were asked to complete a screening questionnaire for each student in their class. The questionnaire contained 18 items associated with oppositional defiant disorder, conduct disorder, attention-deficit/hyperactivity disorder, and indirect aggression

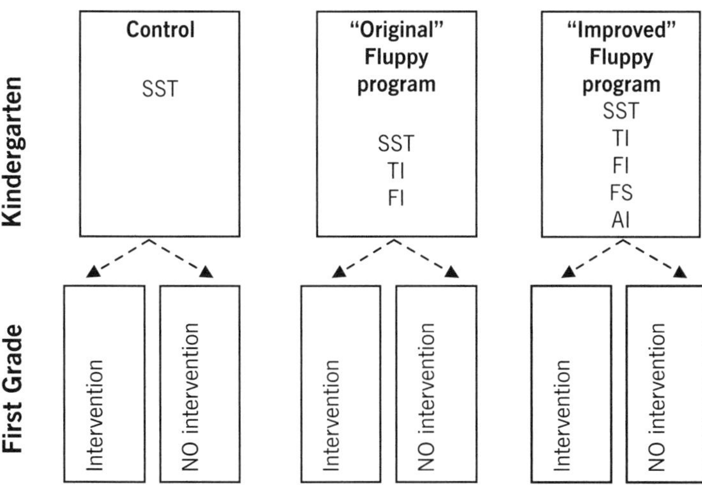

FIGURE 13.1. Design of the effectiveness study. *Note.* SST, social skills training; TI, teacher intervention; FI, family intervention; FS, friendship skills; AI, academic intervention.

(DSM-IV, American Psychiatric Association, 1994; Bjorkvist, Lagerspetz, & Kaukiainen, 1992). The same questionnaire was sent to the parents of each student. Students whose total score on the scale was above the 65th percentile both in class (based on teacher ratings) and at home (based on parent ratings) were identified as being at risk. The majority (90%) of the parents agreed to have their children screened. Almost 4,000 students (n = 3,774) were screened in kindergarten over a 3-year period.

The final sample included 320 at-risk children (69% boys; mean age = 64.98 months; SD = 3.73). With respect to family structure, 71% of these children lived with both biological parents. The average family income was CDN$ 51,200, and 20% of the mothers had received social welfare in recent years. On average, the mothers had completed 14.63 years (SD = 4.10) of schooling and the fathers 15.05 years (SD = 3.68). Most children (95%) were born in Canada and for 94% of them, French was the main language spoken at home.

Research Design and Procedures

The design included three groups to which the targeted children were randomly assigned: (1) the original three-component program; (2) the five-component program, and (3) a comparison group (see Figure 13.1). The children assigned to the comparison group were exposed only to the universal component (social skills and problem-solving training) and received no targeted intervention. A true control group without any intervention could not be used, because implementation data revealed that families assigned to a true control group reported seeking more unplanned professional help both inside and outside school than families in the intervention groups, confounding the evaluation of the school-based prevention services. The evaluation design also provided the opportunity to assess the additional impact of a second year of "booster" intervention sessions in grade 1 compared to a 1-year intervention limited to kindergarten. To achieve this last goal, each group was randomly subdivided into "1 year only" and "2 year" subgroups, so as to test specifically the effect of the duration of the three groups (see Figure 13.1).

Description of Intervention Components

The Fluppy program includes universal and selective components. The universal component takes place in the classroom and is intended for all students in the targeted child's kindergarten class. The selective components are aimed at students with high levels of disruptive behaviors. The detailed content of each component is presented in a manual. These components, as applied in the effectiveness trial, are described briefly below. The professionals responsible for carrying out the interventions in the context of this trial received training and supervision. A 2-day training was provided for the social skills and problem-solving intervention. Teachers also received a 4-day training for the academic intervention. Tearchers received support from the program conceptors thoughout its implementation: Group supervision sessions took place at least four times during the school year. The professionals who conducted the family intervention received a 2-day training, and ongoing supervision was offered by the program conceptors. All the interventions were implemented between November and April.

Social Skills and Problem-Solving Training

In kindergarten, this component was applied as a universal intervention for all children in the classroom. The full program included 15 sessions and aimed to develop social skills, problem-solving skills, and emotion-management skills. However, due to budget constraints of the Québec Educational and Health Services, which was administering the program, a reduced version of nine sessions was used in all classrooms for this trial. Once skills were introduced in a classroom lesson, the teacher provided positive reinforcement for spontaneous use of these skills in naturalistic conflict situations. These kindergarten sessions were co-led by the classroom teacher and a trained therapist.

Teacher Intervention

The program promoters provided the teachers with support in the following areas: (1) teaching social and problem-solving skills; (2) using natural classroom situations to create learning contexts; and (3) developing intervention strategies for students who had problems establishing positive interactions with their peers. The support was specifically provided by the professionals assigned to each classroom, who co-led the classroom sessions. The teacher intervention was not implemented in grade 1.

Family Intervention

This component was designed to include 20 structured sessions in the home, each lasting an average of 90 minutes. These sessions were led by the same therapist who also delivered the classroom social skills component and supported the teacher in positive classroom management. The family intervention aimed specifically at decreasing the level of parents' self-reported stress, changing parental practices associated with the children's behavior problems, reinforcing parental practices associated with the children's positive behaviors, promoting the development of positive parent–child relations, and encouraging the establishment of positive links between the families and the school. Although originally designed to include 20 home visiting sessions in kindergarten, budgetary constraints led to a reduction in the number planned for this effectiveness trial, with a maximum of six sessions in kindergarten.

Friendship Skills

The aim of this component was to foster the formation of positive friendships between at-risk students and their prosocial classmates. The targeted child was paired with a classmate in the context of a series of ten 30-minute dyadic play sessions or handicraft activities under the supervision of a therapist (content drew on Bierman's peer pairing program; 1992).

Academic Intervention

Two academic interventions were implemented. The language intervention provided teacher training and support for the implementation of a systematic phonics teaching program (Kame'enui et al., 2002; adapted by Brodeur, Godard, Vanier, Lapierre, & Messier., 2002). The full program involved 78 lessons, each approximately 30 minutes long, containing a detailed procedure for modeling the names and sounds of letters, as well as letter play and games aimed at developing metaphonological skills. The math intervention was structured around two main themes: (1) numbers (numerical activities); and (2) geometry and measuring. Two types of activities–sequences and capsules–were used in reference to each of the themes (Giroux & St. Marie, 2002). However, the implementation of the full academic program in kindergarten met with resistance from kindergarten education specialists at the schools. After discussion, it was agreed that approximately on- third of the content would be implemented.

Grade 1 Booster Sessions

The Grade 1 booster sessions included small-group sessions held at school for the targeted children and home visit sessions with their parents. There were eight small-group sessions held at school, with groups containing one targeted child and three classmates considered to have good social skills. These grade 1 sessions were administered by a trained therapist, and included content that integrated social skills and problem-solving skills training (parallel to the kindergarten classroom component) with friendship-boosting activities (parallel to the kindergarten dyadic friendship sessions). The same therapist also made home visits, extending the parenting intervention initiated in kindergarten. Eight home visits were planned in grade 1. In addition, in grade 1, on the basis of individual assessments, children who experienced ongoing significant difficulties in reading, writing, or math received academic intervention, delivered by a professional outside the classroom and adapted to the children's specific needs.

Measures

Outcome data were collected before (October of kindergarten) and immediately after the first (May of kindergarten) and second (May of grade 1) year of intervention. Individual testing of the child was conducted at school by trained research assistants. Questionnaires were filled out by teachers and parents.

Individual Testing in French (Kindergarten and Grade 1)

Knowledge of the names of the letters of the alphabet was evaluated using a rapid naming test. The students were asked, within the space of 1 minute, to name as many letters as they could from a list of upper- and lowercase letters presented in random order. A comprehensive assessment of students' knowledge of the letters was also carried out (Brodeur, 2005). Measures of the students' metaphonological ability (Robertson & Salter, 1997), ability to decode words and pseudowords, and reading comprehension (Cormier, Desrochers, & Sénéchal, 2004) were also taken.

Individual Testing in Math (Kindergarten and Grade 1)

This evaluation involved two main categories of tasks. Two of the four tasks in the first category were drawn from the Lollipop Test (Chew & Morris, 1984). The first task, tested using a 4-item measure, involved identifying the cardinality of a set. The second task, tested using a 7-item measure, involved reading numbers. The third task involved comparing numbers: The student was asked to choose the highest number out of two or three numbers. The fourth task involved comparing sets. The second category pertained to numerical problem solving, and was tested using a 2-item measure. For analytical purposes, a global score was calculated by adding up the scores obtained for each of these tasks.

Disruptive Behavior (Kindergarten and Grade 1)

In kindergarten and grade 1, mothers and teachers rated the children's *disruptive behaviors* over the previous month using 35 items from the Social

Behavior Questionnaire (Tremblay et al., 1992). These items covered different aspects of disruptive behaviors in young children: aggression (e.g., gets into fights), opposition (e.g., rebellious, disobedient), hyperactivity (e.g., can't stay still, hyperactive), and inattention (e.g., is easily distracted, can't focus). Ratings for each item ranged from 1 (*does not apply*) to 6 (*applies often*). For each child, individual item scores were added up to compute scale scores. Internal consistency for the disruptive behavior scale was acceptable (Cronbach's alpha = 0.95 at pretest for teachers and 0.94 for mothers).

Academic Readiness (Kindergarten)

Children's *academic readiness* in kindergarten was assessed using the Language and Cognitive Development subscale from the Early Development Instrument (EDI; Janus & Offord, 2007), a multidimensional questionnaire completed by the teacher. In addition to cognitive and language development, it assesses several other aspects of child development (physical health, social competence, emotional maturity, communication skills, and general knowledge). The Language and Cognitive Development subscale was used because it has been shown to predict reliably academic achievement in grade 1 (Forget-Dubois et al., 2007). Its predictive value is comparable to the predictive value of standardized school readiness tests such as the Lollipop Test (Chew & Morris, 1984) and the Peabody Picture Vocabulary Test (Dunn & Dunn, 1997). The Language and Cognitive Development subscale comprises 4 subdomains: basic numeracy skills, basic literacy skills, advanced literacy skills, and memory. The items in the EDI are rated on different scales. Some items are rated as yes–no while others are rated using 3- or 5-point Likert scales. Using this approach, the items from the four subscales were combined into an overall language and cognitive development score (alpha = 0.88).

Academic Achievement in Grade 1

End-of-year school results in reading, writing, and math were collected from students' report cards. Letter-based grades were translated into numbers (A = 4; B = 3; C = 2; D = 1). A mean score was computed (alpha = 0.91).

Findings Regarding Program Implementation

Checklists completed by teachers and therapists indicated that, in kindergarten, the children were exposed to an average of 8.74 social skills sessions (out of nine planned sessions). The average number of home visits was 4.40 (out of six planned visits); 10% of the invited families did not participate (or participated to a very limited extent) in the family intervention component. As for the friendship skills component, the children participated in an average of 9.16 sessions (out of 10 planned sessions); 2% of students did not participate in any sessions at all. Last, with regard to the academic intervention component, just under one-third of the participants benefited from almost the entire program as planned (reduced version of the program), whereas almost all the other children were exposed to at least half of the program content because teachers only taught part of the program.

In grade 1, the students participated, on average, in 6.20 social skills and friendship skills sessions (out of eight planned sessions), while 17% did not take part in these sessions at all. The families received, on average, 4.04 home visits (out of the planned six to eight visits), while 34% did not receive a single visit. Last, with regard to the academic intervention component, 84% of the students concerned underwent a preacademic screening test resulting in a recommendation for individual follow-up in 30% of cases, with these children subsequently receiving, on average, 250 minutes of intervention in math and 673 minutes of intervention in French. This test and the follow-up recommendation were part of the Fluppy preacademic component.

Impact of the Program on Disruptive Behaviors and School Readiness

The impact analyses were carried out in two steps. The first set of analyses examined the effects of the program at the end of kindergarten. A 3 (groups) × 2 (child's gender) factorial design was used. The second set of analyses examined the effects of the program at the end of grade 1. A 3 (groups) × 2 (duration; 1 year vs. 2 years) × 2 (child's gender) factorial design was used. Covariance analyses were conducted on the posttest scores, using the pretest scores as a covariable.

Program Impact after 1 Year of Intervention (End of Kindergarten)

Posttest adjusted means (and standard errors) for each of the dependent variables at the end of kindergarten are presented in Table 13.1. With regard to academic skills, a main effect of the groups was observed in the test evaluating knowledge of the names and sounds of letters, $F(2,187) = 7.43$, $p < .001$; the spelling test, $F(2,187) = 3.66$, $p < .05$; and the school readiness measure completed by the teacher, $F(2,183) = 4.84$, $p < .01$. In all cases, the children in the five-component group (which included the academic intervention component) performed better than the children in the one-component comparison group (i.e., the universal component). No significant effect was observed, however, in the word reading or math tests.

With regard to disruptive behaviors, analyses revealed an interaction effect between the groups and the child's gender. This interaction effect was found for both teacher ratings, $F(2,190) = 3.21$, $p < .05$; and parent ratings, $F(2,176) = 3.27$, $p < .05$. An examination of this effect showed that the girls in both three- and five-component groups presented fewer disruptive behavior problems at posttest than the girls in the control group.

Program Impact after 2 Years of Intervention (End of Grade 1)

Posttest adjusted means (and standard errors) for each of the dependent variables at the end of grade 1 are presented in the lower half of Table 13.1. An interaction effect between the groups and the child's gender was observed, $F(2,151) = 4.55$, $p < .01$, in the test evaluating knowledge of the names and sounds of letters. An examination of this interaction effect revealed that the girls in the five-component group performed better than the girls in the control group. A similar interaction effect was observed in the test evaluating the ability to read numbers. An examination of this interaction effect also revealed that the girls in the five-component group performed better than the girls in the control group. Last, an interaction effect between groups and gender was also observed for academic achievement, $F(2,139) = 5.98$, $p < .005$. The girls in both the five-component and three-component groups performed better than the girls in the control group.

With regard to disruptive behavior, the findings differed according to the source of the assessment (i.e., parents or teachers). Analyses revealed an interaction effect between the groups and the duration of the intervention, $F(2,170) = 4.84$, $p < .01$, in the parents' report. Among the children who were exposed to 2 years of intervention, those in the three- and five-component groups presented fewer disruptive behaviors at the end of grade 1 than those in the control group. In contrast, parent reports showed no intervention effects at the end of grade 1 for children who received intervention in kindergarten only. With regard to teacher report, analyses revealed an interaction effect between the groups and the child's gender, $F(2,184) = 2.85$, $p < .06$. An examination of this interaction effect revealed that the girls in both the three- and five-component groups presented fewer disruptive behavior problems at the end of grade 1 than the girls in the control group, regardless of the duration of the intervention.

TABLE 13.1. Posttest Adjusted Means (and Standard Errors) at the End of Kindergarten and Grade 1 for Each Outcome Variable by Experimental Condition and Gender

	One-component comparison condition		Original three-component condition		New five-component condition	
	Girls	Boys	Girls	Boys	Girls	Boys
Kindergarten						
Names and sounds of letters	4.14 (5.11)	4.22 (2.99)	4.18 (4.07)	4.10 (3.25)	5.82 (4.78)	5.13 (2.88)
Reading of words	0.50 (0.22)	0.27 (0.13)	0.44 (0.17)	0.30 (0.14)	0.77 (0.21)	0.36 (0.12)
Spelling	0.33 (0.22)	0.23 (0.13)	0.50 (0.17)	0.14 (0.14)	0.96 (0.20)	0.44 (0.12)
Math	2.00 (0.67)	1.99 (0.38)	2.04 (0.51)	2.02 (0.41)	2.15 (0.62)	1.98 (0.36)
Academic readiness (teacher)	1.99 (0.08)	2.06 (0.04)	2.14 (0.06)	2.11(0.05)	2.29 (0.07)	2.15 (0.04)
Disruptive behavior (parents)	2.87 (0.14)	2.66 (0.08)	2.29 (0.12)	2.64 (0.09)	2.54 (0.12)	2.63 (0.08)
Disruptive behavior (teacher)	3.06 (0.16)	2.76 (0.09)	2.63 (0.12)	2.85 (0.10)	2.56 (0.14)	2.85 (0.09)
Grade 1						
Names and sounds of letters	8.63 (3.11)	9.61 (1.92)	8.85 (2.53)	9.40 (2.04)	9.71 (2.99)	9.22 (1.77)
Math	22.17 (0.86)	23.30 (0.51)	23.68 (0.66)	22.90 (0.54)	25.41 (0.78)	23.23 (0.47)
Academic achievement	2.47 (0.18)	2.84 (0.11)	3.12 (0.16)	2.93 (0.12)	3.17 (0.16)	2.54 (0.11)
Disruptive behavior (parents)	2.80 (0.14)	2.66 (0.08)	2.48 (0.12)	2.59 (0.09)	2.49 (0.12)	2.72 (0.08)
Disruptive behavior (teacher)	2.49 (0.22)	2.87 (0.12)	2.67 (0.17)	2.68 (0.13)	1.98 (0.19)	2.72 (0.11)

CONCLUSIONS AND RECOMMENDATIONS

The Fluppy program has been implemented across Québec over the last 20 years in an effort to promote school readiness and to prevent violence and other negative outcomes among at-risk kindergartners. In this chapter, we have described the large-scale dissemination of the Fluppy program in Québec, documented the implementation of the program in an effectiveness trial, and reported the findings of this trial with regard to academic and sociobehavioral dimensions of school readiness. Each of these issues is discussed below. Finally, some issues related to the partnership that was established with practitioners are discussed, followed by recommendations concerning the dissemination of programs aimed at promoting school readiness among at-risk kindergartners.

Large-Scale Dissemination of the Fluppy Program

During the years of dissemination following the initial efficacy trial, the way the Fluppy program was administered across Québec varied widely (Capuano et al., 2010). In some schools, the program was implemented in its full form, as recommended by the CPEQ, whereas in other schools, it was implemented in reduced form. In many schools, only the universal component of the program was implemented; alternatively, all the components were implemented, but the number of class sessions or home visits were substantially reduced. This kind of program reduction occurs frequently during the dissemination process (Durlak & DuPree, 2008); Dusenbury et al., 2005; Elias et al., 2003). A number of factors likely contributed to these program modifications: (1) managerial weaknesses, including a lack of recognition and support on the part of managers with regard to the implementation of the program; (2) organizational deficits, including a lack of effective prioritization and a lack of structure with regard to the implementation of the program; (3) personnel weaknesses, such as a lack of supervision of the practitioners who implemented the program; and (4) a lack of human and financial resources.

Fluppy Program Effectiveness Trial

Implementation Issues

The analysis of the implementation of the Fluppy program in the context of our effectiveness trial highlighted several important elements. First, in terms of the number of intervention sessions given for each of the program's components, it became evident that in the schools involved in our trial the program was being implemented less intensively than originally recommended by the team that designed the program. When this effectiveness trial began, the research team urged the schools to increase the intensity of the program's application, in particular, that of the family intervention. However, since the available financial resources were limited, a compromise had to be accepted and an adjustment made in accordance with the on-the-ground reality of the school context.

Second, the implementation of the new academic intervention component presented a number of challenges. Due to resistance on the part of practitioners in the schools, the content of this component had to be cut in half. Among teachers at the kindergarten level, philosophies varied widely regarding preferred pedagogical approaches and learning goals. Some teachers believed that kindergarten should strive to achieve social rather than academic goals. However, given the academic difficulties for which children with disruptive behavior are at risk throughout primary school and beyond, it appears appropriate to give these children a small head start in kindergarten by adjusting the pedagogical approach and providing support for academic learning. Indeed, it should be noted that after the intervention trial was completed, most of the kindergarten teachers were in favor of implementing the entire academic component of the Fluppy program the following year.

Third, the findings regarding program implementation were enlightening with regard to the intensity at which the interventions were actually provided by the schools to children and their families. Thus, it was revealed that the universal component and the component that aimed at fostering the formation of positive friendships were implemented at the recommended intensity. However, it was observed that the academic intervention component was implemented less evenly. Moreover, some families (10%) were not exposed to the family component at all, while 33% of families were only partially exposed to it. This means that 43% of families benefited very little from the family component. This finding is significant, since these families had acknowledged during the screening stage that they were experiencing difficulties with their child at home.

Last, the interventions–in particular the family component–were implemented less successfully in grade 1 than in kindergarten. Several factors could have contributed to this decline. Some families may have decided that a second year of intervention was no longer necessary. In some cases, professionals from outside the Fluppy program were also intervening with the families. Moreover, the family component was not administered by the same practitioner in grade 1 as in kindergarten, and this may have affected the desire of some families to pursue this component. More extensive analyses are needed to determine whether the families who dropped out of this component shared common characteristics (Charlebois, Vitaro, Normandeau, & Rondeau, 2001).

Impact on School Readiness and Early Learning

Overall, the short-term results of the Fluppy program revealed that the interventions had beneficial effects, in particular for the girls. More specifically, as reported by both teachers and parents, the girls who were exposed to either the three-component or the five-component version of the program presented fewer disruptive behaviors than the girls who were only exposed to the universal component. The grade 1 teachers also reported that the girls presented fewer disruptive behaviors at the end of grade 1 whether they had been exposed to 1 or 2 years of intervention. Academically, both the boys and the girls who had been exposed to the five-component version of the program performed better on tests in French and were graded higher by their teachers in terms of academic prerequisites than the children in the comparison group. Last, at the end of grade 1, the girls in both the three- and five-component groups showed higher academic achievement (report card) than the girls in the comparison group.

On the whole, the girls appear to have responded to this prevention program better than the boys. This finding is important, especially in light of the fact that the development path of girls who present disruptive behavior problems is characterized by conflictual relationships, lack of self-esteem, teenage pregnancy, and internalized problems (Fontaine, Carbonneau, Vitaro, Barker, & Tremblay, 2009), and that girls generally benefit from social services later than boys (Conseil Supérieur de l'Éducation, 2001). This finding, in favor of girls, might be explained by the fact that the parents of aggressive girls reported being more at a loss as to how to deal with their child's aggressiveness than the parents of aggressive boys. It is thus possible that the parents of aggressive girls invested more in this prevention program than the parents of aggressive boys. It is also possible that the activities offered by the program were more appropriate for the learning style of girls than for that of boys. Finally, it is possible that girls respond more quickly to positive expectations from their social environment than boys, meaning that longer interventions may be required for boys. A more in-depth examination of the implementation data is needed to explore further the validity of these possible explanations.

The Importance of Collaboration between Researchers and Practitioners

This chapter also illustrates the importance of close collaboration between university researchers and practitioners in the design, implementation, and evaluation of prevention trials. The establishment of such partnerships has been at the heart of the development of the Fluppy program since its inception. The current evaluation research study provides a good illustration of the benefits of such a partnership. A broad evaluation of research study involving a variety of partners with different approaches is neither easy nor economical. It requires rigor and transparency from the outset and throughout the process. It also requires a significant amount of cooperation and respect among the partners. However, the advantages and consequences of such an approach go well beyond the investments and efforts made by each partner.

The application of this partnership-based experimental research design was in itself an important achievement. First, few intervention programs have been subject to effectiveness trials. However, such trials are absolutely essential in order to evaluate the effectiveness of interventions and guide practitioners and decision-makers. As described by Flay and colleagues (Flay et al., 2005), effectiveness trials are more demanding than efficacy trials in terms of methodological rigor; such high standards can only be achieved if researchers and practitioners share a common view of the evaluation process. The current effectiveness trial of the Fluppy program could act as a lever for improving and guiding not only the practices but also the methodological training of teachers and professionals who work with children from the early years of schooling, and whose mandate involves preparing these children to meet the many social and academic challenges they will face throughout their years at school and to assess whether their goals are acheived. Second, applying this rigorous research design in conjunction with practitioners allowed the research team to address research questions related to the challenges posed by implementing exemplary or promising practices in the real school context, with the human and financial resources that are actually available. As argued by Brown Urban and Trochim (2009), the evaluation process may be the key ingredient in linking research and practice. As in the case of other effectiveness trilas (e.g., Fagan & Mihalic, 2003), close monitoring and ongoing efforts to work with schools to identify and overcome problems proved useful in the current context to maximixe the implementation of the multi condition and multicomponent Fluppy trial, and facilitate the multisource assessment of its possible outcomes.

Effectiveness studies are essential at this stage of knowledge development (1) to ensure that children have access to the most effective intervention strategies, implemented rigorously by qualified and supervised practitioners, and (2) to determine whether the intervention strategies being applied will collectively decrease the number of children who present behavior problems along their path through school and improve their graduation rate. A recursive feedback loop system integrating empirical evidence, theoretical constructs, needs and resources from different stakeholders (e.g., funders, practitioners, researchers), and methodological rigor in elaborating, implementing, evaluating, and disseminating the progressive knowledge that is acquired through these trials is required to systematize the process and hopefully increase its effectiveness (Wanderman et al., 2008).

REFERENCES

American Psychiatric Association. (1994). *Diagnostic and statistical manual of mental disorders* (4th ed.). Washington, DC: Author.

Bierman, K. L. (1992). *FAST Track: Manual for peer pairing.* Unpublished manuscript, Pennsylvania State University, University Park.

Bierman, K. L. (2004). *Peer rejection: Developmental processes and interventions strategies.* New York: Guilford Press.

Birsch, S. H., & Ladd, G. W. (1997). The teacher–child relationship and children's early school adjustment. *Journal of School Psychology, 33*, 61–79.

Bjorkqvist, K., Lagerspetz, K. M. J., & Kaukiainen, A. (1992). Do girls manipulate and boys fight?: Developmental trends in regard to direct and indirect aggression. *Aggressive Behavior, 18*, 117–127.

Boisjoli, R., Vitaro, F., Lacourse, E., Barker, E. D., & Tremblay, R. E. (2007). Impact and clinical signifiance of a preventive intervention for disruptive boys: 15 year follow-up. *British Journal of Psychiatry, 191*, 415–419.

Boivin, M., Vitaro, F., & Poulin, F. (2005). Peer relationships and the development of aggressive behavior. In R. E. Tremblay, W. W. Hartup, & J. Archer (Eds.), *Developmental origins of aggression* (pp. 376–397). New York: Guilford Press.

Brendgen, M., Wanner, B., & Vitaro, F. (2006). Verbal abuse by the teacher and child adjustment from kindergarten through Grade 6. *Pediatrics, 117*(5), 1585–1598.

Brodeur, M. (2005). *Évaluation de la connaissance du nom et du son des lettres* [Assessment of the name and sound of letters]. Montréal: University of Quebec at Montreal.

Brodeur, M., Godard, L., Vanier, N., Lapierre, M., & Messier, J. (2002). *French translation of The OPTIMIZE Intervention Program.* Unedited manuscript, University of Quebec at Montreal.

Brown, C. H., Wang, W., Kellam, S. G., Muthen, B. O., Petras, H., Toyinbo, P., et al. (2008). Methods for testing theory and evaluating impact in randomized field trials: Intent-to-treat analyses for integrating the perspectives of person, place, and time. *Drug and Alcohol Dependance, 95*, 74–104.

Brown Urban, J., & Trochim, W. (2009). The role of evaluation in research-practice integration: Working toward the "Golden Spike." *American Journal of Evaluation, 30*, 538–553.

Capuano, F., Poulin, F., Vitaro, F., Verlaan, P., & Vinet, I. (2010). Le programme de prévention Fluppy: Historique, contenu et diffusion au Québec [The Fluppy prevention program: History and dissemination in Quebec]. *Revue de Psychoéducation, 39*, 1–26.

Charlebois, P., Vitaro, F., Normandeau, S., & Rondeau, N. (2001). Predictors of persistence in a longitudinal preventive intervention program for young disruptive boys. *Prevention Science, 2*, 133–143.

Chew, A., & Morris, J. D. (1984). Validation of the Lollipop Test: A diagnostic screening test of school readiness. *Educational and Psychological Measurement, 44*, 987–991.

Conduct Problems Prevention Research Group. (1992). A developmental and clinical model for the prevention of conduct disorders: The Fast Track Program. *Development and Psychopathology, 4*, 509–527.

Conduct Problems Prevention Research Group (CPPRG). (2002). Evaluation of the first 3 years of the Fast Track prevention trial with children at high risk for adolescent conduct problems. *Journal of Abnormal Child Psychology, 30*, 19–35.

Conseil Supérieur de l'Éducation. (2001). *Les élèves en difficulté de comportement à l'école primaire: Comprendre, prévenir, intervenir.* [Students with behavior problems in elemntary school: Understanding, preventing, intervening]. Avis au ministère de l'éducation. Québec, Canada: Ministère de l'Education.

Cormier, P., Desrochers, A., & Sénéchal, M. (2004). *L'élaboration d'une batterie de tests en français pour l'évaluation des compétences en lecture* [The development of a series of tests in French for assessment of readings]. Unpublished manuscrtipt, Laboratory of Cognitive Psychology, University of Ottawa.

DeKlyen, M., & Speltz, M. L. (2001). Attachment and conduct disorder. In J. Hill & B. Maughan (Eds.), *Cambridge monographs in child and cdolescent psychiatry: Conduct disorders in childhood and adolescence* (pp. 320–345). Cambridge, UK: Cambridge University Press.

Dishion, T. J. (2000). Cross-setting consistency in early adolescent psychopathology: Deviant friendships and problem behavior sequelae. *Journal of Personality, 68*, 1109–1126.

Dodge, K. A. (2001). The science of youth prevention: Progressing from developmental epidemiology to efficacy to effectiveness to public policy. *American Journal of Preventive Medecine, 20*, 63–70.

Dodge, K. A. (2006). Translational science in action: Hostile attributional style and the development of aggressive behavior problems. *Development and Psychopathology 18*, 791–814.

Dodge, K. A., Coie, J. D., & Lynam, D. (2006). Aggression and antisocial behavior. In N. Eisenberg (Ed.), *Handbook of child psychology: Social, emotional, and personality development* (Vol. 3., pp. 719–788). New York: Wiley.

Dumas, J. E., Prinz, R. J., Smith, E. P., & Laughlin, J. (1999). The EARLY ALLIANCE prevention trial: An integrated set of interventions to promote competence and reduce risk for conduct disorder, substance abuse, and school failure. *Clinical Child and Family Psychology Review, 2*, 37–53.

Duncan, G. J., Claessens, A., Huston, A. C., Pagani, L. S., Engel, M., Sexton, H. R., et al. (2007). School readiness and later achievement. *Developmental Psychology, 43*, 1428–1446.

Dunn, L. M., & Dunn, L. M. (1997). *Peabody Picture Vocabulary Test.* Circle Pines, MN: American Guidance Service.

Durlak, J. A., & DuPree, E. P. (2008). Implementation matters: A review of research on the influence of implementation on program outcomes and the factors affecting implementation. *American Journal of Community Psychology, 41*, 327–350.

Dusenbury, L., Brannigan, R., Hansen, W. B., Walsh, J., & Falco, M. (2005). Quality of implementation: Developing measures crucial to understanding the diffusion of preventive interventions. *Health Education Research, 20*, 308–313.

Elias, M., Zins, J. E., Graczyk, P. A., & Weissberg, R. P. (2003). Implementation, sustainability and scaling-up of social-emotional and academic innovations in public schools. *School Psychology Review, 329*(3), 303–319.

Ensminger, M. E., & Slusarcick, A. L. (1992). Paths to high school graduation or dropout: A longitudinal study of a first-grade cohort. *Sociology of Education, 65*, 95–113.

Evans, G. D., Rey, J., Hemphill, M. M., Perkins, D. F., Austin, W., & Racine, P. (2001). Academic-community collaboration: An ecology for early childhood violence prevention. *American Journal of Preventive Medicine, 20*, 22, 30.

Fagan, A. A., & Mihalic, S. (2003). Strategies for enhancing the adoption of school-based prevention programs: Lessons learned from the Blueprints for Violence Prevention replications of the Life Skills Training Program. *Journal of Community Psychology, 31*, 235–254.

Flay, B. R., Biglan, A., Boruch, R. F., Castro, F. G., Gottfredson, D., Kellam, S., et al. (2005). Standards of evidence: Criteria for efficacy, effectiveness and dissemination. *Prevention Science, 6*, 151–175.

Fontaine, N., Carbonneau, R., Vitaro, F., Barker, E. D., & Tremblay, R. E. (2009). Research review : A critical review of studies on the developmental trajectories of antisocial behavior in females. *Journal of Child Psychology and Psychiatry, 50*(4), 363–385.

Forget-Dubois, N., Lemelin, J.-P., Boivin, M., Dionne, G., Séguin, J. R., Vitaro, F., et al. (2007). Predicting early school achievement with the EDI: A longitudinal population-based study. *Early Education and Development, 18*, 405–426.

Giroux, J., & St. Marie, A. (2002). *Volet mathématique: Projet Fluppy* [Math intervention. Fluppy program]. Unpublished manuscript, University of Quebec at Montreal.

Henry, D., Farrell, A. D., & the Multisite Violence Prevention Project. (2003). The study design by a committee: Design of the Multisite Violence Prevention Project. *American Journal of Preventive Medicine, 26*, 12–19.

Hill, J., & Maughan, B. (2001). *Cambridge Monographs in Child and Adolescent Psychiatry*. Cambridge, UK: Cambridge University Press.

Hinshaw, S. P. (1992). Externalizing behavior problems and academic underachievement in childhood and adolescence: Causal relationships and underlying mechanisms. *Psychological Bulletin, 111*, 127–155.

Janus, M., & Offord, D. R. (2007). Development and psychometric properties of the Early Development Instrument (EDI): A measure of children's school readiness. *Canadian Journal of Behavioral Science, 39*, 1–22.

Kame'enui, E. J., Simmons, D. C., Good, R., Harn, B., Chard, D., Coyne, M., et al. (2002). *Big ideas in beginning reading*. Retrieved from *http://reading.uoregon.edu/index.php*.

Ladd, G. W., & Dinella, L. M. (2009). Continuity and change in early school engagement: Predictive of children's achievement trajectories from first to eighth grade? *Journal of Educational Psychology, 101,* 190–206.

Lochman, J. E., Whidby, J. E., & FitzGerald, D. P. (2000). Cognitive-behavioral assessment and treatment with aggressive children. In P. C. Kendall (Ed.), *Child and adolescent therapy: Cognitive-behavioral procedures* (pp. 31–87). New York: Guilford Press.

Meehan, B. T., Hugues, J. N., & Cavell, T. A. (2003). Teacher–student relationships as compensatory resources for aggressive children. *Child Development, 74,* 1145–1157.

Metropolitan Area Child Study Research Group. (2002). A cognitive–ecological approach to preventing aggression in urban settings: Initial outcomes for high-risk children. *Journal of Consulting and Clinical Psychology, 70*(1), 179–194.

National Institute of Public Health. (2003). *Plan d'action ministériel de santé publique 2004–2007* [Minsiteral action plan of public health 2004–2007]. Author.

National Longitudinal Survey of Children and Youth (NLSCY). (1999). *Grandir au Canada: Enquête longitudinale nationale sur les enfants et les jeunes* [National Longitudinal Survey of Children and Youth]. Ottawa: Développement des Resources Humaines Canada. Statistique Canada.

Patterson, G. R., (2002). The early development of coercive family process. In J.B. Reid, G.R. Patterson, & J. Snyders (Eds.), *Antisocial behavior in children and adolescents: A developmental analysis and model for intervention* (pp. 25–44). Washington: American Psychological Association.

Patterson, G. R., Reid, J. B., & Dishion, T. J. (1992). *A social learning approach: IV. Antisocial boys.* Eugene, OR: Castalia.

Robertson, C., & Salter, W. (1997). *The Phonological Awareness Test.* East Moline, IL: LinguiSystems.

Snyder, J., Schrepferman, L., Oeser, J., Patterson, G., Stoolmiller, M., Johnson, K., et al. (2005). Deviancy training and association with deviant peers in young children: Occurrence and contribution to early-onset conduct problems. *Development and Psychopathology, 17,* 397–413.

Tremblay, R. E. (2004). Why socialization fails: The case of chronic physical aggression. In B. B. Lahey, T. E. Moffitt, & A. Caspi (Eds.), *Causes of conduct disorder and juvenile delinquency* (pp. 182–226). New York: Guilford Press.

Tremblay, R. E., Hartup, W. W., & Archer, J. (2005). *Developmental origins of aggression.* New York: Guilford Press.

Tremblay, R. E., Pagani-Kurtz, L., Masse, L., Vitaro, F., & Pihl, R. O. (1995). A bimodal preventive intervention for disruptive kindergarten boys: Its impact through mid adolescence. *Journal of Consulting and Clinical Psychology, 63,* 560–568.

Tremblay, R. E., Vitaro, F., Bertrand, L., LeBlanc, M., Beauchesne, H., Boileau, H., et al. (1992). Parent and child training to prevent early onset of delinquency: The Montréal longitudinal-experimental study. In J. McCord & R. E. Tremblay (Eds.), *Preventing deviant behavior from birth to adolescence: Experimental approaches* (pp. 117–138). New York: Guilford Press.

Tremblay, R. E., Vitaro, F., Gagnon, C., Piché, C., & Royer, N. (1992). A prosocial scale for the Preschool Behavior Questionnaire: Concurrent and predictive correlates. *International Journal of Behavioral Development, 15*, 227–245.

Véronneau, M.-H., Vitaro, F., Brendgen, M., Dishion, T. J., & Tremblay, R. E. (2010). Transactional analysis of the reciprocal links between peer experiences and academic achievement from middle childhood to early adolescence. *Developmental Psychology, 46*, 773–790.

Véronneau, M.-H., Vitaro, F., Pedersen, S., & Tremblay, R. E. (2008). Do peers contribute to the likelihood of secondary school graduation among disadvantaged boys? *Journal of Educational Psychology, 100*, 429–442.

Vitaro, F., Brendgen, M., Larose, S., & Tremblay, R. E. (2005). Kindergarten disruptive behaviors, protective factors, and educational achievement by early adulthood. *Journal of Educational Psychology, 97*(4), 617–629.

Vitaro, F., & Tremblay, R. E. (2008). Clarifying and maximizing the usefulness of targeted preventive interventions. In M. Rutter & J. Stevenson (Eds.), *Rutter's child and adolescent psychiatry* (5th ed., pp. 989–1008). Oxford, UK: Blackwell.

Wandersman, A., Duffy, J., Flaspohler, P., Noonan, R., Lubell, K., Stilman, L., et al. (2008). Bridging the gap between prevention research and practice: The interactive systems framework for dissemination and implementation. *American Journal of Community Psychology, 41*, 171–181.

CHAPTER 14

Informing Policy to Support Evidence-Based School Readiness Programs and Practices

Rob Santos

What will long bedevil the eminent editors and distinguished contributors to this book (present company excluded) is that most policymakers will never read this book. But the good news is that this book can (and should) inform and influence policy in order to improve school readiness. The goal of this chapter is to help in getting from here to there. This chapter summarizes the issues involved in using evidence-based research to inform policy. It describes the kind of research information needed by policymakers, suggests implications for policymakers based upon available school readiness research, and recommends future research directions to improve the translation of research to policy. To facilitate use, acronyms that relate to early childhood development (ECD) and other memory aids are suggested, as well as the need for scientists to practice the other ECD: "elevator conversation development." If you happened to share the proverbial elevator ride with a policymaker, what would you say about school readiness? It is important to recognize at the outset that values predominate public policy and politics. What matters to voters, by definition, will matter to politicians. Public opinion drives public priorities. Researchers need to keep these foremost in mind. Understanding the budget cycle, the public mood, political pressures, and fiscal realities is essential to influencing public policy. Detailed discussion of these areas is beyond the scope of this chapter (for further reading and excellent reviews in the Canadian provincial and federal context, see Blakeney & Borins, 1998; Savoie, 1999, 2003; for excellent reviews in an American context, see Radin, 2000, 2013; the classic by Wildavsky, 1979; for child development and U.S. policy, see Meyers & Wilcox, 1998; Zigler & Hall, 2000). "Scientists who expect to see their latest research findings transformed intact into public policy are likely to be disappointed. In contrast, scientists who adjust their expectations may be surprised to discover how powerful science can be" (Gormley, 2011, p. 981).

THE CURRENT CONTEXT: EVIDENCE MEETS POLITICS

Politically across North America, it has been a busy time of late. In Canada, 2011 was a year of elections: A federal election gave the Prime Minister his first majority government, as well as six provincial/territorial elections. In the United States, 2012 marked the reelection of the President, 33 Senate elections, elections for all 435 seats in the 113th Congress, as well as 13 state and territorial governors' races. The electorate has spoken—returning or giving sweeping powers to governments at national and local levels. These governments will have to act in the wake of global economic challenges and growing government deficits. It is a timely moment in history to consider how best to influence the decisions that our Premiers and Prime Minister, our Governors, Senators, Congressmen and Congresswomen, and President will make in the months and years ahead. For better or worse, these decisions will affect all of us, and our children most of all. It is also a timely moment, because we now have over 40 years of longitudinal evidence on the lifetime effects of early childhood intervention (Campbell et al., 2012; Schweinhart et al., 2005; Shonkoff, 2012), and over 40 years of hard-won lessons in bringing evaluation evidence to decision-makers (McCartney & Weiss, 2007; Radin, 2013).

Forty years or so ago also marked the debut of a short animated film that provides a useful analogy to keep in mind when speaking truth to power (Wildavsky, 1979), offering scientific evidence to policymakers and decision-makers. This film was brief and unforgettable. A young fawn (in retrospect reminiscent of emerging evidence on early childhood development) stands placidly grazing in the grass. Suddenly, he is completely crushed by an enormous, scaly reptilian foot. The End: roll credits. The title: *Bambi Meets Godzilla* (Newland, 1969). The late Morris Parloff (1982), a prominent and eminent psychologist at the U.S. National Institute of Mental Health, published a paper 30 years ago with this as its subtitle. The paper was about bringing psychotherapy research evidence to reimbursement decisions. He offered recommendations "prompted by the reluctantly accepted conclusion that currently available research findings . . . standing alone will be insufficient to the task. Research findings can be expected to exert all the impact of a quixotic Bambi planted firmly in the path of the onrushing Godzilla of cost-containment policies" (p. 725).

Bambi Meets Godzilla could easily be the subtitle to the present chapter. Decades later to the present day, politics continues to loom large in comparison to scientific evidence when it comes to influencing policy decisions. This reality raises some key questions for the readers of this book and to everyone who wants to improve the lives of our youngest children: How can we reduce the odds of the evidence being crushed by more powerful forces influencing policy? What evidence do policymakers want (if any)? This chapter offers a framework for informing policy to support evidence-based school readiness programs and practices. It draws on other chapters in this volume, the larger scientific literature, a decade and a half of experience in advising elected officials and senior bureaucrats in government, and learning directly from giants in the field like the late Fraser Mustard (see Packham, 2010) the late Dan Offord, and the late Clyde Hertzman, three eminent Canadian ECD scientists who battled their way in political corridors to promote an ECD agenda among policymakers. To illustrate key concepts, I draw from published evidence and personal experience from the province of Manitoba, and discuss the dissemination of a population-based measure of school readiness, the Early Development Instrument (EDI; Janus & Offord, 2007).

The worlds of science and policy have long been divided by a cultural gap (Shonkoff, 2000; see also Gormley, 2011), perhaps even akin to a cross-species gap (cf. *Bambi Meets Godzilla*). Bridging this gap requires cross-cultural tools: translators, tour guides, ambassadors, and their analogues in scientific and policy settings. Cultural appropriateness, sensitivity, and safety are no less important between and within the cultures of science and policy. And, as in most human efforts to improve the human condition, a recurrent message is the importance of the personal relationships between the people involved. In the end, this relationship may be all that matters.

Issues in Using Evidence to Inform Policy

Forty years ago, in a now-classic article, Carol Weiss (1973) argued that politics impinges on evaluation research and evidence in three ways: (1) through the political nature of the policies and programs that researchers study, (2) through the political nature of the decision-making arena wherein researchers report their findings, and (3) through the inherently political stance of the research enterprise itself. This view has held up remarkably well decades later, perhaps colored by greater optimism at the potential for evidence to influence policy (Weiss, 1993). Nonetheless, more recently, Weiss and colleagues have likened the desires of researchers to be heard by policy makers to wishing for a "Fairy Godmother who would make decision makers pay attention to evaluation findings when choosing programs to implement" (Weiss, Murphy-Graham, Petrosino, & Gandhi, 2008, p. 29). Politics is about influence—the fundamental power of persuasion (for recent Canadian examples in the federal government, see Geddes, 2012). There is an extensive and instructive empirical literature on this topic (e.g., Cialdini, 2009) that scientists wishing to influence policy need to understand and implement.

Policy can be defined as the "authoritative exposition of values . . . defining and pursuing the right course of action in a particular context, at a particular time, for a particular group of people and with a particular allocation of resources" (Greenhalgh & Russell, 2005, p. 35). It is essential for scientists to realize that policymaking involves *all* three forms of Aristotelian argumentation:

> . . . *analytic* (logical argument using premises based on certain knowledge), *dialectic* (debating moves to argue for and against a standpoint), and *rhetoric* (influencing by reference to laws, documents, etc., or by appeal to emotions, authority or previously acceded premises). Most modern-day scientists (including those in the evidence-based [policy] movement) hold that "rationality" is restricted to analytic argument. But for the ancient Greeks, all three dimensions of argumentation were seen as rational, and a respectable scholar was expected to achieve competence in all of them. (Greenhalgh & Russell, 2005, pp. 38–39)

This chapter makes the case for this foregoing "three-dimensional approach" to informing policy, as it can help explain why evidence is not always used ("If you build it, they still may not come"; Driedger et al., 2010, p. 1)) and why evidence in which policymakers request and invest is more likely to be used ("If they build it, they will come"; Martens & Roos, 2005, p. 74). Distilling the messages from research is becoming a specialized role for at least three reasons (Lomas, 2007): (1) enormous growth in research makes it impossible for fellow researchers, never mind practitioners, to keep up; (2) skills are required to sort the research wheat from the chaff before "making the 'summary loaf' from the best ingredients" (p. 16); and (3) countering "spin doctors of research" who do partial summaries that favor their own product or ideology, which requires impartial summaries of all the relevant research, favorable or not. Lomas (p. 16) asks: "Is summarizing research for use in [policy] a technical exercise reserved for skilled specialists in the research world? Or is it a social change exercise where the world of ideas learns to dance with the world of context and values?" This distinction between *knowledge support* (descriptive summarizing of evidence) and *decision support* (prescriptive synthesis of evidence for action) (Lomas, 2007; Mays, Pope, & Popay, 2005; Pope, Mays, & Popay, 2005) is also highly relevant to the issue at hand.

The literature on effective knowledge translation indicates that context matters, especially the characteristics of knowledge, providers, participants, and organizations (i.e., the different cultures, as noted earlier; LaRocca, Yost, Dobbins, Ciliska, & Butt, 2012). When there is a single clear message to convey in a context in which the policy or practice change is relatively simple to accomplish, and knowledge users are aware that a change is required, then simply mass-mailing a printed bulletin summarizing the results of a systematic review can improve evidence-based practice (Murthy et al., 2012). However, in the more common scenario in which more complex messages are required, identifying strategy effectiveness and recommending one strategy over another is a challenge; the evidence base for doing "evidence-based" knowledge translation needs much more work (Mitton, Adair, McKenzie, Patten, & Waye Perry, 2007; Scott et al., 2012). These challenges will grow, as knowledge translation is now beginning to include a wider range of participants, beyond researchers and policymakers, and to increase the valuing of experiential knowledge (Goldner et al., 2011). In the meantime, researchers must find their way in the social drama that is policymaking (Greenhalgh & Russell, 2005). Two mentors and colleagues from Manitoba, both with extensive experience in bringing research findings to governments, said it well:

> Sometimes the "tectonic plates" of researchers and decision-makers move slowly past each other with little noticeable change in the landscape for decades. Other times there is a great deal of friction, resulting in major tidal waves or volcanic eruptions on the policy scene, or in the relationships between these two groups (Martens & Roos, 2005, p. 73)
>
> It is debatable whether the relationship between researchers and policy makers has changed over time. It is even debatable if we can measure whether better relationships change the quality of decisions made.
>
> Easing the friction at the "tectonic plate" means ensuring research credibility within the real-world realm of policy making, and it is only through this frictional contact that we increase the probability that our evidence will be understood and will lead to policy action. (Martens & Roos, 2005, p. 83).

What Do They Need?: A Top-10 List for Informing Policy in ECD

In "speaking truth to power" (Wildavsky, 1979), it can be helpful to have heuristics. In this spirit, a "top-10 list" is discussed in this section. Using the abbreviation ECD, I list four E's, three C's, and three D's, for a total of 10.

What Evidence Do Policymakers Need?: The Four Elements

Policymakers need at least four types of evidence (four E's): epidemiology, explanation, evaluation/effectiveness, and expense/efficiency (an alternative mnemonic is the four P's of prevalence, predictors, policies/programs, and prices; Brownell, Kozyrskyj, Fuchs, & Santos, 2011). In providing for these four E's, meta-analytic evidence is especially useful, particularly for developmental and longitudinal research (van IJzendoorn, Bakermans-Kranenburg, & Alink, 2012). Researchers are generally familiar and comfortable with each of these areas, so they will not be elaborated here, apart from noting particular interests of policymakers in each.

Epidemiology

How widespread is the problem (internationally, nationally, and most importantly, locally)? Evidence on the prevalence and incidence of poor school readiness, particularly in vulnerable subgroups, is of major interest to policymakers. For example, a recent longitudinal, population-based study, commissioned by the Government of Manitoba's Healthy Child Committee of Cabinet, reported on the school readiness outcomes of three vulnerable subgroups: children in families on income assistance, children in the care of child protective services, and children born to mothers who were teenagers at their first childbirth (Santos, Brownell, Ekuma, Mayer, & Soodeen, 2012). The odds of these children being vulnerable was up to four times higher than the odds for children not in any of these subgroups, and the prevalence of vulnerability was considerably higher for children in one or more of these subgroups (33–54%), compared to children who were not (23%). The report contrasted these outcomes with those for a separate cohort, with longitudinal data to young adulthood (Brownell et al., 2010), wherein the odds of poor outcomes rapidly increased over time, indicating a pressing need for earlier intervention. The distribution of vulnerability by socioeconomic status (i.e., SES gradient) is important epidemiological information for policymakers, calling attention both to targeted groups that are in greater need and to the universality of need (Wade, Prime, Browne, & Jenkins, Chapter 4, and Peters & Howell-Moneta, Chapter 12, this volume), and to the need for proportionate universalism (Boivin & Hertzman, 2012a; Commission on the Social Determinants of Health, 2008), which specifies resource allocation proportionate to the level of needs.

Explanation

The independent (or explanatory) variables in our analyses are of great interest to policymakers. Accordingly, variables for which we have the strongest longitudinal or causal evidence are the ones most important to emphasize (see the "Determinants" section below). This is not to say that other independent variables are unimportant. For example, it matters to many Ministers and Secretaries whether outcomes differ for boys and girls, or for children in different ethnic groups. As researchers, we need to help policymakers distinguish between the different kinds of risk (and protective) factors that are commonly included but not always specified in school readiness research (e.g., fixed markers vs. causal factors; Kraemer et al., 1997).

Evaluation/Effectiveness

Perhaps the most common question asked by policymakers is "What works?" In providing relevant information, it is important to help policymakers distinguish between evidence of efficacy (finding that a program works under controlled laboratory conditions) and evidence of effectiveness (finding that a program works under real-world conditions of service delivery). The latter is most often assumed to be the case, when the former is in fact much more common. Because of this, it is important for researchers to encourage policymakers to include an evaluation component even for instances in which the policymaker has decided to invest in an evidence-based program. Not only are all early childhood interventions not equally efficacious (Barnett, 2011; Welsh, Bierman, & Mathis, Chapter 11, this volume), but efficacious programs are also sometimes not as effective under real-world service delivery conditions, especially when scaled up (Barnett, 2011). This important issue is revisited in the concluding section of this chapter.

Expense/Efficiency

Perhaps the second most common question asked by policymakers is "What will it cost?" This is an important opportunity for researchers to highlight cost-effectiveness (efficiency) data, estimated return on investment, and comparative data. where available. It is important for researchers to remind policy-makers that a program that "breaks even" (i.e., the monetary costs of the program are roughly equal to the monetary value of the benefits) is already a success, at least in financial terms, and more so when benefits exceed costs. The cost-effectiveness analyses of the Washington State Institute of Public Policy (Aos et al., 2011; Lee et al., 2012) are exemplary. They thoroughly review the literature, apply strong cost-effectiveness methodology, and summarize their findings in simple (but not simplistic) ways that are understandable to policymakers (e.g., easy-to-read tabular data, easy-to-use effect sizes, executive summaries). Still, it is also important to remind policymakers of the limitations of cost-effectiveness analyses (e.g., some important outcomes may not have been measured and are excluded from monetized benefits), especially when comparing the results of different programs.

What Do Policymakers Need from Scientists?: The Three Capabilities

To influence policymakers effectively, scientists need at least three capabilities (three C's): communication, collaboration, and credibility. It can be noted that these three C's are consistent with the factors that influence research use and their controllability as listed by Gormley (2011, Table 1): comprehensibility and framing (related to *communication*), trust (related to *collaboration*), and *credibility*. These factors operate in both political and scientific contexts (Gormley lists fragmentation, quality of legislative debate, economic conditions, and scholarly consensus). Because the focus of this chapter is on informing policymakers, I primarily discuss communication.

Communication

Personalize and localize the science! There is a considerable literature on how our brains process information, and on reasons why personal, emotional stories are so powerful in their influence on our thinking and decision making (Kahneman, 2011). Rather than dismissing stories outright as scientifically impoverished, researchers may do well by developing the art of telling the evidence-based anecdote, an approach itself based in the evidence about how our brains typically process information. The more personal and local the evidence, the more powerful, because it is literally closer to home, to the constituents who matter most to the policymaker. It is much easier to dismiss troubling data that come from afar, published in some arcane journal, than to dismiss troubling data about those with and for whom we live and work. One of the most powerful benefits of population-based data on children's school readiness outcomes, such as those collected using the Early Development Instrument (EDI; Janus & Offord, 2007), is that they are about *our* children, in our own neighborhood or community, our own province or state or territory, our own country. What is most personal to us is indeed what is most political to us. For elected decision-makers, it will be far more influential to learn that one in four of the kindergarten children in their constituency is vulnerable, than to learn about similar findings at the national level.

The old adage "Know your audience" applies to informing policy. Most politicians and policy-makers are not scientists, nor do they have the requisite training to approach information with the requisite critical analysis and synthesis that are hallmarks of a scientific approach. However, scientists are prone to the same pitfalls in reasoning as nonscientists (Kahneman, 2011). This should give us pause when we consider the enormity of the communication challenges inherent in bringing science to policy. Perhaps the major value of the scientific method is that it is an explicit attempt to be accountable for what we claim to be true about the world. It is this accountability that can add immense value to the policy-making process, which must be accountable to the people whom it affects, indeed, is charged to serve.

An amended version of the KISS principle, "Keep It Simple, Scientists," pertains. It can be challenging to jettison our jargon and impart our information without sacrificing their scientific integrity. But it must be done. A useful format has been the 1:3:25 approach of the Canadian Health Services Research Foundation (Canadian Health Services Research Foundation [CHSRF], 2001; now the Canadian Foundation for Healthcare Improvement). This comprises a 1-page summary of main messages, a 3-page executive summary, and a 25-page report in brief. A major new Canadian report on early childhood development (Boivin & Hertzman, 2012a) recently adopted this approach (Boivin & Hertzman, 2012b, 2012c, 2012d).

Because policymakers are people too, it is essential to consider how most people typically receive information, in what format, and from whom. What do they read? To whom do they listen? Most policymakers, like most people, will never read a scholarly journal article or major scientific report. Neither will most of the people who are most likely to influence policymakers personally. Science is usually filtered (e.g., by interest groups, mass media, political parties) before it reaches policymakers (Gormley, 2011).

Public sources of information (magazines, newspapers, radio, television, the Internet) and public opinion leaders that frequently appear therein, all provide important opportunities for science to influence policy. Communicated well, science can have a much greater impact on policy in the pages of *The Globe and Mail* in Canada, or *The Wall Street Journal* in the United States, and even more so when covered in local outlets such as *The Winnipeg Free Press* in Manitoba, because of the power of the "closer to home" principle. When certain people talk, many people will listen. For example, economists have long held significant influence in North American societies. When these economists also happen to be Nobel Laureates (Heckman, 2006, 2007) or the Chairman of the U.S. Federal Reserve (Bernanke, 2012), policymakers will be listening. These prominent economists have emerged as some of our greatest allies in using science to influence policy for early childhood development. And when they are covered by the mass media, such as *The New York Times* (Rampell, 2011) or *The Wall Street Journal* (Peterson, 2012), many people will listen. And although few scientists will have the opportunity to influence these public opinion leaders directly, they can and should make use of these same mass media to bring science to policy. A Cabinet Minister or a senior official is much more likely to read an article from the mass media that we send them than they are to read an article from the scientific journal that is cited in the mass media article. This is simply because the former is written for them (because they are people too), while the latter more often is not. Some policymakers will want to read more, and there is value in first giving them easier-to-read articles from *The New York Times* about, for example, epigenetics and executive functions (Kristof, 2012), instead of the latest scholarly works on these topics (e.g., Barkley, 2012; Petronis, 2010; Vohs & Baumeister, 2011). Another good option is books written by experts in evidence-based anecdotes, in telling personal, emotional stories based on sound science, such as Paul Tough's (2012) newest book on the importance of self-regulation and executive function for children's lifelong success. Scientists can learn a great deal from such examples, and many scientists are themselves exemplars, as adept at publishing in *Science* as they are at publishing in the popular press for the everyday reader (e.g., Kahneman, 2011).

Last, scientists can and should learn more from the science of communications itself. For example, perhaps surprisingly, it appears that one of the *least* effective ways to translate the science of school readiness to the public and its policymakers is to use the term *school readiness* (Aubrun & Grady, 2002). Telling a core story of early childhood development grounded in deeply held values (e.g., health and prosperity) using simplifying models (i.e., metaphors) such as "brain architecture" and "toxic stress" has proven much more effective in influencing policymakers (Shonkoff & Bales, 2011). In Canada, this approach led by the FrameWorks Institute has proven useful in Alberta (e.g., Kendall-Taylor, 2010) and in my own province of Manitoba, as well as in a newly released report on ECD commissioned by the Royal Society of Canada and the Canadian Academy of Health Sciences (Boivin & Hertzman, 2012a).

Collaboration

Today, good policymaking requires a collaborative approach that involves two key steps: (1) identifying the right constellation of causes, and (2) mobilizing a range of organizations and people who can work together to develop and implement a comprehensive plan (Lenihan, 2011). Herein, government is not the only decision-maker. It can convene and help to lead collaborators (Lenihan, 2011). Within governments, especially in the Westminster models of cabinet government used in Canada and the United Kingdom, good policymaking also requires the "test of consensus" among Cabinet Ministers, at least in provincial or territorial governments (Vogt, 2010).

Almost without exception, every leading scholar in knowledge translation and exchange emphasizes the importance of researchers developing personal relationships with decision-makers (e.g., Lavis, 2005; Lavis, Davies, Gruen, Walshe, & Farquhar, 2005; Lomas, 2005a, 2005b; Martens & Roos, 2005; Straus, Tetroe, & Graham, 2009; Waddell et al., 2005; Wathen, Sibbald, Jack, & MacMillan, 2011; see also Poulin et al., Chapter 13, this volume). Relationships must be defined by respect, responsiveness, and reciprocity (Brownell et al., 2011); they need talk, trust, and time (Wathen et al., 2011). Establishing formal institutions of science–policy relationships and collaboration has become increasingly important (Gormley, 2011), and several models now offer exemplars with a decade or more of experience (e.g., the Centre of Excellence for Early Childhood Development in Canada, the Manitoba Centre for Health Policy, and the Washington State Institute of Public Policy).

Credibility

It should go without saying that scientists must establish, enhance, and always protect their credibility. Inspired by Dante's *Inferno*, a recent summary of "scientific sins," ranging from the commonplace to the unforgivable, provides a humorous but useful heuristic of the "Nine Circles of Scientific Hell" (Neuroskeptic, 2012):

- First Circle: Limbo (passively or actively enabling the other scientific sins)
- Second Circle: Overselling (exaggerating importance of findings)
- Third Circle: Post-Hoc Storytelling (implying random results were anticipated)

- Fourth Circle: *p* Value Fishing (running analyses until a statistically significant result is found)
- Fifth Circle: Creative Use of Outliers (e.g., excluding inconvenient data points from analysis)
- Sixth Circle: Plagiarism
- Seventh Circle: Nonpublication of Data
- Eighth Circle: Partial Publication of Data
- Ninth Circle: Inventing Data

Like the protagonists in Dante's *Inferno*, scientists must be aware of, and beware of, personally descending through each of these circles (i.e., committing scientific sins), lest their credibility begin to erode at the First Circle, until it becomes irretrievably lost by the Ninth Circle. For science to influence public policy, credibility is crucial: "Scientists and policymakers alike need to work within established rules of the evaluation game, rules that reflect 40 years of hard-won lessons . . . in a way that minimizes . . . politicization. Otherwise, evaluation research has no added value to values" (McCartney & Weiss, 2007, p. 73). What are these rules? According to McCartney and Weiss, researchers should (1) use mixed-methods designs, (2) interpret effect size in a research context, (3) synthesize all research findings, (4) adopt fair and reasonable scientific expectations, and (5) encourage peer and public critique of the data. All of these are safeguards against the Nine Circles.

Part of the power of public opinion leaders, as well, rests in their credibility. Ben Bernanke's (2012) recent speech on the importance of early childhood education is influential because of who he is as much as how many public media outlets cover his comments.

What Do Scientists Need to Emphasize to Policymakers?: The Three Deliverables

As the chapters in this volume all attest, achieving school readiness is one of the most important developmental tasks facing our children. Policymakers will benefit most if we deliver three D's regarding school readiness: developmental trajectories, determinants, and demonstrations of interventions.

Developmental Trajectories

Extensive meta-analytic evidence and recent longitudinal studies (Vitaro, Brengden, & Tremblay, Chapter 2, and Boivin, Desrosiers, Lemelin, & Forget-Dubois, Chapter 3, this volume) indicate that school readiness predicts later achievement in school. The strongest specific predictors include math, reading, and attention skills (Duncan et al., 2007; Grimm, Steele, Mashburn, Burchinal, & Pianta, 2010; Hooper, Roberts, Sideris, Burchinal, & Zeisel, 2010; Lemelin et al., 2007; Pagani, Fitzpatrick, Archambault, & Janosz, 2010; Romano, Babchishin, Pagani, & Kohen, 2010), fine motor skills (Grissmer, Grimm, Aiyer, Murrah, & Steele, 2010; Pagani et al., 2010); social and emotional behaviors (Grimm et al., 2010; Pagani et al., 2010; Romano et al., 2010), and general knowledge (Grissmer et al., 2010). In recent longitudinal studies using the EDI to predict later achievement, the physical health and well-being domain and the language and cognitive development domain are especially strong predictors (Boivin et al., Chapter 3, this volume; Forget-Dubois et al., 2007; Lloyd, Li, & Hertzman, 2010); as is overall vulnerability in one or more domains of the EDI (Brownell et al., 2012; Lloyd & Hertzman, 2009; Lloyd, Irwin, & Hertzman, 2009).

Determinants

Identifying the early life determinants or predictors of school readiness is a top cross-sectoral priority for policymakers. Recent evidence indicates a substantial environmental contribution to school readiness, after accounting for the genetic contribution to school readiness (Boivin et al., Chapter 3, this volume; Lemelin et al., 2007). Identifying specific environmental determinants of school readiness that are amenable to policy intervention is essential for improving school readiness in the population. Cross-sectional evidence indicates that low family income is associated with poor school readiness outcomes at both individual and neighborhood levels (Cushon, Vu, Janzen, & Muhajarine, 2011; Janus & Duku, 2007; Kershaw, Forer, Irwin, Hertzman, & Lapointe, 2007; Lapointe, Ford, & Zumbo, 2007; Lesaux, Vukovic, Hertzman, & Siegel, 2007; Puchala, Vu, & Muhajarine, 2010), as is poor health status (Janus & Duku, 2007). Longitudinal evidence indicates that the neighborhood socioeconomic conditions of kindergarten children predict their development 4 years (Lloyd & Hertzman, 2010) and 7 years later (Lloyd et al., 2010), over and above their outcomes in kindergarten. A recent population-based, longitudinal study of two birth cohorts (N = 18,398) in Manitoba found that policy-modifiable variables such as children's health status at birth, family income during early childhood, and breastfeeding initiation predicted children's school readiness at age 5 years in kindergarten (Santos et al., 2012). In exploratory analyses, children who were more biologically vulnerable at birth (low Apgar score) appeared to respond more strongly to breastfeeding initiation in terms of their later school readiness outcomes in kindergarten (Santos et al., 2012). Related recent work on biological sensitivity to context (Boyce & Ellis, 2005) and differential susceptibility

(Belsky & Pluess, 2009; van IJzendoorn & Bakermans-Kranenburg, 2012) represent important developments for policy.

Demonstrations

Science can influence policy by providing real-world demonstrations of putting evidence into action. For some policymakers, a more immediate question is whether any other jurisdiction is doing it (whatever the "it" may be; e.g., implementing a model ECD program). And hearing that the answer is yes often provides immediate comfort, for several reasons. At times, many policymakers prefer to avoid setting precedents, especially if the stakes are high and available resources are low. But hearing that others, especially in high-profile settings, are "already doing it" can often increase the chances of doing the same or something similar. Hearing that Mayor Bloomberg is opening a new "cradle-to-kindergarten" preschool in Brooklyn can be very influential, just as hearing that 17 other cities had previously done so was likely influential in his own decision to act (Baker, 2012). Demonstrations are precedents. After them, no one can say "It can't be done," because it has been done. And moving scientific demonstrations into real-world demonstrations moves the science that much closer to policy, even if not done formally as effectiveness or dissemination studies per se. It is powerful to be able to point to the work in Washington State that is building evidence-based prevention investment portfolios, or to the prevention legislation enacted in Connecticut, or to the large-scale rollout of early childhood intervention in Ontario. The private sector also has considerable influence over public policy. Thus, having private sector demonstrations of evidence into action, such as the Ounce of Prevention Fund in Chicago, the work of the Buffet Early Childhood Fund, the Bill and Melinda Gates Foundation in the United States (Baker, 2012), and the Norlien Foundation in Canada also serve as powerful public demonstrations.

At other times, some policymakers will want to be leaders and precedent-setters. These times provide unprecedented opportunities for simultaneous scientific and real-world demonstrations. For example, the Government of Manitoba was so influenced by the evidence base for the PAX Good Behaviour Game (see Embry, 2002, 2011; Kellam et al., 2008, 2011) that it moved quickly to launch a provincewide pilot, the first of its kind in Canada. Because community demand from schools exceeded the available supply, a desire for equity (giving every interested school an equal chance to participate in the pilot) led to the use of a lottery to determine which schools would implement the program. Over 200 schools reaching over 5,000 grade 1 children are currently participating in what amounts to the largest cluster randomized field trial of the program to date. The immediate and longitudinal results will add much-needed evidence to the literature on effectiveness, program scale-up and dissemination, as discussed further in a later section of this chapter.

With sufficient skill, and a dose of good timing and good luck, using this "top-10 list" (four Elements, three Capabilities, three Deliverables) for ECD can lead to The Big D . . . Dollars. These drive policy, for better and worse (Meyers & Wilcox, 1998; Savoie 1999, 2003). In the current post–Great Recession era, as every government struggles with financial deficits, there may be increased opportunities for evidence to drive dollars. While it exerts significant personal and societal costs, we live in a time when economics is the dominant cultural narrative, what Michaels (2011) has called the *monoculture*; recognizing this reality has implications for how science can influence school readiness policy and practice.

Implications for Policymakers: Providing the Three R's

So, for all the policymakers who will never (have the time, interest, or capacity to) read this (entire) book, what might be our elevator conversation with them, if we had only a few minutes to tell them what they most need to know about the contents of this book? What points would or should we convey if they asked for more information in written form?

However long we have in the proverbial elevator, and however many pages we may have to fill, we have to cover the three R's: the Reasons, a Range of policy options, and Recommendations (at least one). In other words, we have to tell them *why* school readiness is important, what policy *can* do about it and, of the available options (whenever possible), what policy *should* do about it (cf. Shonkoff in Institute of Medicine & National Research Council, 2012). Using the knowledge translation terms of Mays et al. (2005) and Pope et al. (2005), the first R is a form of *knowledge support*, whereas the second and third R's are forms of *decision support*. The following is a generic example that could (and should) be tailored to specific policymakers, depending on the scientist's sense of the policymaker's specific knowledge needs.

The Reasons: *Why* Is School Readiness a Policy Priority? ("So What?")

School readiness is essential for almost everything that matters to you and your department, and the people you serve, your constituents. It predicts later achievement (Boivin et al., Chapter 3, this volume), including high school graduation (Vitaro et al., Chapter 2, this volume). In turn, it will contribute, for better or worse, to the future productivity and prosperity of your community and your country, as well as its lifelong health and well-being. Inequalities in children's school readiness pervade your community. For many children, these inequalities begin very early, in fact, before birth. Many children lack the opportunities necessary for school readiness. The good news is that science can offer some potential solutions.

A Range of Options: What *Can* We Do about School Readiness? ("What Now?")

You have a range of evidence-based options to improve the school readiness of children in your community. We know that in early life, before children start school, their language skills (Dionne, Mimeau, & Mathieu, Chapter 5, this volume), self-regulation skills such as attention and self-control (Li-Grining, Lennon, Marcus, Flores, & Haas, Chapter 9, this volume), early parenting and family experiences (Wade, Prime, Browne, & Jenkins, Chapter 4, this volume), and early child care experiences (Côté, Geoffroy, & Pingault, Chapter 6, this volume) influence children's school readiness. There are evidence-based interventions to improve early literacy skills such as children's vocabulary (Wasik & Hindman, Chapter 7, this volume), early math skills (Starkey, Klein, & DeFlorio, Chapter 8, this volume), and early social-emotional and cognitive skills (Bierman, Domitrovich, Nix, Welsh, & Gest, Chapter 10, this volume), as well as to support parents (Welsh, Bierman, & Mathis, Chapter 11, this volume), communities (Peters & Howell-Moneta, Chapter 12, this volume), and the most vulnerable families (Poulin et al., Chapter 13, this volume).

Recommendations: What *Should* We Do about School Readiness? ("Which Now?")

We will need to review this range of options in the context of your current pressures, challenges, and available resources. At any given time you have four general options: do nothing (status quo), increase/enhance something you're currently doing, decrease/cease something you're currently doing, and/or do something new that you aren't currently doing. If you don't currently have measures of school readiness in place, the good news is that there are relatively simple and inexpensive measures you can implement (e.g., Boivin et al., Chapter 3, this volume). If possible, you should build in an evaluation component and use the school readiness measure to monitor outcomes. You should develop collaborative partnerships to implement and evaluate the best available options that you choose (Poulin et al., Chapter 13, this volume), using as rigorous a methodology as possible (Welsh et al., Chapter 11, this volume). It is likely that, relative to cognitive skills (e.g., reading and math, which are very important), there is an underrecognition of the importance of social-emotional skills (Bierman et al., Chapter 10, this volume) and early mental health, and what are known as the executive function skills (e.g., self-regulation; Li-Grining et al., Chapter 9, this volume). What you choose should strengthen as many of these as possible and also buffer toxic stressors (things such as poverty, child abuse, parental mental illness and addictions, family and community violence) that damage the child's developing brain, which is at the center of all of these skills. Whatever you choose to do must strengthen the impacts of early childhood education and intervention by (1) enhancing the capabilities of families, caregivers, and educators to mitigate the effects of toxic stress; and (2) build executive function skills, enhance self-regulation, and strengthen mental health (Diamond & Lee, 2011; Shonkoff, 2011). As much as possible, it is essential to do so in an integrated manner across the silos of health policy, child care policy, education policy, and child welfare policy, to name a few (Shonkoff, Richter, van der Gaag, & Bhutta, 2012).

Current Challenges and Future Directions

Recommendations to Improve the Translation of Research to Policy

No single book can do it all, and this volume is no exception, notwithstanding its many exceptional contributions from some of the best developmental scientists in the business. What's missing in this book? Several school readiness policy-relevant areas of science are noted only briefly or not at all (e.g., physical health, nutrition, income). As noted earlier, cost and cost-effectiveness data are of perennial importance to policymakers. A number of promising programs are described in this book, but there is next to no information on what they would cost to implement, or what the estimated return on investment might be. It is also clear that ECD and school readiness need primary studies and systematic reviews of knowledge translation strategies, similar to mental health (Goldner et al., 2011; Waddell et al., 2005), public health (LaRocca et al., 2012) and allied health (Scott et al., 2012), to improve the evidence base for helping base policy on evidence.

Even more challenging, as hopefully was evident earlier in the "Recommendations" section, is the limited ability to recommend specific programs, let alone which specific combination(s) of programs. This limitation is only partly related to the need to take context into account. Regardless of the particular pressures, challenges, and available resources in a given policymaking setting, the empirical reality is that we currently lack key evidence to inform making specific policy choices to address multiple needs. As described in several chapters in this book, some programs affect some important school readiness outcomes (e.g., behavior), but not others (cognitive skills). Some improve outcomes in some groups (e.g., girls) but less so in others (e.g., boys). Even before the Great Recession, it was unlikely that any government could financially afford to implement a different program for each desired outcome, especially with the knowledge that "crossover effects" for outcomes do not happen as often as desired (cf. Bierman et al., Chapter 10, this volume). In the current fiscal environment, it will be a challenge for all governments to implement even a single new program. The evidence base for the range of policy and program options is even more important now. So what could (or should) be next?

Scale-Up and Innovation

The current research frontier is about designing and scaling up, innovating, and evaluating. The big question for the big payoff is whether large-scale public programs can replicate the effects of small-scale research programs, and under what conditions (Barnett, 2011). There is an empirical reason to believe the answer can be yes, as shown by Starkey and colleagues (Chapter 8, this volume) in scaling up and sustaining the positive effects of a public preschool mathematics program, and by Poulin and colleagues (Chapter 13, this volume) in their effectiveness trial of a kindergarten program to promote school readiness and prevent disruptive behaviors, albeit with more positive effects for girls.

Effective Ingredients

At the same time, it is clear that we also need to move beyond existing brand-name programs. A recent meta-analysis of 123 studies from 1960 to 2000 brings both the good news that early childhood intervention is indeed efficacious, and the bad news that little evidence is available for designing the structure and process of these interventions at multiple levels with multiple components (Camilli, Vargas, Ryan, & Barnett, 2010). The mixing and matching of programs and their components is often the rule rather than the exception in the real world of service delivery, evidence aside (and frequently so). Balancing program fidelity with program adaptation will likely remain the major challenge when going to scale. One of the necessary conditions for data to influence public policy is that "evaluation data need to support innovation and continuous improvement" (McCartney & Weiss, 2007, p. 74). Moving forward will mean using evidence-based ingenuity to design and test early childhood intervention innovations (Shonkoff, 2012), particularly using rigorous multisite, randomized evaluations that systematically vary these design elements (Barnett, 2011; Camilli et al., 2010), that help communities "learn as they go" in ways that preserve both the scientific and frontline credibility of the intervention. Such program improvement research—which should systematically test "big-ticket items" such as duration, length of day, teacher–child ratio, educator qualifications, and inservice educator development—is essential for program scale-up that preserves the cost-effectiveness of small-scale pilot or model programs (Barnett, 2011). Identifying the "effective ingredients" of programs (cf. Li-Grining et al., Chapter 9, and Wasik & Hindman, Chapter 7, this volume) remains as important as ever. Recent work on "evidence-based kernels" or fundamental units of behavior change (Embry & Biglan, 2008; Embry, 2011) can be helpful in this regard.

The Need for Theory

A decade ago, Shonkoff (2003) urged the field of early childhood intervention to move beyond asking *whether* early childhood intervention works to asking *how* its effects can be maximized. Others shared this perspective: "Instead of the typical outcome question 'Does the program work?' a more important set of questions to ask is; 'How did the intervention work? For whom? Under what circumstances?' " (Korfmacher, 2002, p. 283). "Accordingly, the key question for evaluators and for consumers of evaluations—especially policy makers—may be not 'did an intervention work?' but 'for whom and under what circumstances are particular services most effective?' " (Berlin, O'Neal, & Brooks-Gunn, 1998, p. 13). These relatively recent recommendations from leading early childhood intervention researchers (including those in the current volume; e.g., Welsh et al., Chapter 11) are reminiscent of exhortations to psychotherapy researchers that date back at least six decades. For example: "From the point of view of science, the question 'Does psychotherapy do any good?' has little interest because it is virtually meaningless. . . . The question is which people, in what circumstances, responding to what psychotherapeutic stimuli" (Sandford, 1953, pp. 335–336). The most famous and most quoted version came from Gordon Paul (1967, p. 11): "*What* treatment, by *whom*, is most effective for *this* individual with *that* specific problem, under *which* set of circumstances?" After several decades and thousands of studies, it became clear that this atheoretical "matrix of all possible combinations of treatments, therapists, clients, problems, and sets of circumstances" (Omer & Dar, 1992, p. 92) was fatally flawed, with "no clear agreement about even a single cell in this matrix. Clearly, a blind accumulation of comparisons, unrelated to or unanchored in theories, teaches us little. . . . Filling Paul's matrix, therefore, is a Sisyphean task" (p. 92). The lesson for the current volume is clear: Integrated theoretical frameworks for evaluating early childhood interventions to improve school readiness will be essential to advance the science in order to advance policy. Several promising frameworks are now available (e.g., Biglan, Flay, Embry, & Sandler, 2012; Halfon, Barrett, & Kuo, 2010; Shonkoff, Boyce, & McEwen, 2009; Shonkoff et al., 2012).

Evolutionary Perspectives

Few chapters in this book reference an evolutionary perspective on child development (e.g., Hrdy, 2009; Konner, 2010; Narvaez, Panksepp, Schore, & Gleason, 2013). This perspective will likely prove invaluable to better understand and improve school readiness and life course development, for both scientific and sociocultural reasons. Scientifically, if nothing in childhood makes sense except in the light of evolution (Konner, 2010), then nothing we do through policy to improve childhood will make sense without an evolutionary perspective. The parts of our brains that govern our emotions—the joy, love, grief, and sorrow that define our lives—are also the oldest parts of our brains, built from a blueprint billions of years in the making (Panksepp & Biven, 2012). The developmental mismatch between our ancient brains and bodies and our modern lives (Gluckman & Hanson, 2004, 2006; Gluckman et al., 2009; Trevathan, 2010) suggests approaches worth (re)considering for future research, policy, and practice. Many of these approaches have long ancestral traditions of practice in Indigenous and other cultures, including breastfeeding, co-sleeping, alloparenting by extended family, intergenerational peers, and significant emphasis on play, the land and nature, oral history, language, and cultural rites of passage (Diamond, 2012; Hrdy, 1999, 2009; Konner, 2010; Narvaez et al., 2013; Trevathan, 2010; Worthman, Plotsky, Schechter, & Cummings, 2010).

Indigenous Children and Immigrant Children

More (and more culturally appropriate) research is needed regarding the school readiness of Aboriginal children and immigrant children. For Canada, as well as other developed nations, the future health, learning, and prosperity of the country are intertwined with the future of its Indigenous peoples (Giroux, 2012; Jamieson, 2012) and newcomers (Omidvar & Lopes, 2012). The economic implications alone are staggering. For example, "If we closed the education and employment achievement gap between indigenous and other Canadians, we would save more than $115 billion over 15 years while adding more than $401 billion to Canada's GDP" (Jamieson, 2012, p. 49). Data on children's school readiness depicts massive gaps. For example, in Manitoba, 45% of Indigenous kindergarten children and 51% of newcomer kindergarten children are vulnerable, as measured by the Early Development Instrument.

Truth and Reconciliation

Countries such as Canada have started to move forward in understanding and addressing the historical impacts and human suffering that resulted from government policies of colonization, particularly residential schools for Indigenous children (for readers less familiar with this history, see Truth and Reconciliation Commission of Canada, 2012a). An evolutionary perspective grounded in the newest neuroscience holds significant potential for understanding the underlying epigenetics of colonization, intergenerational trauma, and intergenerational transmission of negative outcomes (see Bombay, Matheson, & Anisman, 2009, 2011). Socioculturally, many non-Indigenous people in the general public still struggle to understand how and why the cultural dispossession and child abuse experienced several generations past still continue to affect their children and grandchildren today. Many wonder, "Why can't they just get over it?" For others, the overrepresentation of Indigenous children in the child welfare system (as well as other service delivery systems; e.g., mental and physical health, income assistance, and criminal justice)

> are indivisible from Canada's history of placing First Nations children in residential schools; breaking family continuity and undermining parenting and life course traditions. Although residential schools have been closed for decades, their disruptive effects on First Nations families are still felt across generations. Thus, addressing [adverse childhood experiences] in First Nations populations is difficult to separate from current initiatives being taken to promote reconciliation with the non-First Nations population and to re-build First Nations communities. (Boivin & Hertzman, 2012a, p. 18)

Our new scientific understanding of the lifelong impacts of adverse childhood experiences (Boivin & Hertzman, 2012a; Shonkoff, Garner, et al., 2012; see also Felitti et al., 1998) and the underlying neurobiology (Boyce, Sokolowski, & Robinson, 2012) of how these toxic stressors in the social environment get "under the skin" and biologically embedded (Hertzman, 2012; McEwen, 2012; Rutter, 2012), and transmitted epigenetically and intergenerationally (Boivin & Hertzman, 2012a) can help explain the far-reaching effects of residential schools in Canada and other countries with similar histories of colonizing their Indigenous peoples. For some people, for better or worse, sociocultural understanding will only come fully after being grounded in the terminology of science, particularly the science of early brain development. For some people, hearing the personal, emotional stories of the residential school survivors may or may not be sufficient to understand. Yet this understanding, however it arrives, is essential to move forward. In this way, science can support both truth and reconciliation.

A fundamental teaching of many Indigenous peoples is that in making decisions for the future, "we must focus our attention not on ourselves, not on our children or even our grandchildren, but rather on the Seventh Generation—those yet to be born, children whose faces are still coming toward us" (Jamieson, 2012, p. 49). Emerging evidence on early childhood adversity, epigenetic mechanisms, and intergenerational transmission of parenting may provide a scientific way of understanding the destructive, enduring effects of colonization. It can also provide a scientific frame of reference for an enduring cultural wisdom tradition of the Seventh Generation, bridging one of the most important cross-cultural gaps of our generation. In addition to the latter knowledge support (truth), we can also find decision support (reconciliation). For example, a major recommendation of the Truth and Reconciliation Commission of Canada (2012b) is "that all levels of government develop culturally appropriate early childhood and parenting programs to assist young parents and families affected by the impact of residential schools and historic policies of cultural oppression in the development of parental understanding and skills" (p. 8). As noted earlier, government cannot and should not do this alone.

Partnerships with the Private Sector

A recent article in one of Canada's national newspapers asks, "Can the private sector and market-based models play a bigger role in the traditional turf of charities and government, tackling issues like youth unemployment and childhood obesity? The head of Canada's largest bank thinks so" (Grant, 2012). Gordon Nixon, the head of the Royal Bank of Canada, Canada's largest bank, recently discussed the leadership role of the private sector and is quoted as saying, "The ability to ensure that dollars invested are really generating a social impact is there. If we can get it right, it can be very exciting. We're looking for both a financial and social return" (Grant, 2012). A few weeks later, another one of Canada's largest banks, TD, released a major new report, coauthored by its chief economist, on the excellent economics of early childhood education (Alexander & Ignjatovic, 2012), which was covered widely by both the national and local media (e.g., CBC News Canada, 2012; Winnipeg Free Press, 2012). The report concludes:

> Unfortunately, with governments at all levels currently in deficit fighting mode, increasing spending on large-scale new programs in not in the cards.

Still, given such persuasive evidence of the widespread benefits that early learning promotes, there is scope for further investment and reform in the industry. Hence, once government balance sheets are back in order, they should consider placing investment in early learning as a high priority. (Alexander & Ignjatovic, 2012, p. 8)

LOOKING FORWARD

But perhaps there still is fiscal hope, in the surprising conclusions regarding the future affordability of large-scale public programs, from another eminent economist, William Baumol (2012a):

> The key conclusion that follows from this is that no matter how painful rising medical and educational bills may be, *society can afford them* [emphasis in original], and there is no need to deny them to ourselves or to the less affluent members of our society, or indeed to the world. (Baumol, 2012b, pp. 28–29)
>
> Given this, it is clear that if improvements to health care and education are hindered by the illusion that we cannot afford them, we will all be forced to suffer from self-inflicted wounds. The very definition of rising productivity ensures that the future will offer us a cornucopia of desirable services and abundant products. The main threat to this happy prospect is the illusion that society cannot afford them, with resulting political developments—such as calls for reduced government revenues entwined with demands that budgets always be in balance—that deny these benefits to our descendants. (Baumol, 2012b, p. 30)

Edward Zigler, one of the founding fathers of early childhood development policy, said it best:

> The key to how well and how quickly child-friendly policies evolve is leadership. We need leading researchers in the science of child development who can enhance understanding of the myriad ingredients and principles of human growth and their intricate interactions. We need leaders who can apply the evidence derived from science to develop programs that work in meeting children's needs. Finally, we need leadership in the policy arena, including those who create and pass laws that affect children and those who serve as interpreters of the knowledge needed for effective social policy. (2007, p. 284)

Leadership in science, practice, and policy, and the strength of their relationships, will define, for better or worse, the future of the next generation.

REFERENCES

Alexander, C., & Ignjatovic, D. (2012, November 27). *Special report: Early childhood education has widespread and long lasting benefits*. Toronto: TD Economics. Retrieved from *www.td.com/document/pdf/economics/special/di1112_earlychildhoodeducation.pdf*.

Aos, S., Lee, S., Drake, E., Pennucci, A., Klima, T., Miller, M., et al. (2011, July). *Return on investment: Evidence-based options to improve statewide outcomes*. Olympia: Washington State Institute of Public Policy.

Aubrun, A., & Grady, J. (2002). *Promoting school readiness and early child development: Findings from cognitive elicitations*. Washington, DC: FrameWorks Institute.

Baker, A. (2012, September 24). City to add pre-K efforts in poor areas next year. *The New York Times*. Retrieved from *www.nytimes.com/2012/09/25/nyregion/city-will-extend-hours-for-prekindergarten-in-poor-neighborhoods.html*.

Barkley, R. A. (2012). *Executive functions: What they are, how they work, and why they evolved*. New York: Guilford Press.

Barnett, W. S. (2011). Effectiveness of early educational intervention. *Science, 333*, 975–978.

Baumol, W. (2012a). *The cost disease: Why computers get cheaper and health care doesn't*. New Haven, CT: Yale University Press.

Baumol, W. (2012b, November). We can have it all: Why health care will still be affordable. *Policy Options*, pp. 28–30.

Belsky, J., & Pluess, M. (2009). Beyond diathesis stress: Differential susceptibility to environmental influences. *Psychological Bulletin, 135*, 885–908.

Berlin, L. J., O'Neal, C. R., & Brooks-Gunn, J. (1998). What makes early intervention programs work?: The program, its participants, and their interaction. *Zero to Three, 18*, 4–15.

Bernanke, B. S. (2012, July 24). Early childhood education. Retrieved from *www.federalreserve.gov/newsevents/speech/bernanke20120724a.htm*.

Biglan, A., Flay, B. R., Embry, D. D., & Sandler, I. N. (2012). The critical role of nurturing environments for promoting human well-being. *American Psychologist, 67*, 257–271.

Blakeney, A., & Borins, S. (1998). *Political management in Canada: Conversations on statecraft* (2nd ed.). Toronto: University of Toronto Press.

Boivin, M., & Hertzman, C. (Eds.). (2012a). *Early childhood development: Adverse childhood experiences and developmental health*. Ottawa: Royal Society of Canada & Canadian Academy of Health Sciences Expert Panel (with R. Barr, W. T., Boyce, A. Fleming, H. MacMillan, C. Odgers, M. B., Sokolowski, & N. Trocmé). Retrieved from *http://rsc-src.ca/en/expert-panels/rsc-reports/early-childhood-development-rsccahs*.

Boivin, M., & Hertzman, C. (Eds.). (2012b). *Executive summary: Early childhood development*. Ottawa: Royal Society of Canada & Canadian Academy of Health Sciences Expert Panel (with R. Barr, W. T., Boyce, A. Fleming, H. MacMillan, C. Odgers, M. B., Sokolowski, & N. Trocmé). Retrieved from *http://rsc-src.ca/en/expert-panels/rsc-reports/early-childhood-development-rsccahs*.

Boivin, M., & Hertzman, C. (Eds.). (2012c). *Main messages: Early childhood development*. Ottawa: Royal Society of Canada & Canadian Academy of Health Sciences Expert Panel (with R. Barr, W. T., Boyce, A. Fleming, H. MacMillan, C. Odgers, M. B., Sokolowski, & N. Trocmé). Retrieved from *http://rsc-src.ca/en/expert-panels/rsc-reports/early-childhood-development-rsccahs*.

Boivin, M., & Hertzman, C. (Eds.). (2012d). *Report in brief: Early childhood development*. Ottawa: Royal Society of Canada & Canadian Academy of Health Sciences Expert Panel (with R. Barr, W. T., Boyce, A. Fleming, H. MacMillan, C. Odgers, M. B., Sokolowski, & N. Trocmé). Retrieved from *http://rsc-src.ca/en/expert-panels/rsc-reports/early-childhood-development-rsccahs*.

Bombay, A., Matheson, K., & Anisman, H. (2009, November). Intergenerational trauma: Convergence of multiple processes among First Nations peoples in Canada. *Journal of Aboriginal Health*, pp .6–47.

Bombay, A., Matheson, K., & Anisman, H. (2011). The impact of stressors on second generation Indian residential school survivors. *Transcultural Psychiatry, 48*, 367–391.

Boyce, W. T., & Ellis, B. J. (2005). Biological sensitivity to context: I. An evolutionary-developmental theory of the origins and functions of stress reactivity. *Development and Psychopathology, 17*, 271–301.

Boyce, W. T., Sokolowski, M. B., & Robinson, G. E. (2012). Toward a new biology of social adversity. *Proceedings of the National Academy of Sciences, 109*(Suppl. 2), 17143–17148.

Brownell, M., Chartier, M., Santos, R., Ekuma, O., Au, W., Sarkar, J., et al. (2012). *How are Manitoba's children doing?* Winnipeg: Manitoba Centre for Health Policy.

Brownell, M., Kozyrskyj, A., Fuchs, D., & Santos, R. (2011). Using administrative data to study child health [Special issue]. *Healthcare Policy, 6*, 91–93.

Brownell, M., Roos, N. P., MacWilliam, L., Leclair, L., Ekuma, O., & Fransoo, R. (2010). Academic and social outcomes for high-risk youths in Manitoba. *Canadian Journal of Education, 33*, 804–836.

Camilli, G., Vargas, S., Ryan, S., & Barnett, W. S. (2010). Meta-analysis of the effects of early education interventions on cognitive and social development. *Teachers College Record, 112*, 579–620.

Campbell, F. A., Pungello, E. P., Burchinal, M., Kainz, K., Pan, Y., Wasik, B. H., et al. (2012). Adult outcomes as a function of an early childhood educational program: An Abecedarian project follow-up. *Developmental Psychology, 48*, 1033–1043.

Canadian Health Services Research Foundation. (2001). *Reader-friendly writing–1:3:25*. Ottawa: Author. Retrieved from *http://www.cfhi-fcass.ca/migrated/pdf/communicationnotes/cn-1325_e.pdf*.

CBC News Canada. (2012, November 27). Early childhood education pays for itself, TD says. Retrieved from *www.cbc.ca/news/canada/story/2012/11/27/td-early-childhood-education.html*.

Cialdini, R. B. (2009). *Influence: The psychology of persuasion*. New York: HarperCollins.

Commission on Social Determinants of Health. (2008). *Closing the gap in a generation: Health equity through action on the social determinants of health: Final report of the Commission on Social Determinants of Health*. Geneva: World Health Organization.

Cushon, J. A., Vu, L. T. H., Janzen, B. L., & Muhajarine, N. (2011). Neighbourhood poverty impacts children's physical health and well-being over time: Evidence from the Early Development Instrument. *Early Education and Development, 22*, 183–205.

Diamond, A., & Lee, K. (2011). Interventions shown to aid executive function development in children 4 to 12 years old. *Science, 333*, 959–964.

Diamond, J. (2012). *The world until yesterday: What can we learn from traditional societies?* New York: Viking.

Driedger, S. M., Kothari, A., Graham, I. D., Cooper, E., Crighton, E. J., Zahab, M., et al. (2010). If you build it, they still may not come: Outcomes and process of implementing a community-based integrated knowledge translation mapping innovation. *Implementation Science, 5*, 1–13. Retrieved from *www.implementationscience.com/content/5/1/47.*

Duncan, G. J., Dowsett, C. J., Claessens, A., Magnuson, K., Huston, A. C., Klebanov, P., et al. (2007). School readiness and later achievement. *Developmental Psychology, 43*, 1428–1446.

Embry, D. D. (2002). The Good Behavior Game: A best practice candidate as a universal behavioral vaccine. *Clinical Child and Family Psychology Review, 6*, 273–297.

Embry, D. D. (2011). Behavioral vaccines and evidence-based kernels: Nonpharmaceutical approaches for the prevention of mental, emotional, and behavioural disorders. *Psychiatric Clinics of North America, 34*, 1–34.

Embry, D. D., & Biglan, A. (2008). Evidence-based kernels: Fundamental units of behavioral influence. *Clinical Child and Family Psychology Review, 11*, 75–113.

Felitti, V. J., Anda, R. F., Nordenberg, D., Williamson, D. F., Spitz, A. M., Edwards, V., et al. (1998). Relationship of childhood abuse and household dysfunction to many of the leading causes of death in adults: The Adverse Childhood Experiences (ACE) Study. *American Journal of Preventive Medicine, 14*, 245–258.

Forget-Dubois, N., Lemelin, J., Boivin, M., Dionne, G., Séguin, J. R., Vitaro, F., et al. (2007). Predicting early school achievement with the EDI: A longitudinal population-based study. *Early Education and Development, 18*, 405–426.

Geddes, J. (2012, December 3). The power list: 25 most important people in Ottawa. *Macleans*, pp. 17–40.

Giroux, D. (2012, August). Closing the gap in First Nations education. *Policy Options*, pp. 50–53.

Gluckman, P. D., & Hanson, M. A. (2004). Living with the past: Evolution, development, and patterns of disease. *Science, 305*, 1733–1736.

Gluckman, P. D., & Hanson, M. A. (2006). *Mismatch: Why our world no longer fits our bodies*. New York: Oxford University Press.

Gluckman, P. D., Hanson, M. A., Bateson, P., Beedle, A. S., Law, C. M., Bhutta, Z. A., et al. (2009). Towards a new developmental synthesis: Adaptive developmental plasticity and human disease. *Lancet, 373*, 1654–1657.

Goldner, E. M., Jeffries, V., Bilsker, D., Jenkins, E., Menear, M., & Petermann, L. (2011). Knowledge translation in mental health: A scoping review. *Healthcare Policy, 7*(2), 83–98.

Gormley, W. T. (2011). From science to policy in early childhood education. *Science, 333,* 978–981.

Grant, T. (2012, November 12). Corporate Canada begins the search for (social) returns. *The Globe and Mail.* Retrieved from *www.theglobeandmail.com/report-on-business/economy/economy-lab/corporate-canada-begins-the-search-for-social-returns/article5195048.*

Greenhalgh, T., & Russell, J. (2005). Reframing evidence synthesis as rhetorical action in the policy making drama. *Healthcare Policy, 1*(2), 34–42.

Grimm, K. J., Steele, J. S., Mashburn, A. J., Burchinal, M., & Pianta, R. C. (2010). Early behavioral associations of achievement trajectories. *Developmental Psychology, 46,* 976–983.

Grissmer, D., Grimm, K. J., Aiyer, S. M., Murrah, W. M., & Steele, J. S. (2010). Fine motor skills and early comprehension of the world: Two new school readiness indicators. *Developmental Psychology, 46,* 1008–1017.

Halfon, N., Barrett, E. S., & Kuo, A. (2010). Translations from human development to public policy. In C. M. Worthman, P. M. Plotsky, D. S. Schechter, & C. A. Cummings (Eds.), *Formative experiences: The interaction of caregiving, culture, and developmental psychobiology* (pp. 505–530). New York: Cambridge University Press.

Heckman, J. J. (2006). Skill formation and the economics of investing in disadvantaged children. *Science, 312,* 1900–1902.

Heckman, J. J. (2007). The economics, technology, and neuroscience of human capability formation. *Proceedings of the National Academy of Sciences, 104,* 13250–13255.

Hertzman, C. (2012). Putting the concept of biological embedding in historical perspective. *Proceedings of the National Academy of Sciences, 109*(Suppl. 2), 17160–17167.

Hooper, S. R., Roberts, J., Sideris, J., Burchinal, M., & Zeisel, S. (2010). Longitudinal predictors of reading and math trajectories through middle school for African American versus Caucasian students across two samples. *Developmental Psychology, 46,* 1018–1029.

Hrdy, S. B. (1999). *Mother nature: A history of mothers, infants, and natural selection.* New York: Pantheon.

Hrdy, S. B. (2009). *Mothers and others: The evolutionary origins of mutual understanding.* Cambridge, MA: Belknap Press of Harvard University Press.

Institute of Medicine & National Research Council. (2012). *From neurons to neighborhoods: An update: Workshop summary.* Washington, DC: National Academies Press.

Jamieson, R. (2012, August). Realizing Canada's promise in partnership with Indigenous peoples. *Policy Options,* pp. 46–49.

Janus, M., & Duku, E. (2007). The school entry gap: Socioeconomic, family, and health factors associated with children's school readiness to learn. *Early Education and Development, 18,* 375–403.

Janus, M., & Offord, D. R. (2007). Development and psychometric properties of the Early Development Instrument (EDI): A measure of children's school readiness. *Canadian Journal of Behavioural Science, 39*, 1–22.

Kahneman, D. (2011). *Thinking, fast and slow.* Toronto: Doubleday Canada.

Kellam, S. G., Brown, C. H., Poduska, J. M., Ialongo, N. S., Wang, W., Toyinbo, P., et al. (2008). Effects of a universal classroom behaviour management program in first and second grades on young adult, behavioural, psychiatric, and social outcomes. *Drug and Alcohol Dependence, 95S*, S5–S28.

Kellam, S. G., Mackenzie, A. C. L., Brown, C. H., Poduska, J. M., Wang, W., Petras, H., et al. (2011, July). The Good Behavior Game and the future of prevention and treatment. *Addiction Science and Clinical Practice*, pp. 73–84.

Kendall-Taylor, N. (2010). *Experiences get carried forward: How Albertans think about early child development: A FrameWorks research report.* Washington, DC: FrameWorks Institute and Norlien Foundation.

Kershaw, P., Forer, B., Irwin, L. G., Hertzman, C., & Lapointe, V. (2007). Toward a social care program of research: A population-level study of neighborhood effects on child development. *Early Education and Development, 18*, 535–560.

Konner, M. (2010). *The evolution of childhood: Relationships, emotion, mind.* Cambridge, MA: Belknap Press of Harvard University Press.

Korfmacher, J. (2002). Early childhood interventions: Now what? In H. E. Fitzgerald, K. H. Karraker, & T. Luster (Eds.), *Infant development: Ecological perspectives* (pp. 273–294). New York: RoutledgeFalmer.

Kraemer, H. C., Kazdin, A. E., Offord, D. R., Kessler, R. C., Jensen, P. S., & Kupfer, D. J. (1997). Coming to terms with the terms of risk. *Archives of General Psychiatry, 54*, 337–343.

Kristof, N. D. (2012, October 20). Cuddle your kids! *The New York Times.* Retrieved from *www.nytimes.com/2012/10/21/opinion/sunday/kristof-cuddle-your-kid.html.*

Lapointe, V. R., Ford, L., & Zumbo, B. D. (2007). Examining the relationship between neighborhood environment and school readiness for Kindergarten children. *Early Education and Development, 18*, 473–495.

LaRocca, R., Yost, J., Dobbins, M., Ciliska, D., & Butt, M. (2012). The effectiveness of knowledge translation strategies used in public health: A systematic review. *BMC Public Health, 12*, 1–28. Retrieved from *www.biomedcentral.com/1471-2458/12/751.*

Lavis, J. (2005). Moving forward on both systematic reviews and deliberative processes. *Healthcare Policy, 1*(2), 59–63.

Lavis, J., Davies, H., Gruen, R., Walshe, K., & Farquhar, C. (2005). Working within and beyond the Cochrane Collaboration to make systematic reviews more useful to healthcare managers and policy makers. *Healthcare Policy, 1*(2), 21–33.

Lee, S., Aos, S., Drake, E., Pennucci, A., Miller, M., & Anderson, L. (2012, April). *Return on investment: Evidence-based options to improve statewide outcomes.* Olympia: Washington State Institute of Public Policy.

Lemelin, J., Boivin, M., Forget-Dubois, N., Dionne, G., Séguin, J. R., Brendgen, M., et al. (2007). The genetic–environmental etiology of cognitive school readiness and later academic achievement in early childhood. *Child Development, 78*, 1855–1869.

Lenihan, D. (2011, December). Rescuing policy: The case for collaboration. *Policy Option*, pp. 42–45.

Lesaux, N. K., Vukovic, R. K., Hertzman, C., & Siegel, L. S. (2007). Context matters: The interrelatedness of early literacy skills, developmental health, and community development . *Early Education and Development, 18*, 497–518.

Lloyd, J. E. V., & Hertzman, C. (2009). From Kindergarten readiness to fourth-grade assessment: Longitudinal analysis with linked population data. *Social Science & Medicine, 68*, 111–123.

Lloyd, J. E. V., & Hertzman, C. (2010). How neighbourhoods matter for rural and urban children's language and cognitive development at Kindergarten and grade 4. *Journal of Community Psychology, 38*, 293–313.

Lloyd, J. E. V., Irwin, L. G., & Hertzman, C. (2009). Kindergarten school readiness and fourth-grade literacy and numeracy outcomes of children with special needs: A population-based study. *Educational Psychology, 29*, 583–602.

Lloyd, J. E. V., Li, L., & Hertzman, C. (2010). Early experiences matter: Lasting effect of concentrated disadvantage on children's language and cognitive outcomes. *Health & Place, 16*, 371–380.

Lomas, J. (2005a). Using research to inform healthcare managers' and policy makers' questions: From summative to interpretive synthesis. *Healthcare Policy, 1*(1), 55–71.

Lomas, J. (2005b). Whose views count in evidence synthesis? And when do they count? *Healthcare Policy, 1*(2), 55–57.

Lomas, J. (2007). CHRSF knowledge transfer decision support: A new approach to making the best healthcare management and policy choices. *Healthcare Quarterly, 10*(3), 16–18.

Martens, P. J., & Roos, N. P. (2005). When health services researchers and policy makers interact: Tales from the tectonic plates. *Healthcare Policy, 1*(1), 72–86.

Mays, N., Pope, C., & Popay, J. (2005). Systematically reviewing qualitative and quantitative evidence to inform management and policy-making in the health field. *Journal of Health Services Research and Policy, 10*(Suppl. 1), 6–20.

McCartney, K., & Weiss, H. B. (2007). Data for a democracy: The evolving role of evaluation in policy and program development. In J. L. Aber, S. J. Bishop-Josef, K. T. McLearn, & D. A. Phillips (Eds.), *Child development and social policy: Knowledge for action* (pp. 59–76). Washington, DC: American Psychological Association.

McEwen, B. S. (2012). Brain on stress: How the social environment gets under the skin. *Proceedings of the National Academy of Sciences, 109*(Suppl. 2), 17180–17185.

Meyers, J. C., & Wilcox, B. L. (1998). Public policy applications of research on violence and children. In P. K. Trickett & C. J. Schellenbach (Eds.), *Violence against children in the family and the community* (pp. 465–478). Washington, DC: American Psychological Association.

Michaels, F. S. (2011). *Monoculture: How one story is changing everything.* Vancouver: Red Clover Press.

Mitton, C., Adair, C. E., McKenzie, E., Patten, S. B., & Waye Perry, B. (2007).

Knowledge transfer and exchange: Review and synthesis of the literature. *Milbank Quarterly, 85*, 729–768.

Murthy, L., Shepperd, S., Clarke, M. J., Garner, S. E., Lavis, J. N., Perrier, L., et al. (2012). Interventions to improve the use of systematic reviews in decision-making by health system managers, policy makers and clinicians. *Cochrane Database of Systematic Reviews, 9*, CD09401.

Narvaez, D., Panksepp, J., Schore, A. N., & Gleason, T. R. (Eds.). (2013). *Evolution, early experience and human development: From research to policy and practice.* New York: Oxford University Press.

Neuroskeptic. (2012). The nine circles of scientific hell. *Perspectives on Psychological Science, 7*, 643–644.

Newland, M. (Producer & Director). (1969). *Bambi Meets Godzilla* [motion picture]. Los Angeles, CA: Art Center of Design.

Omer, H., & Dar, R. (1992). Changing trends in three decades of psychotherapy research: The flight from theory into pragmatics. *Journal of Consulting and Clinical Psychology, 60*, 88–93.

Omidvar, R., & Lopes, S. (2012, August). Canada's future success closely linked to a successful immigration program. *Policy Options*, pp. 54–57.

Packham, M. A. (2010). *J. Fraser Mustard: Connections and careers.* Toronto: University of Toronto Press.

Pagani, L. S., Fitzpatrick, C., Archambault, I., & Janosz, M. (2010). School readiness and later achievement: A French Canadian replication and extension. *Developmental Psychology, 46*, 984–994.

Panksepp, J., & Biven, L. (2012). *The archaeology of mind: Neuroevolutionary origins of human emotions.* New York: Norton.

Parloff, M. B. (1982). Psychotherapy research evidence and reimbursement decisions: *Bambi Meets Godzilla. American Journal of Psychiatry, 139*, 718–727.

Paul, G. L. (1967). Strategy of outcome research in psychotherapy. *Journal of Consulting and Clinical Psychology, 31*, 109–118.

Peterson, K. (2012, July 24). Bernanke champions early childhood education. *The Wall Street Journal.* Retrieved from *http://blogs.wsj.com/economics/2012/07/24/bernanke-champions-early-childhood-education.*

Petronis, A. (2010). Epigenetics as a unifying principle in the aetiology of complex traits and disease. *Nature, 465*, 721–727.

Pope, C., Mays, N., & Popay, J. (2005). Informing policy making and management in healthcare: The place for synthesis. *Healthcare Policy, 1*(2), 43–48.

Puchala, C., Vu, L. T. H., & Muhajarine, N. (2010). Neighbourhood ethnic diversity buffers school readiness impact in ESL children. *Canadian Journal of Public Health, 101*(Suppl. 3), S13–S18.

Radin, B. A. (2000). *Beyond Machiavelli: Policy analysis comes of age.* Washington, DC: Georgetown University Press.

Radin, B. A. (2013). *Beyond Machiavelli: Policy analysis reaches midlife* (2nd ed.). Washington, DC: Georgetown University Press.

Rampell, C. (2011, March 3). Bernanke for early childhood education? *The New York Times.* Retrieved from *http://economix.blogs.nytimes.com/2011/03/03/bernanke-for-early-childhood-education.*

Romano, E., Babchishin, L., Pagani, L. S., & Kohen, D. (2010). School readiness and later achievement: Replication and extension using a nationwide Canadian survey. *Developmental Psychology, 46,* 995–1007.

Rutter, M. (2012). Achievements and challenges in the biology of environmental effects. *Proceedings of the National Academy of Sciences, 109*(Suppl. 2), 17149–17153.

Sandford, N. (1953). Clinical methods: Psychotherapy. *Annual Review of Psychology, 4,* 317–342.

Santos, R., Brownell, M., Ekuma, O., Mayer, T., & Soodeen, R. (2012). *The Early Development Instrument (EDI) in Manitoba: Linking socioeconomic adversity and biological vulnerability at birth to children's outcomes at age 5.* Winnipeg: Manitoba Centre for Health Policy.

Savoie, D. J. (1999). *Governing from the centre: The concentration of power in Canadian politics.* Toronto: University of Toronto Press.

Savoie, D. J. (2003). *Breaking the bargain: Public servants, ministers, and Parliament.* Toronto: University of Toronto Press.

Schweinhart, L. J., Montie, J., Xiang, Z., Barnett, W. S., Belfield, C. R., & Nores, M. (2005). *Lifetime effects: The High/Scope Perry Preschool study through age 40* (Monographs of the High/Scope Educational Research Foundation, No. 14). Ypsilanti, MI: High/Scope Press.

Scott, S. D., Albrecht, L., O'Leary, K., Ball, G. D. C., Hartling, L., Hofmeyer, A., et al. (2012). Systematic review of knowledge translation strategies in the allied health professions. *Implementation Science, 7,* 1–32. Retrieved from *www.implementationscience.com/content/7/1/70.*

Shonkoff, J. P. (2000). Science, policy, and practice: Three cultures in search of a shared mission. *Child Development, 71,* 181–187.

Shonkoff, J. P. (2003). Still waiting for the right questions. *American Journal of Preventive Medicine, 24*(3S), 4–5.

Shonkoff, J. P. (2010). Building a new biodevelopmental framework to guide the future of early childhood policy. *Child Development, 81,* 357–367.

Shonkoff, J. P. (2011). Protecting brains, not simply stimulating minds. *Science, 333,* 982–983.

Shonkoff, J. P. (2012). Leveraging the biology of adversity to address the roots of disparities in health and development. *Proceedings of the National Academy of Sciences, 109*(Suppl. 2), 17302–17307.

Shonkoff, J. P., & Bales, S. N. (2011). Science does not speak for itself: Translating child development research for the public and its policymakers. *Child Development, 82,* 17–32.

Shonkoff, J. P., Boyce, W. T., & McEwen, B. S. (2009). Neuroscience, molecular biology, and the childhood roots of health disparities: Building a new framework for health promotion and disease prevention. *Journal of the American Medical Association, 301,* 2252–2259.

Shonkoff, J. P., Garner, A. S., the Committee on Psychosocial Aspects of Child and Family Health, Committee on Early Childhood Adoption and Dependent Care, & Section on Developmental and Behavioral Pediatrics, (2012). The lifelong effects of early childhood adversity and toxic stress. *Pediatrics, 129,* e232–e246.

Shonkoff, J. P., Richter, L., van der Gaag, J., & Bhutta, Z. A. (2012). An integrated scientific framework for child survival and early childhood development. *Pediatrics, 129*, e460–e472.

Straus, S. E., Tetroe, J., & Graham, I. (2009). Defining knowledge translation. *Canadian Medical Association Journal, 181*, 165–168.

Tough, P. (2012). *How children succeed*. Boston: Houghton Mifflin/Harcourt.

Trevathan, W. (2010). *Ancient bodies, modern lives: How evolution has shaped women's health*. New York: Oxford University Press.

Truth and Reconciliation Commission of Canada. (2012a). *They came for the children: Canada, Aboriginal peoples, and residential schools*. Winnipeg: Author. Retrieved from *www.trc.ca/websites/trcinstitution/index.php?p=580*.

Truth and Reconciliation Commission of Canada. (2012b). *Truth and Reconciliation Commission of Canada: Interim report*. Winnipeg: Author. Retrieved from *www.trc.ca/websites/trcinstitution/index.php?p=580*.

van IJzendoorn, M. H., & Bakermans-Kranenburg, M. J. (2012). Integrating temperament and attachment: The differential susceptibility paradigm. In M. Zentner & R. L. Shiner (Eds.), *Handbook of temperament* (pp. 403–424). New York: Guilford Press.

van IJzendoorn, M. H., Bakermans-Kranenburg, M. J., & Alink, L. R. A. (2012). Meta-analysis in developmental science. In B. Laursen, T. D. Little, & N. A. Card (Eds.), *Handbook of developmental research methods* (pp. 667–686). New York: Guilford Press.

Vogt, P. (2010). The Manitoba Cabinet. In P. G. Thomas & C. Brown (Eds.), *Manitoba politics and government: Issues, institutions, traditions* (pp. 181–204). Winnipeg: University of Manitoba Press.

Vohs, K. D., & Baumeister. R. F. (Eds.). (2011). *Handbook of self-regulation: Research, theory, and applications* (2nd ed.). New York: Guilford Press.

Waddell, C., Lavis, J. N., Abelson, J., Loma, J., Shepherd, C. A., Bird-Gayson, T., et al. (2005). Research use in children's mental health policy in Canada: Maintaining vigilance amid ambiguity. *Social Science and Medicine, 61*, 1649–1657.

Wathen, C. N., Sibbald, S. L., Jack, S. M., & MacMillan, H. L. (2011). Talk, trust and time: A longitudinal study evaluating knowledge translation and exchange processes for research on violence against women. *Implementation Science, 6*, 1–15. Retrieved from *www.implementationscience.com/content/6/1/102*.

Weiss, C. H. (1973). Where politics and evaluation research meet. *Evaluation, 1*(3), 37–45.

Weiss, C. H. (1993). Politics and evaluation: A reprise with mellower overtones. *American Journal of Evaluation, 14*, 107–109.

Weiss, C. H., Murphy-Graham, E., Petrosino, A., & Gandhi, A. G. (2008). The fairy godmother—and her warts: Making the dream of evidence-based policy come true. *American Journal of Evaluation, 29*, 29–47.

Wildavsky, A. (1979). *Speaking truth to power*. Boston: Little, Brown.

Winnipeg Free Press. (2012, November 26). Make early childhood education a priority when books balanced, TD report urges. Retrieved from *www.winnipegfreepress.com/business/make-early-childhood-education-a-priority-when-books-balanced-td-report-urges-180929411.html*.

Worthman, C. M., Plotsky, P. M., Schechter, D. S., & Cummings, C. A. (Eds.).

(2010). *Formative experiences: The interaction of caregiving, culture, and developmental psychobiology*. New York: Cambridge University Press.

Zigler, E. F. (2007). Epilogue: Combining basic and applied science in constructing sound social policy. In J. L. Aber, S. J. Bishop-Josef, K. T. McLearn, & D. A. Phillips (Eds.), *Child development and social policy: Knowledge for action* (pp. 281–284). Washington, DC: American Psychological Association.

Zigler, E. F., & Hall, N. W. (2000). *Child development and social policy: Theory and applications*. New York: McGraw-Hill.

CHAPTER 15

School Readiness in a Developmental Perspective

Summary of Findings and Implications for Future Research and Practice

Karen L. Bierman and Michel Boivin

In recent years, interest in school readiness has increased dramatically. Developmental studies linking early school performance to long-term school outcomes have amplified concerns about children who start school poorly prepared for the academic and social demands of formal schooling. Growing awareness of the long-term costs of poor school readiness has, in turn, fueled interest in early interventions that can address initial developmental disparities. The prevailing hope and expectation is that reducing the gap in school readiness at school entry will set at-risk children on a positive learning trajectory and put them on track for later school attainment and success (Zaslow, Tout, Halle, Vick, & Lavelle, 2010).

Effectively reducing the impact of early disadvantage and improving the school readiness of at-risk children requires a good understanding of the developmental processes associated with delays in school readiness, as well as a keen appreciation of effective intervention approaches. Promising new research provides insights into how early disadvantage delays learning and offers hope that early disparities may be reversed with effective early education and intervention. School readiness is now being conceptualized more broadly than knowing one's letters and numbers, with greater attention being paid to the biological and socialization factors that influence the diverse dimensions of cognitive, social, and emotional development that motivate and support school success. Most importantly, an increasing set of rigorous randomized controlled evaluations document evidence-based programs and practices that effectively reduce the disparities in school readiness associated with poverty. Yet a very large gap exists between the research base and the quality of early childhood practice. There is a great need to promote the dissemination of research on school readiness and its implications for early childhood programs and policies.

This volume was designed to bring together interdisciplinary perspectives on the current state of knowledge regarding the foundations of school readiness and the opportunities for wide-ranging policy and program enrichment that might reduce school inequalities and position all children on a trajectory to success at school entry. A key goal was to harness the power of developmental science to inform efforts to promote school readiness, and to convene research addressing theory, research, practice, and policy associated with school readiness and early learning.

Longitudinal Studies: Early Predictors of Later School Success

Population-based longitudinal studies that examine the long-term school outcomes associated with early childhood skills and socialization provide a critical guide for defining school readiness and strategically positioning effective preventive interventions. This book began with an introduction and two chapters that focused on the prediction of school success, examining child characteristics, as well as school, family, and community risk and protective factors that were linked longitudinally with later achievement. Although these developmental links do not necessarily represent causal relations, they identify indices of school readiness that may function as early developmental markers of the capacity to succeed in school, and characteristics of the socializing context that are associated with long-term success or risk.

In Chapter 2, Vitaro, Brengden, and Tremblay examined the early elementary school predictors of high school graduation, and found that it was best predicted by a complex interplay of behavioral, motivation, and achievement factors, each affecting the others in a transactional manner throughout elementary school. Specifically, children who entered school with higher school motivation (e.g., those who liked school more and were more interested in learning) showed an accelerated pace of achievement during elementary school, and similarly, children with higher levels of initial academic achievement showed increased school motivation over time. Behavior problems played a significant part in a negative school process, with early inattention–hyperactivity predicting decreases over time in achievement and motivation, and similarly, low achievement and low school motivation predicting escalations in children's inattention–hyperactivity problems over the course of elementary school. Both behavioral and academic factors predicted high school graduation, as children (especially boys) who entered school with elevated inattention–hyperactivity tended to underachieve, lose interest in school, then drop out. Overall, the longitudinal findings described in this chapter illustrate an interplay of school attitudes, behaviors, and achievement that operate over time to create a "Mathew effect," increasing the gap in school adjustment and attainment separating children who entered school with protective characteristics (e.g., positive school attitudes and motivation, behavioral control, and academic knowledge) from those who entered school with attitudinal, behavioral, or academic risks. At the same time, it is noteworthy that in the transactional models presented by Vitaro and his colleagues, the stability coefficients dwarfed the change estimates, indicating that most of the individual differences in the behavioral and motivational dimensions were already established at school entry. The implication of these findings is that effective strategies to promoting school success should start early (i.e., in preschool or early in elementary school) and be multifaceted, attending to the promotion of positive attitudes, behavioral and emotional self-regulation skills, as well as cognitive skills acquisition.

In Chapter 3, Boivin, Desrosiers, Lemelin, and Forget-Dubois described findings from two other longitudinal studies, the Québec Longitudinal Study of Child Development and the Québec Newborn Twin Study, examining a set of child characteristics (cognitive, language, motor, social-emotional skills, and academic knowledge) and family and social variables, assessed at school entry, as predictive antecedents of later academic and social outcomes. Latent profile analyses identified four developmental trajectories of academic achievement across early elementary school (grades 1–4). Academic knowledge in preschool (e.g., knowing letters, numbers, and colors/shapes) and preschool teacher ratings of children's adaptive skills (e.g., communication skills, social competence, and physical independence) each differentially predicted children's placement in elementary school achievement trajectories, particularly distinguishing those in the highest and lowest achievement groups. Although using different samples and a different methodology than Vitaro and colleagues (Chapter 2), Boivin and colleagues came to a similar conclusion, namely, that elementary school achievement is predicted by a variety of preschool cognitive and social-behavioral components, including academic knowledge and basic skills (e.g., literacy, numeracy), as well as interpersonal skills and behaviors, thus validating the multidimensional approach to school readiness.

Using the Québec Newborn Twin Study, Boivin and colleagues also estimated the contribution of socialization factors, relative to genetic factors, as determinants of these multifaceted dimensions of school readiness. They concluded that genetic factors contributed both to children's school readiness and early achievement, but environmental experiences, especially those shared by children of the same family, played a larger role. These results validate the importance of attending to the home environment and family socialization experiences in developmental models of school readiness, as well as examining effects on social-emotional, behavioral, attitudinal, and cognitive dimensions of child development. They also suggest that there is ample room to promote school readiness and academic achievement by intervening at the level of malleable factors in children's early environments, as these contribute in significant ways to children's academic outcomes.

Taken together, these longitudinal studies provide important information for the field of school readiness, identifying early specific markers of child and contextual risk (and resilience) associated with future school performance and attainment. Complementing these longitudinal studies that took a broad examination of prediction in the school readiness domain, this volume also included a set of studies that tested specific mechanisms of change, with the goal of elucidating developmental processes, dynamics, and determinants in particular domains of school readiness.

Developmental Processes and Potential Determinants of Readiness in Specific Domains

Understanding developmental processes in the early childhood years is particularly important. In early childhood, rapid development occurs in areas of neural, cognitive, and social-emotional growth, and children appear particularly vulnerable to the negative effects of early adversity and exposure to associated risks of poverty during this time (Gershoff, 2003). Long-term school success depends heavily on the child's acquisition of a set of central competencies that allow him or her to succeed and learn in the school environment, many of which have their roots in developmental processes that occur during the first 5 years of life. The skills that influence school success are not purely cognitive, as they also include the capacity to focus and persist on goal-oriented learning tasks and to control impulses and resist distractions, along with the social-emotional skills that allow children to develop good working relationships with peers and teachers (Blair, 2002; Farrington et al., 2012). During the early childhood years, social environments, including interactions within the family and experiences in child care and early school contexts, have a powerful impact on the development of these noncognitive skills, thereby affecting school readiness in direct ways (via their impact on language skills and cognitive development) and indirect ways (via their impact in areas broadly considered to be "state regulating" factors). Recent advances in developmental neuroscience have particularly illuminated the importance of the early childhood years for the development of the "neural architecture for learning" (e.g., the cognitive structures that support the regulation of attention, behavior, and emotion). Developmental scientists are just beginning to document the dynamics of early experiences that "get under the skin" and influence the developing structure and functioning of basic neurobiological systems, including stress responding, arousal modulation, and learning processes, which affect cognitive functioning and underlie the development of the noncognitive factors associated with academic success. With the goal of articulating developmental models associated with school readiness, Chapters 4–6 in this volume have examined developmental dynamics in core areas of language, emergent literacy, and behavioral development, testing the association between developing child skills and environmental experiences at the level of the parent–child relationship, the family, child care settings, and the broader neighborhood.

In Chapter 4 of this volume, Wade, Prime, Browne, and Jenkins examined the developmental dynamics of early language development. Focusing on the early years (e.g., 0–3), they documented family and neighborhood characteristics, and their associations with later child expressive language and emerging reading skills. Wade and colleagues argued that, in addition to the proximal developmental context (family experiences, parent–child interactions), the broader developmental context operating at the level of the neighborhood might also show unique associations with child school readiness. Using data from Kids, Families and Places, a longitudinal study of 501 newborns and their older siblings, they found that age 3 oral language skills and early reading were predicted by both the family context (maternal sensitivity, mother's use of English in the home) and the neighborhood context (collective efficacy), measured during infancy. Maternal sensitivity appeared to compensate for economic disadvantage, leading the authors to recommend maternal sensitivity as a possible key target for preventive interventions during the first 3 years of life (a topic also addressed in Chapters 11 and 12). The unique association of neighborhood collective efficacy also suggests greater attention should be paid to community-level factors in the design of early intervention and parenting programs (a topic also addressed in Chapter 12).

In Chapter 5, Dionne, Mimeau, and Mathieu also took a close look at associations between language development in the family context, focusing on the first years of life, and predicting children's readiness to read at school entry. Using data from the Québec Longitudinal Study of Child Development, and the Québec Newborn Twin Study, they found that family factors, particularly parent–child reading, predicted variation in children's language development (accounting for 8–9% of the variance). It was by way of these improved oral language skills that parent–child reading in early childhood was linked with later reading skills in second grade. In this chapter, Dionne and colleagues also attempted to unpack the relative and unique associations between maternal education, frequency of parent–child reading, and the development of oral language skills during early childhood. Higher levels of maternal education were associated with better child oral language skills development, but the frequency of mother–child book reading moderated this association. Frequent mother–child book reading, particularly when it started at an early age, compensated somewhat for the lack of maternal education, enhancing child language skills acquisition even at the lowest level of maternal education studied. Overall, this study suggests that maternal education and frequent, early parent–child reading are linked with enhanced oral language development. Furthermore, although reading is more heavily linked to genetic factors than to oral language development, the quality of parent–child language and reading at home may enhance child reading skills development indirectly, by way of its positive association with oral language skills development.

In Chapter 6, Côté, Geoffroy, and Pingault examined associations between early child care experiences and later cognitive school readiness. Intuitively, improving the quality of early learning experiences within child care settings may be a valuable prevention strategy for reducing the socioeconomic gap that exists at school entry. But this approach rests on the assumption that the quality of early child care experienced by children is associated with their school readiness. Côté and colleagues noted that many of the studies on this topic examining the school readiness of children who received child care compared with children who received maternal care in the early years have garnered mixed findings. Citing their analyses of the Québec Longitudinal Study of Child Development, the authors noted that children from socioeconomically disadvantaged backgrounds, but not children from well-off families, benefited from regular child care in their first year of life (Geoffroy et al., 2007). Similar findings emerged when the authors performed the same type of comparison with data from the British Millennium Cohort Study in the United Kingdom, with substantial, positive associations between formal and center-based child care and school readiness among children of mothers with low levels of education but attenuated or nonsignificant effects for children of mothers with higher levels of education. The authors suggested that early formal child care may benefit children from disadvantaged homes by enriching their early environments in areas of language and cognitive stimulation, whereas children with more well-educated mothers receive sufficient stimulation and support in the home setting, reducing the value-added aspect of child care relative to school readiness.

Côté and colleagues also suggested that studies focusing on children's participation in child care may not adequately characterize the associations between child care experiences and school readiness, because they do not assess the quality of child care (i.e., crucial elements that may substantially affect child development). Accordingly, they reviewed findings from the Cost, Quality, and Child Outcomes in Child Care Centers Study and the National Institute of Child Health and Human Development Study of Early Child Care and Youth Development (NICHD ECCRN, 2005; Peisner-Feinberg et al., 2001). Key take-home points were that (1) quality of child care predicted the pace of development during early childhood, with sustained contributions evident in areas of cognitive (e.g., math and language) and noncognitive skills (e.g., learning engagement, problem behaviors, peer relations) into the early elementary school years; (2) quality of child care was associated with developmental and school readiness outcomes for children from a wide range of family backgrounds, but (3) disadvantaged children appeared to benefit to a greater extent from the quality of child care experiences than other children (see also Peisner-Feinberg et al., 1999). In the NICHD study, the degree to which child care was sensitive–responsive and cognitively stimulating was still significantly associated with the child's school functioning in adolescence (Vandell, Belsky, Burchinal, Steinberg, & Vandergrift, 2010), suggesting possible long-term benefits of enriching the quality of early child care to promote school readiness and school attainment, particularly for children growing up in socioeconomically disadvantaged families. Côté and colleagues (Chapter 6, this volume) also provided evidence suggesting that too many children (up to 75%) receive low-quality child care, increasing the relevance of further, rigorous study of child care quality and impact, including experimental trials examining the impact of improving child care quality with evidence-based practices.

Testing the Efficacy of Early Childhood Interventions to Improve School Readiness

The developmental studies described in this volume contribute to a growing base of knowledge regarding the importance of the early childhood years for the development of cognitive and noncognitive skills associated with school readiness. They highlight risk and protective factors at the level of the family, child care, school, and neighborhood context that are potentially malleable, and thereby hold promise as potential targets for intervention. However, these developmental studies examined patterns of covariation, which may or may not be causal. There is a critical need for experimental studies that use interventions to change the features of the child's early environment, and then evaluate whether those changes promote child school readiness and attainment. Only through such experimental methods can causality be determined and the effectiveness of an intervention approach clearly evaluated.

In developmental studies, interpreting causality is complicated by unmeasured factors that might account for the observed association. For example, when child care quality predicts improved school readiness for children, one cannot be sure whether it is the quality of child care per se that is the causal ingredient in that association or whether school readiness is improved by a host of other factors that accompany child care quality, such as teacher education levels, neighborhood resources, more skilled peers in the classroom, higher levels of parent involvement, and so forth. Although some studies do measure, and provide statistical control for some of these factors, one cannot be sure that all relevant potentially confounding variables have been taken into account. In addition, selection biases occur when certain kinds of parents elect to place their children in certain kinds of care settings, creating a host of factors that may differentiate children in one child care setting from another, and that might affect child school readiness outcomes. For this reason, strong causal conclusions about the impact of a particular early childhood experience are most confidently made in the context of rigorous randomized designs, in which teachers, parents, or children are randomly assigned to receive different kinds of intervention that involve the systematic manipulation of the child's experience. The goal of random assignment is to create groups that are equivalent on selection factors and other unmeasured factors, so that the "true" impact of the dimension of schooling, parenting, or child care quality on child outcomes is more clearly delineated.

This volume included five chapters describing randomized controlled studies of early intervention strategies designed to improve child school readiness. Each focused on samples of children at risk due to socioeconomic disadvantage, although they differed in the particular focus of intervention and domain of child school readiness skills targeted.

In Chapter 7, Wasik and Hindman described an intervention that provided intensive professional development support to preschool teachers. This intervention, the *Ex*ceptional *C*oaching for *E*arly *L*anguage and *L*iteracy (ExCELL), used evidence-based curriculum components to promote children's vocabulary growth, phonological sensitivity, alphabet knowledge, and emergent writing skills. It also included intensive training for teachers in the form of workshop training, weekly coaching, detailed manuals with lesson plans and learning activities for teachers to deliver, and tools for progress monitoring of teachers and children. Multiple types of professional development activities were used, including didactic instruction, reflective discussion, coach modeling, and videotaping teacher practice with coach-supported review and explicit feedback. A series of randomized controlled trials has documented improvements in teaching quality and enriched language use (more frequent conversations, more open-ended questions, better use of vocabulary words), as well as improved book-reading practices in the classroom among teachers in ExCELL compared to "usual practice" control groups (see also Wasik & Hindman, 2011). Importantly, ExCELL also produced significant changes in children's school readiness, promoting the vocabulary and phonological sensitivity of children in intervention classrooms relative to those in the control group. Additional analyses suggested that children who entered ExCELL with the lowest language skills experienced greater gains over the course of the intervention year than children with higher initial language skills.

In Chapter 8, Starkey, Klein, and DeFlorio first described developmental studies that document the unique predictability of math skills at school entry to later math achievement and school success. They then documented the effectiveness of their intervention program, Pre-K Mathematics, in promoting the early math skills among socioeconomically disadvantaged children. Pre-K Mathematics includes 26 small-group math activities and learning games designed for prekindergarten children, and organized with a developmental scope and sequence that moves children from easier to more difficult math challenges. Teachers are asked to schedule small-group math activity sessions three times per week, adjusting their pace and the difficulty level of the learning activities according to children's responses. Teachers are also taught how to scaffold learning and provide support to children who experience difficulty, tracking individual children's learning of specific math content over the course of the year. The intervention also includes synchronized math activities for parents to do with children at home. Starkey and colleagues described positive findings when Pre-K Mathematics was evaluated in a randomized, multisite trial. At the end of the year, multilevel models of posttest assessments revealed that children in the intervention classrooms outperformed children in the "usual practice" control classrooms on two standardized tests of math performance. Furthermore, significant treatment effects persisted into kindergarten. The team was also able to document significant sustained effects on teaching practices associated with mathematics instruction, as well as continued implementation of the curriculum and learning games. Children showed improved math achievement scores at the end of the sustainability year, relative to children in the control group. Interestingly, teachers also rated children in the intervention group as making more progress in following directions in the classroom, compared with children in the control group. These effects persisted over the transition into kindergarten, with significant treatment effects still evident on children's math knowledge and teacher-rated mathematical ability. The study documented that teachers could be trained to implement a curricular math intervention, Pre-K Mathematics, with fidelity and sustain the intervention at least 1 year after training, producing significant effects on children's school readiness and kindergarten in areas of math achievement. These effects were particularly impressive because they were attained in the context of a large-scale effectiveness trial.

In Chapter 9, Li-Grining, Lennon, Marcus, Flores, and Haas described the Chicago School Readiness Project (CSRP), which focused on improving the quality of teacher–student interactions, positive classroom management, and the quality of classroom emotional support, in order to foster child self-regulation skills and thereby enhance the school readiness of economically disadvantaged children attending Head Start. Consistent with the developmental study results reported in Chapters 2 and 3 in this volume, the CSRP design was based on the hypothesis that improvements in classroom order and teacher support in preschool would reduce child behavior problems, strengthen emotion regulation and social competencies, and improve academic motivation and persistence, thereby promoting the noncognitive skills associated with learning success. The CSRP further hypothesized that classroom order and teacher support were malleable aspects of the preschool environment and could be improved by the use of a positive professional development (e.g., the Incredible Years Teacher Training Program) along with in-class behavioral management support from a mentor and social support for teacher stress management (see Raver et al., 2011). The randomized trial evaluating the CSRP revealed that classroom order and teacher support were successfully improved by the intervention, demonstrating the malleability of these environmental factors. Observers documented increases in positive classroom climate, teacher warmth and sensitivity, and reductions in negative classroom climate in intervention compared with control classrooms, with moderate to large effect sizes. As noted by Li-Grining et al., further analyses showed significant positive effects of the intervention on children's self-regulation and executive function skills, reductions in behavior problems (by teacher and observer report), and improved academic skills (see Raver et al., 2011, for more details). In addition to documenting these positive effects, Li-Grining and colleagues described mediational analyses showing that improvements in child self-regulation skills over the course of the preschool year accounted for the treatment effects on child academic gains (Raver et al., 2011). This intervention study suggests that a concentrated focus on improving teachers' provision of positive classroom management and emotional support can have significant benefits for preschool children, evident in both cognitive and noncognitive skill domains associated with school readiness.

The findings described in Chapters 7–9 are encouraging, because they illustrate that evidence-based curriculum components combined with professional development supports can significantly improve the quality of teaching and opportunities for learning in preschool programs serving socioeconomically disadvantaged children. Each intervention was able to document significant improvements in the targeted domain: CSRP improved the social-emotional climate for learning in the classroom, Pre-K Mathematics increased support for emergent numeracy and math skills, and ExCELL improved teachers' language use and support for emergent literacy skills. These findings raise the question of whether teachers can incorporate evidence-based practices in multiple areas at one time, increasing the cross-domain impact on their students.

In Chapter 10, Bierman, Domitrovich, Nix, Welsh, and Gest described the Head Start REDI (Research-Based, Developmentally Informed) program, which addressed this question by providing simultaneous enrichment curriculum components and professional support in the dual domains of social-emotional learning and language/emergent literacy skills. On the one hand, such cross-domain integration could have significant synergistic benefits for children, potentially supporting changes in both motivational and cognitive systems that would combine to improve academic success. On the other hand, intervening across domains raises a risk of overwhelming teachers or diluting intervention components in ways that might limit their effectiveness. To support children's social-emotional skills development, the REDI intervention utilized the Preschool PATHS Curriculum (Domitrovich, Greenberg, Cortes, & Kusche, 1999), which includes 33 classroom lessons and coordinated extension activities to promote child competencies in areas of friendship skills, emotional understanding, self-control, and problem-solving skills. To promote children's oral language and emergent literacy skills, REDI included an interactive reading program based on the work of Wasik and Hindman (see Chapter 7, this volume), "sound games" to promote phonological awareness, and print center activities to teach letter knowledge. Detailed curriculum manuals and intensive professional development for teachers (e.g., workshops, classroom observations, and weekly mentoring) supported high-fidelity program implementation, and take-home materials were provided to help parents provide support for child skills development at home.

The randomized trial evaluation of REDI revealed positive benefits for teachers who showed improved teaching practices (e.g., positive and proactive classroom management, enriched language use) relative to the "usual practice" control groups. In addition, hierarchical linear models (accounting for children nested in classrooms) revealed positive REDI effects on child outcomes in areas of both emergent literacy (vocabulary, phonemic awareness, print knowledge) and social-emotional competence (emotion knowledge, social problem-solving skills, social competence, learning engagement, and reduced aggression). These findings suggest that when teachers are provided with empirically supported curricula and sufficient professional development support, they can successfully improve their practice in both social-emotional and cognitive domains of school readiness, promoting cross-domain gains in socioeconomically disadvantaged children that may enhance learning trajectories in later school years.

Although the majority of interventions designed to promote children's school readiness have focused on preschool settings, a smaller set of interventions have attempted to intervene with parents to improve family supports for school readiness development. In Chapter 11, Welsh, Bierman, and Mathis provided a critical review of the extant empirical literature on parent education and home visiting programs, focusing on those that utilized randomized trial evaluations and included specific assessments of child school readiness outcomes. Although one might expect that any program that improves early parenting skills should have benefits for child school readiness, this is not always the case: Some parenting programs have benefits for parents and children, but these do not translate into substantial improvements in child school readiness outcomes. For example, Welsh et al. reviewed programs that start early (during pregnancy or early in the child's life) and focus broadly on educating and supporting parents to enhance their feelings of efficacy and problem-solving skills. Some of the children in these programs demonstrated gains in preschool cognitive or behavioral school readiness, but in general (and despite other benefits for parents), program effects on child school readiness per se were not as large or as consistent as the impacts attained with preschool-based early interventions. Hence, although these early parent-focused interventions have value, they are not likely to reduce substantially the socioeconomic gap in children's school success without additional programming. A second group of parent-focused interventions described in this chapter focused on improving the quality of parent–child interactions, particularly maternal sensitivity–responsiveness, and reducing coercive parenting and harsh punishment. Randomized trials documented the efficacy of three such programs to improve parenting practices and the quality of parent–child interactions, with corresponding improvements documented in child functioning in areas associated school functioning (e.g., enhanced social competence, reduced behavior problems), although only one of these programs (the Incredible Years) collected preschool measures. None of the studies collected cognitive outcomes, making it unclear whether improvements in parent–child interaction quality alone might enhance cognitive readiness for school. Finally, Welsh et al. reviewed studies that focused on parents as teachers. In these interventions, parents were taught how to play and talk with children in cognitively stimulating ways. Each of these programs showed some evidence of effectiveness, but results were more positive in quasi-experimental trials and relatively weak in randomized trials, suggesting that the programs are underperforming and may not be cost-effective compared with alternative preschool-based interventions (Gomby, 2005). Some parent intervention programs described in this chapter used parents as a supplement to a school-based intervention, which may enhance parent–teacher collaboration and amplify school-based intervention effects. Additional programs described in the chapter provided parents with specific learning support activities and instructions, such as teaching parents how to read in a dialogic manner and tutor their children in emergent reading skills. Welsh and colleagues concluded that child school readiness outcomes are generally more positively affected when intervention programs give parents specific guidelines for how to read with or work with their children on learning activities, rather than focus more generally on promoting positive parent–child interactions. However, the authors also cautioned that the social-emotional and motivational outcomes associated with positive school adjustment have not been well-studied in the evaluations of parenting programs and deserve closer scrutiny. It may also be the case that certain subgroups of children, such as those with early disruptive behaviors, benefit from parenting programs focused on improved parenting practices and positive discipline strategies in ways that nondisruptive children do not (Reid, Webster-Stratton, & Baydar, 2004). Welsh and colleagues (Chapter 11, this volume) make several recommendations for future research on parenting interventions designed to enhance child school readiness. They suggest that future research should (1) articulate and test the hypothesized mechanisms of action in order to clarify how they are working (or not working); (2) examine issues of intensity and dose, and consider individualized interventions in order to reduce attrition, which tends to be high in parent-focused programs for young children; and (3) consider the conditions under which (and subgroups for whom) different parenting interventions do (or do not) have an impact on child school readiness outcomes.

The randomized efficacy studies described in Chapters 7–11 provide a foundation for optimism regarding the potential of evidence-based practices to improve the early learning environments and school readiness of children at risk. These studies demonstrate that the quality of adult–child interactions can be improved in preschool and family settings in ways that enrich the language exposure, cognitive stimulation, and social-emotional support that promote positive school readiness. In addition, these studies document the value of providing children with developmentally appropriate learning materials that are organized according to a developmental scope and sequence, supporting learning progressions that allow children who are delayed in areas of emergent literacy and numeracy skills to catch up with their more advantaged peers. At the same time, these studies raise important questions about the feasibility of "going to scale" with effective, evidence-based early childhood interventions. The successful programs each provided substantial professional development support and carefully designed learning materials in order to achieve the fidelity of implementation and "dose" of intervention necessary to promote substantial gains in critical areas of child school readiness. In order to promote these kinds of gains at a population level, several challenges must be solved. In the next chapters of this volume, investigators addressed the challenges of "going to scale" with evidence-based practices, clarifying the challenges and identifying possible areas of potential solutions.

Going to Scale with Evidence-Based Programs

In Chapter 12, Peters and Howell-Moneta describe Better Beginnings, Better Futures (BBBF), a large-scale, community-based prevention program designed to facilitate school readiness and successful transition into school. This program took a different approach than the programs described in Chapters 7–11. In recognition of evidence that cultural and community level factors affect school readiness and may also affect the attractiveness and effectiveness of different intervention approaches, BBBF used an ecological approach, giving the community a role in intervention design. Operating in eight disadvantaged neighborhoods in Ontario, Canada, BBBF is more of a framework for action than a specific program. In BBBF, each community decides which specific programs to deliver, while attending to factors associated with high-quality implementation and positive impact on child outcomes. Five sites focused on providing programs for children from birth to age 4 and implemented an average of 26 different programs, including home visiting programs, and interventions to increase child care quality. Three sites focused on providing programs for children ages 4 to 8 years and averaged 16 different programs, including school-based programs, and supports to enrich out-of-school time (e.g., before school and afterschool care, homework support, and recreation programs). The evaluation of program impact involved a quasi-experimental control, with selection of comparison sites similar to intervention communities on demographic features. Short-term outcomes included significant improvements in teacher-rated anxiety, self-control, and parent involvement, as well as reduced maternal smoking and positive changes in parent reports about their neighborhoods. Follow-up assessments conducted 4 years later revealed no lasting impact for children and families at the five BBBF *younger child* sites, but sustained effects at the three BBBF *older child* sites. At the *older child* sites, teacher ratings revealed sustained improvements in student self-control, hyperactivity and inattention, fewer school suspensions and special education services, and higher math achievement. Several of the effects on school adjustment remained significant through high school for children at the *older child* sites, including less need for special education, higher adaptive functioning in school, and fewer grade retentions. The authors suggest that the programs for older children may have been more successful because they were able to use the school as a scaffold for service delivery, thereby offering more program sessions and recruiting a larger segment of the targeted child and family population into their interventions.

The BBBF findings suggest that there may be advantages of activating community involvement during the process of program selection and implementation, although the findings also suggest that long-term impact occurs only when high-quality programs are implemented with fidelity at a sufficient dose to build child skills.

In Chapter 13, Poulin, Capuano, Vitaro, Verlaan, Brodeur, and Giroux also describe an effort to diffuse and implement an evidence-based program, the Fluppy program, on a large scale, providing the multifaceted program services throughout the entire Canadian province of Québec. In the original efficacy trial, the Fluppy program, which included universal social-emotional lessons delivered by a teacher in early elementary school, along with three intervention components delivered to children with high levels of aggression (academic tutoring, social skills training with peer pairing, and parent management training), proved effective at improving behavioral adjustment and academic learning. Like many of the programs described in Chapters 7–11, during the efficacy trial, the program was delivered by highly qualified professionals with a high-fidelity implementation. However, in order to implement the program at a larger scale, a number of compromises were made in order to fit a reduced budget and gain acceptance by a large number of teachers. The program modifications, as described in Chapter 13, required reducing all program components substantially. Implementation fidelity suffered as well, as the abridged program was rolled out at scale, but the budget allowed for only a small level of training and professional development support for the program implementers. The evaluation revealed reduced effects for children, which likely reflected the abbreviated intervention dose they received relative to the original efficacy trial.

The Fluppy program large-scale diffusion illustrates one of the greatest challenges that we, as a society, face in terms of substantially reducing the gap in school readiness associated with socioeconomic disadvantage and early adversity. That is, evidence-based interventions with proven power make a substantial difference and close the gap, but these efforts require an intensity of exposure and quality of implementation that are very difficult to achieve without the financial and professional supports available within an efficacy trials. Effects tend to fade as programs go to scale, because levels of financial support and professional development support are often lower, resulting in reduced fidelity and reduced dose.

Finally, in Chapter 14, Rob Santos provides sage advice to help researchers bridge the communication gap with policymakers whose support is needed for the sustainable incorporation and funding of evidence-based programs as "usual practice." Santos clarifies the kinds of research information that policymakers want and need, and urges researchers to consider a list of "top-10" factors when communicating with policymakers about programming to enhance school readiness. Topping the list are four types of evidence that policymakers need in order to make decisions about evidence-based programs: (1) the scope of the problem addressed by the program (epidemiology); (2) the nature and cause of the problem, including the early risk indicators (explanation); (3) the evidence of a program's effectiveness at addressing the problem (evaluation/effectiveness); and (4) the cost of the program and the value of its impact (cost–benefit efficiency). Next on the list are three characteristics that significantly influence the degree to which policymakers will find the evidence provided (points 1–4) compelling: (5) the skill with which the information is expressed (the clarity of the communication); (6) the trustworthiness of the communication source (collaboration); and (7) the credibility of the evidence, including the quality of the scientific method upon which it is based. Finally, the list includes three areas of documentation that may increase the degree to which school readiness programming becomes a priority for policymakers, relative to the host of other pressing issues they face: (8) evidence documenting the long-term value of investing in early childhood programming (and the long-term costs of failing to do so); (9) descriptions of the underlying determinants of school readiness, with an emphasis on how early childhood experiences affect core processes of brain development and regulatory functioning (e.g., how disadvantage "gets under the skin"; Shonkoff, 2010) in ways that have large downstream costs for individual and societal functioning; and (10) illustrations that demonstrate how early, evidence-based interventions can reverse the effects of early adversity and promote substantial improvements in children's early school success and future life course.

FUTURE DIRECTIONS

The studies described in this volume testify to the importance of focusing efforts on enriching early learning environments to promote the school readiness of children growing up under conditions of socioeconomic disadvantage or exposed to other risk factors that delay their school readiness. The chapters demonstrate the developmental predictability of early learning environments. They document that the pace of early development in areas of cognitive and social-emotional domains has implications for long-term school achievement and attainment. The importance of the early childhood years may reflect both the rapid development that occurs during the first 2,000 days of life in the areas of the brain that represent the fundamental building blocks for later learning. In addition, the early years may be particularly important because of the way they affect later learning experiences, through developmental cascades in which the gap between prepared and unprepared children widens after school entry.

This book has focused on what we know about school readiness, what we should be doing in earlier stages of development, and how effective intervention strategies are at creating positive changes in early learning environments and accelerating early learning. Several take-home points are clear: The development of school readiness is affected by multifaceted variables that affect each other over time. Contextual factors that influence the pace and scope of early learning and school readiness operate from multiple levels, including parenting and family experiences, teacher and school experiences, as well as experiences occurring at the more distal broader neighborhood and community levels. The quality of parent–child and teacher–child interactions play an important role in early learning, as does the quality of learning materials to which the child is exposed. Efficacy trials demonstrate the significant potential of evidence-based programs and practices to improve school readiness, particularly for disadvantaged children. However, going to scale remains a substantial challenge with potential hurdles, including the effective engagement of communities, schools, teachers, and parents, and the insufficient funding to train intervention deliverers and support high-fidelity program implementation.

What is left to be done? More research is needed to identify further the nature and processes of early experiences as they relate to school readiness, including the interactions with adults and peers, and the early childhood education experiences (teaching methods and curricula) most effective at accelerating early development, particularly for children from diverse backgrounds and those exposed to early adversity. This research should examine the multiple domains of development of relevance for school readiness, including cognitive and language development, emergent literacy and numeracy skills, social-emotional competence, self-regulation, and motivation to learn. Especially important are theoretically driven attempts to test mechanisms of action and examine the mediating processes accounting for the predictive relations between early learning experiences and outcomes in child learning and development, particularly with a view that these processes may differ across children and families in different communities or cultural settings.

Individual differences in learning are the hallmark of human development and should be the object of persistent attention, especially as they relate to experiences in the early years. As recently summarized in the Royal Society of Canada Expert Panel on Early Childhood Development, it is clear that children vary greatly in their response to early childhood experiences and that developmental pathways are moderated by a wide range of factors, from genes to community-level support:

> Clearly, the inequalities in physical, social/emotional, and cognitive development that emerge early in life are largely accounted for by the interplay of genetic factors and early environments. Early childhood is a sensitive period during which the environment may modify the brain circuitry, especially that governing the emotion, attention, self-control and stress systems of the child; and it is increasingly clear that the environment may change the way genes are expressed through epigenetic processes. Early childhood is a period of high plasticity in brain development, a period that progressively gives rise to the consolidation of individual differences. . . . Clearly, any serious prevention "system" needs to start strong in that period, and more than at any later time in development. (Boivin & Hertzman, 2012, pp. 118–119)

The contributions of this volume have to be comprehended within this overarching view. They bring good news. This volume makes it clear that a variety of early interventions and intervention approaches show significant promise as strategies that can mitigate the early effects of socioeconomic disadvantage, promote positive changes in environmental influences associated with early learning, and positively impact the school readiness of at-risk children (and their parents and teachers). However, there is still substantial work to be done in the area of intervention design and evaluation. Central questions include the degree to which interventions targeting specific domains of school readiness can be integrated without diluting their effectiveness, and how the professional development support needed to implement these programs with fidelity can be delivered in cost-effective and sustainable ways. Some early childhood experiences with adults and peers, and with certain kinds of early childhood curricula or programs, may be more effective for some children than others, raising important research questions about which intervention strategies are most effective for which children, and under what conditions.

There is a particular need to address mechanisms and strategies that can enhance the effective diffusion of evidence-based practices into early learning programs. Relatedly, it is important to understand better the nature of the gap that exists between the research on evidence-based practices and the "usual practice" programming that exists in the field. To some extent, this gap reflects a lack of accessibility of the research to practitioners, but it also likely reflects differences in the priorities that inform the research and those that affect practitioners in the field. Processes of effective (and ineffective) diffusion should be studied in order to understand better "what works" in the field of practice. To facilitate "going to scale" with evidence-based early intervention strategies, more cost-effective strategies are needed that will allow teacher-training and parent-training interventions to achieve diffusion at scale without loss of fidelity. Innovative strategies and careful evaluation studies are needed to expand the current toolkit in areas of the preparation, education, training, and professional development of persons involved in the care and education of young children. The need to individualize this support requires exploration, as different levels or approaches to professional development may be needed depending upon the characteristics of the parents, teachers, or child care providers. A critical, yet underexplored, issue involves strategies to elicit administrative support for the investment and sustained monitoring of evidence-based practice, which is likely critical to promoting change at scale. The gap in translation from research to practice will likely only be solved by a better understanding of the factors that affect the decision-making processes of practitioners, policymakers, teachers, and parents, so that evidence-based practices appear interesting, appealing, and feasible to these important consumers. Partnerships between researchers, policymakers, and school administrators may be critical in order to ensure that programs that have a documented evidence base are designed in a way that maximizes their translation into use in the field.

The advances in conceptualization and methodology, the discovery of malleable antecedents and mediators of school readiness, and the new data on the efficacy of evidence-based practice all create a solid foundation for improving current early childhood programs and practices. If we can surmount the challenges of going to scale, we have the potential to close the achievement gap associated with poverty and promote the school readiness of all children, giving them a strong starting base for future achievement.

REFERENCES

Blair, C. (2002). School readiness: Integrating cognition and emotion in a neurobiological conceptualization of child functioning at school entry. *American Psychologist, 57,* 111–127.

Boivin, M., & Hertzman, C. (Eds.). (2012). *Early childhood development: Adverse experiences and developmental health.* Royal Society of Canada–Canadian Academy of Health Sciences Expert Panel (with Ronald Barr, Thomas Boyce, Alison Fleming, Harriet MacMillan, Candice Odgers, Marla Sokolowski, & Nico Trocmé). Ottawa: Royal Society of Canada. Available from *http://rsc-src.ca/sites/default/files/pdf/ecd%20report_0.pdf.*

Domitrovich, C. E., Greenberg, M. T., Cortes, R., & Kusche, C. (1999). *Manual for the Preschool PATHS Curriculum.* University Park: The Pennsylvania State University.

Farrington, C. A., Roderick, M., Allensworth, E., Nagaoka, J., Keyes, T. S., Johnson, D. W., et al. (2012). *Teaching adolescents to become learner: The role of noncognitive factors in shaping school performance: A critical literature review.* Chicago: University of Chicago Consortium on Chicago School Research.

Geoffroy, M.-C., Côté, S. M., Borge, A., Larouche, F., Séguin, J. R., & Rutter, M. (2007). Association between nonmaternal care in the first year of life and children's receptive language skills prior to school entry: The moderating role of the socioeconomic status. *Journal of Child Psychology and Psychiatry, 48*(5), 490–497.

Gershoff, E. T. (2003). Low income and the development of America's kindergartners. National Center for Children in Poverty. Retrieved from *http://nccp.org/publications/pdf/text_533.pdf.*

Gomby, D. (2005). *Home visitation in 2005: Outcomes for children and parents.* Committee for Economic Development: Invest in Kids Working Group: *www.ced.org/projects/kids.shtml.*

National Institute of Child Health and Human Development Early Child Care Research Network (NICHD ECCRN). (2005). Early child care and children's development in the primary grades: Follow-up results from the NICHD study of early child care. *American Educational Research Journal, 42*(3), 537–570.

Peisner-Feinberg, E. S., Burchinal, M. R., Clifford, R. M., Culkin, M. L., Howes, C., Kagan, S. L., et al. (1999). *The children of the Cost, Quality, And Outcomes Study go to school: Public report.* Chapel Hill: University of North Carolina at Chapel Hill, Frank Porter Graham Child Development Center.

Peisner-Feinberg, E. S., Burchinal, M. R., Clifford, R. M., Culkin, M. L., Howes, C., Kagan, S. L., et al. (2001). The relation of preschool child-care quality to children's cognitive and social developmental trajectories through second grade. *Child Development, 72*(5), 1534–1553.

Raver, C. C., Jones, S. M., Li-Grining, C., Zhai, F., Bub, K., & Pressler, E. (2011).

CSRP's impact on low-income preschoolers' preacademic skills: Self-regulation as a mediating mechanism. *Child Development, 82*(1), 362–378.

Raver, C. C., Jones, S. M., Li-Grining, C., Zhai, F., Metzger, M. W., & Solomon, B. (2009). Targeting children's behavior problems in preschool classrooms: A cluster-randomized controlled trial. *Journal of Consulting and Clinical Psychology, 77*(2), 302–316.

Reid, M. J., Webster-Stratton, C., & Baydar, N. (2004). Halting the development of conduct problems in Head Start children: The effects of parent training. *Journal of Clinical Child and Adolescent Psychology, 33*, 279–291.

Shonkoff, J. P. (2010). Building a new biodevelopmental framework to guide the future of early childhood policy. *Child Development, 81*, 357–367.

Vandell, D. L., Belsky, J., Burchinal, M., Steinberg, L., & Vandergrift, N. (2010). Do effects of early child care extend to age 15 years? Results from the NICHD Study of Early Child Care and Youth Development. *Child Development, 81*(3), 737–756.

Wasik, B. A., & Hindman, A. H. (2011). Low-income children learning language and early literacy skills: The effects of a teacher professional development model on teacher and child outcomes. *Journal of Educational Psychology, 103*, 455–469.

Zaslow, M., Tout, K., Halle, T., Vick, J., & Lavelle, B. (2010). *Toward the identification of features of effective professional development for early childhood educators: A review of the literature*. Washington, DC: U.S. Department of Education.

Index

An *f* following a page number indicates a figure;
a *t* following a page number indicates a table.

F

L

M

N

O

P

Q

R

S

T

U

V

W